GOAL WRITING

for the Speech-Language Pathologist and Special Educator

Bridging the Gap Between Assessment and Intervention

Edited by

Terry H. Gozdziewski, MA, CCC-SLP, TSHH, SAS, SDS

Renee Fabus, PhD, CCC-SLP, TSHH

Cindy Geise Arroyo, DA, CCC-SLP, TSHH

J. Reilly Limowski, MA, MS, AA

Julia Yudes-Kuznetsov, MS, CCC-SLP

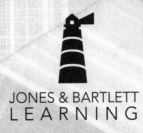

JONES & BARTLETT
LEARNING

World Headquarters
Jones & Bartlett Learning
5 Wall Street
Burlington, MA 01803
978-443-5000
info@jblearning.com
www.jblearning.com

Jones & Bartlett Learning books and products are available through most bookstores and online booksellers. To contact Jones & Bartlett Learning directly, call 800-832-0034, fax 978-443-8000, or visit our website, www.jblearning.com.

Substantial discounts on bulk quantities of Jones & Bartlett Learning publications are available to corporations, professional associations, and other qualified organizations. For details and specific discount information, contact the special sales department at Jones & Bartlett Learning via the above contact information or send an email to specialsales@jblearning.com.

Production Credits
VP, Product Management: David D. Cella
Director of Product Management: Matt Kane
Product Manager: Laura Pagluica
Product Assistant: Rebecca Feeney
Production Manager: Carolyn Rogers Pershouse
Director of Marketing: Andrea DeFronzo
Product Fulfillment Manager: Wendy Kilborn
Composition: codeMantra U.S. LLC
Cover Design: Kristin E. Parker
Rights & Media Specialist: Thais Miller
Media Development Editor: Troy Liston
Cover Image (Title Page, Chapter Opener): © Getty Images
Printing and Binding: Edwards Brothers Malloy
Cover Printing: Edwards Brothers Malloy

Library of Congress Cataloging-in-Publication Data
Names: Gozdziewski, Terry H. (Terry Hausner), editor. | Fabus, Renee Laura,
  1968- editor. | Arroyo, Cindy Geise, editor. | Reilly Limowski, Jeanne,
  editor. | Yudes-Kuznetsov, Julia, editor.
Title: Goal writing for the speech-language pathologist and special educator:
  bridging the gap between assessment and intervention / edited by Terry
  H. Gozdziewski, Renee Fabus, Cindy Geise Arroyo, Jeanne Reilly Limowski,
  Julia Yudes-Kuznetsov.
Description: Burlington, MA: Jones & Bartlett Learning, [2019] | Includes
  bibliographical references and index.
Identifiers: LCCN 2017042562 | ISBN 9781284104806 (paperback)
Subjects: | MESH: Communication Disorders–therapy | Speech-Language
  Pathology–methods | Goals
Classification: LCC RC428.5 | NLM WL 340.2 | DDC 616.85/5–dc23
LC record available at https://lccn.loc.gov/2017042562

6048

Printed in the United States of America
22 21 20 19 18   10 9 8 7 6 5 4 3 2 1

CONTENTS

Unit A: Writing Goals: The Basics   1

Unit B: Writing Goals in Speech-Language Pathology, Aural Rehabilitation and Habilitation, and Special Education   25

PREFACE

Approach to the Text

The importance of well-written goals is emphasized in programs in speech-language pathology and special education throughout the country. Well-written goals are necessary in order to determine and document client progress. There are several assessment and intervention books available to students in programs in speech-language pathology and special education. Although these books are comprehensive and provide students with valuable resources, there is not one book to date that "bridges" the gap between assessment and intervention for the student. Our book offers the crucial element that is missing in most textbooks. How do students derive goals from the assessment data they have obtained? The title of this book includes the word "bridge" because this book helps guide the reader to "bridge the gap" between the ability to assess, interpret, and analyze assessment information in order to derive functional goals for intervention. Instructing students about how to develop functional goals is often difficult and can be a challenging process for the instructor. Our book provides the reader with important elements to consider when writing goals for their client regardless of the therapeutic setting. It provides the (figurative) roadmap to helping the people we serve.

This book is designed to be a reference for how to derive goals from the assessment process. It incorporates the disciplines of speech-language pathology and special education and is intended to be used by instructors in these fields and as a resource for both novice and experienced clinicians.

How to Use This Book

The first section is an all-purpose overview with chapters about the historical perspective on goal writing and the essential elements required for writing a goal. The second section is dedicated to specific areas in the fields of speech-language pathology and special education. Each chapter targets a different disorder and provides the necessary information as to what to look for when assessing the targeted population and then how to develop goals based on the treatment that the clinician decides to employ with the client.

Each chapter of the book consists of the following sections: key terms, introduction, comprehensive assessment, analysis and interpretation of results of assessment data, forming specific goals, types of intervention approaches, summary, two case scenarios, five multiple choice questions, and references. Each of the chapters in the second section discuss formal and informal assessments, as well as various types of interventions that are important to consider when writing goals. These areas must be thoroughly understood by the clinicians and teachers who will be providing services because goals are determined by knowledge of these topics.

The editors chose contributors based on their expertise and experience working with a specific population. Great care was taken to ensure that only experts in their individual fields were chosen to write a chapter in this book.

We hope that university instructors will use this text in their courses to help guide students in developing and writing functional goals for different disorders and populations.

Instructor Support Tools

The following instructor resources are available online at go.jblearning .com/goalwriting:

- Slides in PowerPoint format
- Syllabus
- Answers to End of Chapter Questions

ABOUT THE EDITORS

Terry H. Gozdziewski, MA, CCC-SLP, TSHH, SAS, SDS

Clinical Educator, St. John's University
Adjunct Professor, Long Island University, Post and Adelphi University
Retired Speech-Language Pathologist from the North Bellmore School District, NY

Terry Hausner Gozdziewski, MA, CCC-SLP, TSHH, SDS, SAS, has been a clinical speech-language pathologist for over 40 years. She received her BA from Adelphi University, her MA from The George Washington University, and her educational administration degrees from Long Island University, C.W. Post campus. She is currently an adjunct professor at both LIU-Post and Adelphi University as well as being a clinical educator at St. John's University. Her previous publications include a teaching DVD, along with Dr. Fabus and Mrs. Yudes-Kuznetsov, titled "Clinical Case Studies of Children with Articulation and Phonological Disorders." Prior to working in higher education, she provided speech therapy in several different venues including public schools in New York and Connecticut as an SLP as well as serving as Chairperson of the Committee on Special Education and Preschool Special Education. "Mrs. Goz." has also conceived, created, and taught numerous workshops on the integration of speech and language skills with reading and English language arts to speech-language pathologists, general educators, special educators, administrators, and parents.

Renee Fabus, PhD, CCC-SLP, TSHH

Associate Professor
School of Health Technology and Management
Stony Brook University

Renee Fabus, PhD, CCC-SLP, TSHH, is currently an Associate Professor, Chair of a Proposed Speech-Language Pathology Graduate Program. She received her bachelor's degree from New York University, her master's degree in speech-language pathology from Teachers College, and her PhD from Columbia University. She has been a licensed and certified speech-language pathologist for over 20 years and has practiced in a variety of medical settings. She has taught and supervised in programs in the New York City area and published in the areas of aphasia, dysphagia, speech sound disorders, and stuttering. She has served on various editorial boards and committees at the regional, state, and national level. Additionally, she has served in many positions, including President, of the Long Island Speech-Language-Hearing Association (LISHA).

Cindy Geise Arroyo, DA, CCC-SLP, TSHH

Associate Professor
Department of Communication Sciences and Disorders
Adelphi University

Cindy Geise Arroyo, DA, CCC-SLP, TSHH, is currently an Associate Professor and Graduate Program Director in the Communication Sciences & Disorders Program at Adelphi University. She received her bachelor's, master's, and doctor of arts degrees from Adelphi University. Dr. Arroyo has worked with infants and children with feeding and swallowing disorders for over 37 years in various settings and private practice. She has also conducted augmentative and alternative communication (AAC) evaluations and intervention for individuals with complex communication needs and continues to do so through the AAC lab at Hy Weinberg Center, Adelphi University. Dr. Arroyo has published in the areas of AAC and pediatric feeding.

J. Reilly Limowski, MA, MS, AA

Retired Adjunct Professor from Adelphi University
Retired Special Education Teacher from the North Bellmore School District, NY

Jeanne Reilly Limowski, MA, MS, AA, is a learning specialist and consultant with over 40 years of experience. She completed her undergraduate studies at SUNY Stony Brook with dual majors in English and elementary education. She received a master of arts degree in elementary education and a master of science degree in special education from Long Island University, C.W. Post Campus (LIU-Post). Additionally, she is certified in the Wilson Reading System and she is trained in the Fundations reading and Step Up to Writing programs. She has served as a general education classroom teacher, a teacher in a self-contained classroom, a resource room teacher, a special education evaluator, a member of the Committee on Special Education, an advisor for student teachers, and a mentor for numerous administrators and educators. Ms. Limowski was an adjunct faculty member at Nassau Community College and Adelphi University and guest lectured at Suffolk Community College and LIU-Post. Furthermore, she has created and presented many workshops for parents, teachers, and administrators on a variety of topics.

Julia Yudes-Kuznetsov, MS, CCC-SLP

Senior Adjunct Faculty
Department of Communication Sciences and Disorders
Adelphi University

Julia Yudes-Kuznetsov, MS, CCC-SLP, is a bilingual speech-language pathologist and a senior adjunct instructor at Adelphi University. She received her undergraduate and graduate education in speech-language pathology from Moscow State Pedagogical University in Russia and Teachers College, Columbia University, in the United States. She has been employed in a variety of medical settings for the past 20 years specializing in neurogenic communicative disorders for monolingual and bilingual populations. Currently, she is employed as a speech-language pathologist for adults diagnosed with cognitive-communication disorders and dysphagia secondary to head trauma and stroke. In addition, she teaches undergraduate and graduate courses in neurogenic speech disorders and anatomy and physiology of the speech mechanism.

CONTRIBUTORS

The authors would like to recognize the following individuals who contributed chapters to this text:

Susan Antonellis, AuD, CCC-A/F-AAA
Operations Manager of Center for Hearing Health
Program of Mill Neck Services

Anita W. Frey, MA, SDS, SAS
Clinical Assistant Professor
Ruth S. Ammon School of Education
Adelphi University

Margaret M. Laskowski, PhD, CCC-SLP/TSHH-BE
Assistant Professor
Department of Communication Sciences and Disorders
Long Island University, Post

Ciara Leydon, PhD, CCC-SLP
Associate Professor
Department of Speech-Language Pathology
Sacred Heart University

Florence L. Myers, PhD, CCC-SLP, ASHA Fellow
Professor
Department of Communication Sciences and Disorders
Adelphi University

Elizabeth Stein, MSEd, NBCT
Special Education/Universal Design for Learning Instruction Coach
Smithtown Central School District
Adjunct Lecturer
Stony Brook University

Laurie Wenerholm, MA, CCC-SLP, BCS-S
Board Certified Specialist in Swallowing and Swallowing Disorders
Supervisor, Speech Pathology and Swallowing Center for Cancer Care
White Plains Hospital/Montefiore Health System

ACKNOWLEDGMENTS

This book is dedicated to Tom Gozdziewski, Florence Hausner, and Stan Hausner who still inspire me every day and to Sherry Miller, Roseann Schoen, and Lois Susskind who laugh with me, cry with me, and never fail to tell me the truth. I want to thank Renee Fabus who has encouraged me to reach professional heights I never dreamed possible and to Jeanne Limowski, Cindy Arroyo, and Julie Yudes-Kuznetsov as well as all of our wonderful contributors, without whom this book could never have been written. Sincerest thanks are extended to Rebecca Feeney, Carolyn Pershouse, Laura Pagluica, and Mary Menzemer and their staff from Jones & Bartlett Learning, with special kudos given to Anne Remonde Limowski.

There's an old saying: "All work and no play makes Jack a dull boy." The same is true for this author. The hours of work that were devoted to writing and editing this book had to be balanced. Were it not for the balance, I could not have completed this manuscript. In that vein, I want to thank those who have shared their friendship, support, and love of life with me. They include T.J., Ginger, "Chewy," Beau, and George Gozdziewski, all of whom remind me every day to stay grounded. I also want to acknowledge my newly found family from O.L.O.L., especially Jennifer Milton, Patricia Bambanelli, and Nancy Adamescu, along with every other member of this fabulous group of people who showed me a world I never knew existed and brought me more joy than I had experienced in a very long time. Of course, this could not have been possible without the leadership, humor, knowledge, and belief in me shown by J.C. Laws. For all of this, I will be forever grateful.

–Terry H. Gozdziewski

I would like to thank all of my family, friends, and colleagues. Special thanks go out to my fellow coeditors, our contributing authors, and the staff at Jones & Bartlett Learning.

–Renee Fabus

I would like to dedicate this book to the individuals and families who have experienced feeding and swallowing challenges, and those with augmentative/alternative communication needs. I have learned so much from them and have been privileged to observe their achievements.

—Cindy Geise Arroyo

I wish to thank all those who contributed to my knowledge over the years: my professors, mentors, colleagues, friends, and the students with whom I have had the pleasure to work. A special thank you to my children, Annie, Stephen, and Edward, for their support, opinions, and technologic assistance, which all contributed to allowing me to embark on this endeavor.

—J. Reilly Limowski

I would like to express my gratitude to our wonderful team. Dear Renee, Terry, Cindy, and Jeanne: Thank you for inviting me to be part of this creation. I also want to thank our contributors: Without your professional knowledge and expertise in your various fields, this book could not have been developed. I want to thank my husband Valera, my parents, and my children for their patience and support. Finally, I want to thank my patients who have taught me how life is precious and pushed me to think outside the box.

—Julie Yudes-Kuznetsov

I would like to express gratitude to my parents, Joseph and Norene Laskowski, who instilled in me a passion for learning and education. I also am grateful for the encouragement I received over the years from all the educators and mentors in my life. In particular, I would like to thank Dr. Ronald J. Baken, my master's and doctoral advisor, for his intelligence, dedication to excellence, and not least of all, his sense of humor.

—Margaret Laskowski

I would like to thank Terry Gozdziewski for this amazing opportunity to be part of such a wonderful project.

—Anita Frey

I would like to thank Dr. Christopher Atkins, CCC-SLP, for his thoughtful assistance with writing goals.

—Ciara Leydon

The authors would like to thank the following reviewers for their work on the manuscript:

Joanne L. Abdallah
Bridgewater State University

Diana Almodovar
Lehman College, CUNY

Angela Beckman Anthony
Eastern Illinois University

Donald Aubry
MacMurray College

Sheila H. Bernstein
CUNY Hunter, St. John's University

Nicole Bougie
Eastern New Mexico University

Jill L. Brady
Indiana University of Pennsylvania

Catherine Brumbaugh
Duquesne University

Dave A. Buchanan
Nova Southeastern University

Nancy Carlino
California University of Pennsylvania

Maura DeMilt
Bowling Green State University

Janet L. Dodd
Chapman University

Regina L. Enwefa
Southern University and A&M College

Melissa P. Garcia
Texas A&M International University

Keri P. Gonzalez
University of Texas Rio Grande Valley

Stacie M. Greene
St. Ambrose University

Sharon Jones
Northeastern State University

Erin E.G. Lundblom
University of Pittsburgh

Natalie Neubauer
Seton Hall University

Eusebia Mont
University of Maryland

Wendy J. Pulliam
Longwood University

Julie Raplee
St. Joseph's College

Yolanda Rory
The Ohio State University

Shannon Salley
Longwood University

Laura Schrock
Bowling Green State University

Robert W. Serianni
Salus University

Amanda Solesky
Indiana State University

Betty D. Sutton
Jackson State University

Rosalie Unterman
Touro College

Horabail Venkatagiri
Iowa State University

Shari M. Weisz
University of North Dakota

Unit A

Writing Goals: The Basics

CHAPTER 1

The Elements of Goal Writing

Terry H. Gozdziewski
Cindy G. Arroyo
Renee Fabus

Key Terms

ASHA Code of Ethics
Behavioral objectives
Data collection
Evidence-based practice (EBP)
Individualized education plan (IEP)
Interprofessional collaborative
    practice

Interprofessional practice (IPP)
Long-term goals
Scope of Practice in Speech-
    Language Pathology
Short-term goals
Task analysis

Introduction

Speech-language pathologists and special educators develop and write goals as part of the intervention process after they analyze the assessment data and determine if services are warranted. There is a demand for **evidence-based practice (EBP)**, "treatment efficacy, fiscal accountability" (Guilford, Graham, & Scheuerle, 2007, p. 3), and consumer advocacy and education in speech-language pathology and special education; therefore, developing goals that are specific, measurable, and functional is essential. Guilford and colleagues discuss the importance of clinicians developing interpersonal skills, problem-solving skills, technical skills (including treatment planning and task analysis), and increasing their knowledge and experience so they can make good clinical decisions during the assessment and intervention. Speech-language pathologists must adhere to the **ASHA Code of Ethics** (American Speech-Language-Hearing Association [ASHA], 2016a) and the **Scope of Practice in Speech-Language Pathology** (ASHA, 2016b) when making clinical decisions about their clients. The fields of speech-language pathology and special education continue to evolve in a dynamic process that encompasses working collaboratively with other professionals in health care, education, and other fields, in addition to the individual and family. The American Speech-Language-Hearing Association (ASHA) defines this as **interprofessional practice (IPP)**, also called **interprofessional collaborative practice** (ASHA, 2016b). This collaboration supports the interchange of professional knowledge and information and enhances the quality and breadth of goals and interventions.

Clinicians must use EBP to determine which procedures and intervention approaches provide good clinical efficacy. EBP "reflects recent advancements in quantifying efficacy research. Service delivery has evolved to the point that customary, habitual approaches to intervention can no longer be accepted without proof (evidence) of the anticipated outcome. Nor can professional decisions regarding treatment (goals, hierarchy for assumptions and clinical judgement) rely entirely on assumptions and clinical judgement" (Guilford et al., 2007, p. 5).

ASHA requires all clinicians to incorporate EBP during the assessment and intervention of clients with communication and swallowing disorders. The "goal of EBP is the integration of: (a) clinical expertise/expert opinion, (b) external scientific evidence, and (c) client/patient/caregiver perspectives to provide high-quality services reflecting the interests, values, needs, and choices of the individuals we serve" (ASHA, 2017b, para. 1). ASHA published policy statements that specify the knowledge and skills required for different topic areas. For example, one policy statement addresses dysphonia (ASHA, 2017a).

Historically, an impairment-based model was used as a foundation for developing goals and intervention plans (Bleile, 2004). The International Classification of Functioning, Disability and Health (ICF), developed by World Health Organization (2001), infused a social model into goal development. This model emphasizes life goals developed with input from the individual, family, and other professionals. It encompasses body structures, functions, and performance, as well as environmental and personal factors (Bleile, 2004). This chapter will present the essentials of goal writing. It is assumed that the reader has comprehensive knowledge about assessment in the different communication and swallowing disorders. Additionally, the term *clinician* is used to collectively refer to speech-language pathologists and special educators.

Goals

Clinicians analyze the results of formal and informal testing, which are attained from an assessment, to determine the client's present level of functioning and possible **long-term goals**. Prior to developing long-term goals, the clinician must consider factors such as the client's interests and motivation, the client's current level of functioning, and cultural and linguistic factors.

It is essential that clinicians acquire specific technical skills, including tool and procedure selection, task selection and implementation, and task analysis, to conduct efficacious assessments and interventions. It is essential for clinicians to select appropriate tools and procedures so a comprehensive and thorough assessment can be conducted to determine the client's strengths and weaknesses and to evaluate the need for therapy.

Clinicians need to understand and know how to perform a **task analysis** and task sequence (Paul, 2014). A task analysis is the process of separating the different components of a task to understand how to perform the task. The clinician performs a task analysis and task sequence by breaking down long-term goals into smaller segments to develop **short-term goals**. This is important in goal development because an understanding of how short-term goals will be achieved is required to determine how a long-term goal will be mastered. The clinician helps guide and instruct the client in performing a task analysis and task sequence. Task selection and implementation help the clinician determine which tasks and materials are essential during therapy to help the client master goals.

In most situations, different clinicians will conduct the evaluation and the treatment. If the clinician does not conduct the assessment, he or she may not have access to the evaluation and results. For example, in a school setting, the clinician will receive a copy of the **individualized education plan (IEP)**, which contains the long-term (annual) goals and short-term goals (benchmarks) for the student.

In some situations, after receiving the diagnostic, assessment, or evaluation report, the clinician may perform baseline testing to assess the client's current level of functioning because the client's skills could have matured or regressed since the evaluation was completed.

Pretreatment baseline goals are designed by the clinician and are not written with a criterion component (discussed later in this chapter in the "Components of a Goal" section).

Roth and Worthington (2016) recommend including 20 stimuli for baseline testing. After the clinician obtains baseline data, he or she needs to determine the accuracy percentage that was achieved for the target behavior. If the client achieves 75 percent or higher, the clinician will likely not address that target behavior at that level in therapy because the skill (at that level) is within the client's repertoire. If the client achieves between 50 and 75 percent, the clinician may choose to address this target behavior at this level in therapy. If the client achieves less than 50 percent, the clinician should not address this target behavior at this level. Instead, the clinician may choose to address the target behavior at an easier level (Roth & Worthington, 2016).

For example, suppose a clinician is obtaining baseline data for a child with a speech sound disorder. The clinician provides 20 pictures of items with the /s/ phoneme in the initial position (prevocalic) of words. If the child produces the /s/ correctly when shown 10 of the 20 pictures, the score is 50 percent correct. In this case, correctly pronouncing the /s/ phoneme in the initial position of words may be a therapy goal. However, if the child produces the /s/ phoneme correctly when shown 5 of the 20 pictures, the score is 25 percent. In this scenario, correctly pronouncing the /s/ phoneme in the initial position of words should not be a therapy goal because it is too difficult for the child. Instead, the clinician may address the /s/ phoneme at the syllable level, which would be easier to master, before progressing to the word level.

In different texts, the terms *long-term goals* and *long-term objectives* are synonymous. Long-term goals or objectives relate to the outcome the client will achieve at the time of discharge (Moon Meyer, 1998) and should indicate what the client will functionally be able to achieve. Paul says the "achievement of these goals will be justification for terminating therapy" (2014, p. 177), whereas Moon Meyer says long-term goals "might or might not be the same as terminal objectives that are the final objectives that need to be mastered prior to discharge" (1998, p. 21). A clinician usually indicates the length of time for the long-term goal to be accomplished. The length of time usually varies depending on the setting where the services are being provided. For example, in a university clinic, the long-term goal may be a semester, and in a school setting it may be a year.

Similarly, the terms *short-term goals* and *short-term objectives* are synonymous. Both terms indicate that the goals or objectives are usually "attainable in a short period of time" (Moon Meyer, 1998, p. 20). The clinician must complete a task analysis to discern the short-term goals from the long-term goals. Short-term goals are developed and "arranged hierarchically" (Goldfarb & Serpanos, 2014, p. 276) so that the client will achieve the long-term goal by mastering the short-term goals. The following example illustrates a possible hierarchy of short-term goals that are necessary to achieve a long-term goal.

- Long-term goal:
  - The client will use functional communication skills for social interactions (e.g., greetings, social etiquette, and short questions or simple sentences) with both familiar and unfamiliar partners.

- Short-term goals:
  - The client will name functional objects in the environment to make requests for wants and needs with 80 percent accuracy, given minimum verbal cues.
  - The client will perform sentence completion to communicate daily wants and needs (or basic, medical, or social wants and needs) with 80 percent accuracy, given minimum verbal cues.
  - The client will formulate three-word utterances to communicate daily needs in a picture description task with 80 percent accuracy, given minimum verbal cues.
  - The client will be trained on strategy of circumlocution to improve word-finding ability and will demonstrate its use during simple conversational speech related to activities of daily living (ADLs) 80 percent of the time, given minimal verbal cues.

Components of a Goal

Long-term and short-term goals are written in the form of **behavioral objectives** (Moon Meyer, 1998). Roth and Worthington (2016), Paul (2014), and Moon Meyer (1998) state that a behavioral objective contains three components: do statement, condition, and criterion. The do statement "identifies the specific action the client is expected to perform" (Roth & Worthington, 2016, p. 12). The condition provides information about "which performance is to be done" and specifies "what you will provide to the individual in order to help him do the task" (Moon Meyer, 1998, p. 7). Moon Meyer goes on to say that a condition is "not obligatory" (1998, p. 8) in all behavioral objectives. A criterion is a standard that is used to evaluate performance. It is often expressed as a percentage (e.g., Sherry will recite the alphabet with 80 percent accuracy).

The elements that are included in goals may vary, particularly in situations where guidelines are established by a facility, agency, or school. Therefore, some general considerations for developing goals will be addressed in this discussion, using the framework *what, how, who, where,* and *when.* The *who, where,* and *when* elements are important in the process of developing goals, but they are not always written in the behavioral objective.

What Skill Will Be Targeted?

The first element to be considered is what skill will be targeted. Roth and Worthington (2016) say this is the do statement component of the behavioral objective, whereas Moon Meyer (1998) says this is the performance component of the behavioral objective. A targeted skill may be identified from information such as formal and informal assessments; dynamic observations; client, parent, or family input; developmental norms; cultural or linguistic factors; and clinical judgment. Whatever skill is targeted in therapy, it should be realistic, relevant, and specific. According to Paul, the do statement "contain(s) verbs that name observable actions, such as point, label, repeat, say, match, write, name, or ask" (2014, p. 178).

How Will Success Be Measured?

The second element is to determine how success will be measured. Roth and Worthington (2016), Paul (2014), and Moon Meyer (1998) say this is the criterion component of the behavioral objective. Determining how success will be measured is accomplished by setting accuracy levels then collecting data in a consistent, systematic manner. **Data collection** may be defined as a "systematic measurement of client/student performance and treatment efficacy" (Roth & Worthington, 2016, p. 6). It is an objective way to determine if a client has demonstrated progress or achieved a goal.

Percentages used in goals may be expressed as a range, such as 75–90 percent, because it may be unrealistic to set a goal at 100 percent. It may not be appropriate or realistic to measure some targeted skills or goals in percentages; rather, the number of trials may be used (e.g., Johnny will demonstrate a controlled, sustained bite on a hard cookie in three out of five trials). Goldfarb and Serpanos say that sometimes "an interval (temporal) goal is more appropriate than a ratio (numerical) goal" (2014, p. 276). Data collection may also include other valuable information, such as the number of self-corrections and the need for prompts and cues.

Who Will Collect the Data?

Because goals should be measurable, it should be determined who will collect the data. Typically, the speech-language pathologist or the special educator may collect data but sometimes it is efficacious for another individual to record the client's responses and behaviors. For example, an educational paraprofessional or a teacher's aide may record the number of conversational interactions a child makes using his or her augmentative communication device in the classroom. Or a parent or guardian may be asked to record data if the goal is for the child to improve his or her fluency in the home environment. If the client is an adult and the objective is to generalize (carry over) skills for safe swallowing, the client's significant other, a hospital aide, or a home health aide may record the data.

Where Will Services Occur?

The location where the services will occur may be dictated, or it may be decided by the client or family. In early intervention, services are typically provided in the child's home as prescribed in the individualized family service plan (IFSP). However, services may need to be provided in a babysitter's house, grandparent's house, or a day care center. Within a school, services may be provided in the classroom, a separate speech room, or a resource room. Services may also be delivered in the cafeteria or the playground, where pragmatic skills and interactions with peers may be facilitated. In a hospital or rehabilitation facility, services may be provided at a patient's bedside, in a separate lounge area, or in a location that is designated for speech services.

Varying the location where goals are targeted may be an important part of the intervention. For example, children with autism spectrum disorders may have difficulties generalizing their communication skills outside the therapy room, so practicing skills in other settings with different communication partners may be beneficial. In some cases it may be appropriate to include peers in the setting as part of the goal; for example, Johnny will initiate a request to peers using Picture Exchange Communication System (PECS) three times during lunch in the cafeteria.

When Will the Goal Be Attained?

The last element to be considered is when goals are expected to be met. This may be determined by the setting or the placement. If services are being delivered in or through a school, goals are often set to be completed at the time report cards are distributed or at the end of the academic year. If services are being delivered at a college or university clinic, the completion date is often the end of the academic semester. If services are delivered through early intervention, the goals are generally set for 6-month intervals.

Prompts and Cues

Prompts and cues may help clients achieve their goals. The terms *prompts* and *cues* are often used synonymously, but there are differences. Prompts are supplementary strategies or reminders to support or elicit the targeted skill (Fisher & Frey, 2013; West & Billingsley, 2005). Cues are more specific and direct than prompts because they shift the client's attention (Fisher & Frey, 2013). Prompts and cues may be delivered through various sensory modalities, including visual, auditory, kinesthetic, tactile, or a combination.

The intensity and consistency of the prompts and cues may vary depending on the individual, context, and goal. It may be appropriate to include information regarding prompts and cues in the goals. Clinicians may also need to consider the consistency in the delivery of prompts and cues. Consistent cues are delivered in a predetermined way, such as every time or every other time a response is expected. Inconsistent (also called intermittent) prompts and cues do not follow a predetermined pattern and are used only as needed. The ultimate goal is for the prompts to be internalized, through fading, so the client responds to natural cues (Fisher & Frey, 2013; West & Billingsley, 2005).

Prompting and prompt-fading procedures are based on the applied behavior analysis literature (MacDuff, Krantz & McClannahan, 2001). The following models have been implemented in goals and interventions and are discussed in the literature:

- Increasing assistance: With increasing assistance, the least to the most prompts are provided; for example, verbal prompts, gestures, modeling, manual prompts or physical assistance.
- Decreasing assistance: With decreasing assistance, the most to the least prompts are provided; for example, physical prompts or assistance, modeling, gestures, verbal prompts.

- Delayed prompts: Fading is accomplished by inserting a time delay between the stimulus and the implementation of a prompt or cue.
- Graduated guidance: Full physical guidance (e.g., hand over hand) is initially provided, then the intensity fades (e.g., a prompt at the elbow or wrist).
- Stimulus fading: A physical aspect (e.g., color, size) of a stimulus is exaggerated to facilitate a desired response, and the intensity is gradually faded.

It is essential to shift the emphasis from prompted responses to unprompted responses through fading in a systematic and consistent process to avoid prompt dependence (MacDuff et al., 2001).

Documenting Progress and Evaluating Objectives

Clinicians are required to maintain an accurate representation of data collected during the intervention sessions. They are accountable for the effectiveness of the intervention services. Data collection permits the documentation of a given treatment strategy (Roth & Worthington, 2016) because intervention is a dynamic process that requires the clinician to constantly reevaluate the goals to determine if modifications in the therapy are necessary.

Data recording sheets should be designed prior to the start of the intervention. The notation system that is used to collect the data should be specific to the client's needs and goals, and it should indicate the types of cues and prompts being used. With simple written notation, the clinician can note additional significant information, such as self-corrections and the need for cues and prompts. Maintaining data is imperative to determine if the client mastered a goal. Various data sheets are available in textbooks, but clinicians can design data sheets that are specific to the client and his or her goals. The data sheet can be used to record the number of stimulus presentations, correct and incorrect productions, and the types of cues and prompts that were used during a session.

The clinician provides probes intermittently during the intervention process to determine if a client is achieving his or her goals (Roth & Worthington, 2016). The clinician may need to reevaluate the goals if the client is not achieving them or progressing toward mastery. Clinicians need to reflect on the interventions and use the collected data to determine if the therapy objectives were met (Kersner & Wright,

2012). If the objectives were not met, the clinician needs to evaluate if they were realistic for the client. The clinician may want to consider the influence of the client's cognitive-linguistic skills, evaluate whether the materials or stimulus items were appropriate or motivating for the client, consider using a different teaching strategy, or contemplate using prompts and cues in the session. At the same time, the clinician may need to modify a component of the goal (do statement, condition, or criterion) if the client is not making progress toward mastery of the goals.

General Elements to Consider When Developing and Writing Goals

The clinician may want to consider additional factors when developing and writing goals for a client, including the client's current level of functioning, age-appropriate speech-language skills, and the client's cultural and linguistic diversity. Additionally, the clinician needs to consider the facility where the intervention is provided (for example, a healthcare facility, school, or private practice). Additionally, if the client is receiving services in a school, the clinician must be knowledgeable about the Common Core State Standards (CCSS) and response to intervention (RTI). If a client is receiving services in a skilled nursing facility, hospital, rehabilitation center, or private practice, the clinician should be knowledgeable about the ICF and insurance carriers, including their guidelines for the provision of therapy services.

The clinician should consider developing functional goals. According to the ICF model, a clinician needs to consider how the client's diagnosis and signs and symptoms affect his or her body structures and functions. Additionally, the clinician should note how they affect the client's activity and participation in various activities.

An acronym that may be helpful in developing goals is SMART (Torres, 2013). Goals should be *specific* and identify the client's strengths, preferences, and areas of need; in addition, targeted skills should be prioritized. Goals should be *measurable* and *attainable*, with appropriate criterion levels. Goals should be *relevant* and functional for the client's communication environments and interactions with communication partners. Finally, goals should be attainable in a *timely* manner within a reasonable time frame.

Summary

Because there is a demand for EBP and treatment efficacy, it is essential for clinicians to develop goals that are specific, measurable, and functional (Guilford et al., 2007). Developing and writing goals is an important part of the intervention process.

REVIEW QUESTIONS

1. The goal of EBP is to integrate which of the following?
   a. Client, patient, and caregiver perspectives only
   b. External scientific evidence only
   c. The newest treatment program available on the market
   d. Clinical expertise and expert opinion; external scientific evidence; and client, patient, and caregiver perspectives
   e. None of the above

2. Why do clinicians need to perform a task analysis?
   a. It allows the clinician to formulate short-term goals, which are essential to master the long-term goal.
   b. It allows the clinician to attain an Award for Continuing Education (ACE) from ASHA.
   c. It allows the clinician to obtain observation hours.
   d. Both B and C are correct.
   e. None of the above are correct.

3. Which of the following is not an example of a goal with a criterion?
   a. The client will produce /s/ in the initial position of words with 8/10 correct.
   b. The client will produce the present progressive form of verbs in sentences with 80 percent accuracy.
   c. The client will use prolonged speech every time he or she stutters.
   d. The client will name functional objects with 80 percent accuracy.
   e. None of the above are correct.

4. What are the three components of a behavioral objective?
   a. Do statement, condition, and where the services are being provided
   b. Do statement, SMART goals, and ICF
   c. CCSS, RTI, and ICF
   d. Do statement, condition, and criterion
   e. None of the above

5. How is a prompt defined?
   a. A data collection system for clinicians
   b. Part of the do statement
   c. A supplementary strategy or reminder to support or elicit the targeted skill
   d. Both A and B
   e. None of the above

REFERENCES

American Speech-Language-Hearing Association. (2016a). Code of ethics. Retrieved from http://www.asha.org/Code-of-Ethics

American Speech-Language-Hearing Association. (2016b). Scope of practice in speech-language pathology. Retrieved from http://www.asha.org/policy/SP2016-00343

American Speech-Language-Hearing Association. (2017a). ASHA practice policy. Retrieved from http://www.asha.org/policy

American Speech-Language-Hearing Association. (2017b). Evidence-based practice (EBP). Retrieved from http://www.asha.org/Research/EBP

Bleile, K. (2004). The ICF: A framework for setting goals for children with speech impairment. *Child Language Teaching and Therapy, 20,* 199–219.

Fisher, D., & Frey, N. (2013). *Better learning through structured teaching: A framework for the gradual release of responsibility.* Alexandria, VA: Association for Supervision and Curriculum Development.

Goldfarb, R., & Serpanos, Y. (2014). *Professional writing in speech-language pathology and audiology* (2nd ed.). San Diego, CA: Plural.

Guilford, A., Graham, S., & Scheuerle, J. (2007). *The speech-language pathologist: From novice to expert.* Upper Saddle River, NJ: Pearson Education.

Kersner, M., & Wright, J. (2012). *Speech and language therapy: The decision making process when working with children.* New York, NY: Routledge.

MacDuff, G., Krantz, P., & McClannahan, L. (2001). Prompts and prompt-fading strategies for people with autism. In C. Maurice, G. Green, & R. M. Foxx (Eds.), *Making a difference: Behavioral intervention for autism* (pp. 37–50). Austin, TX: PRO-ED.

Moon Meyer, S. M. (1998). *Survival guide for the beginning speech-language clinician.* Gaithersburg, MD: Aspen.

Paul, R. (2014). *Introduction to clinical methods in communication disorders* (3rd ed.). Baltimore, MD: Paul H. Brooks.

Roth, F., & Worthington, C. (2016). *Treatment resource manual for speech-language pathology* (5th ed.). Clifton Park, NY: Cengage Learning.

Torres, I. (2013). Make it work: Write targeted treatment goals. *The ASHA Leader, 18,* 26–27.

West, E., & Billingsley, F. (2005). Improving the system of least prompts: A comparison of procedural variations. *Education and Training in Developmental Disabilities, 40*(2), 131–144.

World Health Organization. (2001). *ICF: International classification of functioning, disability and health.* Geneva, Switzerland: Author.

ADDITIONAL RESOURCES

Academy of Neurologic Communication Disorders and Sciences. www.ancds.org

Agency for Healthcare Research and Quality. www.ahrq.gov

Agency for Healthcare Research and Quality. AHRQ's National Guideline Clearinghouse is a public resource for summaries of evidence-based clinical practice guidelines. www.guideline.gov

American Speech-Language-Hearing Association. ASHA/N-CEP Evidence-Based Systematic Reviews. www.asha.org/Research/EBP/EBSRs

American Speech-Language-Hearing Association. ASHA Practice Policy. www.asha.org/policy

American Speech-Language-Hearing Association. National Outcomes Measurement System (NOMS). www.asha.org/NOMS

American Speech-Language-Hearing Association. Writing Measurable Goals and Objectives. www.asha.org/uploadedFiles/Writing-Measurable-Goals-and-Objectives.pdf

Centre for Evidence-Based Medicine. www.cebm.net

Cochrane. www.cochrane.org

World Health Organization. International Classification of Functioning, Disability and Health (ICF). www.who.int/classifications/icf/en

CHAPTER 2

Historical Perspective of Goal Writing and Contemporary Practice

Terry H. Gozdziewski

Key Terms

Appropriate education
Brown v. Board of Education
Committee on Special Education
Due process
Free appropriate public education
(FAPE)
Individualized education program
(IEP)
Individuals with Disabilities
Education Act (IDEA)
Individuals with Disabilities
Education Improvement Act
(IDEIA)

Least restrictive environment
No Child Left Behind (NCLB) Act
*PARC v. Commonwealth of
Pennsylvania*
Public Law (PL) 94-142
Public Law (PL) 99-457
Section 504 of the Rehabilitation
Act of 1973
Separate but equal
Zero reject

Introduction

The mere mention of the word *history* often elicits moans and groans from students and adults alike. It is only with a thorough understanding

...

of the evolution of federal and state regulations that students will comprehend why goal writing is critical. It is important, therefore, to understand the history of special education law, which encompasses teaching communication skills and academic skills.

In his book *The Law and Special Education*, Yell (2012) claims that our country views education as a birthright. He says that "a common misconception regarding public education is that it is guaranteed by the U.S. Constitution. In fact, education is not (even) mentioned in the Constitution" (2012, p. 45). As professionals in our chosen fields, we believe that all children, no matter if they have disabilities or not, should be given as many educational opportunities as possible (Walker, Brooks, & Wrightsman, 1999).

It may be surprising that not so long ago, the term *special education* did not even exist. Children with obvious learning problems, and even those with subtle learning issues, were ignored and either sent off to institutions or labeled slow and unteachable. Even worse, some children were viewed as being lazy or having behavioral problems. The thought process began to change with a 1954 Supreme Court ruling that became known as **Brown v. Board of Education**, or simply the Brown case.

The Brown Case

The Brown case was actually four cases that were consolidated into one. It involved the doctrine of **separate but equal** and involved the question of whether or not segregation of students of color allowed for equal educational opportunities. Arguments focused on the 14th Amendment of the U.S. Constitution, which states that all citizens are guaranteed equal protection under the law.

The unanimous ruling was delivered by the chief justice himself, the Honorable Earl Warren. The final ruling by the court acknowledged the importance of education for everything from learning what good citizenship means to understanding cultural values to professional training. It ended with the statement that education "is a right that must be made available to all on equal terms" (Yell, 2012, p. 45).

The final judgment made it clear that the idea of separate but equal was inherently unequal: "We conclude that in the field of public education the doctrine of 'separate but equal' has no place. Separate educational facilities are inherently unequal (and) deprived of the equal protection of the laws guaranteed by the Fourteenth Amendment" (Turnbull, 1990, p. 295).

Obviously, the Brown case had an enormous impact on the civil rights movement, and it also had an enormous effect on the lives of educationally handicapped children. In short, since the government decreed that schools cannot discriminate due to a child's ethnicity, they also cannot discriminate due to a child's educational abilities or disabilities. This was the beginning of special education law.

The PARC Case

"Prior to 1975, children with disabilities were routinely excluded from public education, while others were placed in inadequate segregated programs or left in regular education without any accommodations or support" (Cohen, 2009, p. 13). This very obvious inequality led to other class action lawsuits. One of these suits, **PARC v. Commonwealth of Pennsylvania**, or the PARC case, became a landmark case that made its way to the Supreme Court. Similar to the Brown case, it was actually a compilation of several cases. The primary litigant was a student named Nancy Beth Brown who was severely cognitively impaired. At the time, the State of Pennsylvania had established criteria for attending public school. Nancy and other children who did not meet the criteria were not allowed to participate in the public school educational system.

The plaintiffs were Nancy's parents and the parents of other children who were refused entrance into the public school system due to their low cognitive abilities. These parents claimed that by not allowing their children to go to school, the State of Pennsylvania was violating the children's 14th Amendment rights guaranteed by the U.S. Constitution, specifically their right to due process and equal protection. The parents based their claim on the Brown case, citing the part of the ruling that said all children are entitled to equal educational opportunity.

The court found in favor of the plaintiffs, ruling that children with disabilities were being denied access to an education and that the denial constituted a violation of the 14th Amendment. Furthermore, the PARC case established several important ideas that formed the basis of the Education of the Handicapped Act (EHA) several years later. These ideas included the following:

1. the "**zero reject**" principle—all children are capable of learning and should not be excluded from educational programs.
2. "**least restrictive environment**"—students with disabilities should, when appropriate, be educated alongside their peers.
3. **due process** procedures must be followed in all placements

- ◆ due process includes notification to the parent, the right to a hearing, the right to examine records and to cross examine witnesses, and the right to an independent evaluation.
4. **appropriate education**—the education provided must be appropriate to the learning capacities of the student (Northern Arizona University, n.d., para. 4)

In essence, the Supreme Court ruled that "education was essential to enable a child to function in society and that ALL children can benefit from education" (Turnbull, 1990, p. 30). What does this have to do with writing goals? Everything.

Public Law (PL) 94-142

Soon after the PARC case, another class action lawsuit was filed. It was brought to the judicial system because the parents and guardians of children with several different disabilities (including behavioral issues, hyperactivity, epilepsy, and other physical impairments) were also being denied access to a public school education (Yell, 2012). The outcome was a ruling guaranteeing procedural safeguards and due process rights for students in special education.

The results of these cases revealed that the education of all children, no matter their abilities or disabilities, is of paramount importance not just to their families, but to American society as a whole. Being directly responsible for the education of these youngsters, we must prove to families, school personnel, and the students themselves that the best course of action will be taken. This includes what we plan to accomplish and how we plan to accomplish it so the child can reach his or her full potential. This can be done only with the establishment of appropriate goals.

Federal special education laws do not derive strictly from judicial system decisions; they are also derived from federal regulations and statutes. As a result of the PARC case, arguably the most important federal law that specifically addressed special education (including speech therapy) was written. It was officially called the Education for All Handicapped Children Act but is better known as **Public Law (PL) 94-142**. In short, this education law came with the promise of federal financial incentives (Yell, 2012). It was signed into law by then-president Gerald Ford. PL 94-142 mandated that students with disabilities were to be guaranteed fair and nondiscriminatory assessments and a free and appropriate education in what has become known as the least restrictive environment. It also mandated that educationally handicapped children be provided an **individualized education program (IEP)** (Yell, 2012).

Two of the main purposes of PL 94-142 were as follows (Education for All Handicapped Children Act of 1975):

1. "To assure that all children with disabilities have available to them a free and appropriate education."
2. "To assure that the rights of children with disabilities and their families are protected."

It is interesting to note that PL 94-142 incorporated many of the principles established in the PARC case. Among the provisions were the following principles:

- All children have the right to an education that addresses their individual needs.
- All parents have the right to participate in educational decisions.
- All parents have the right to disagree with decisions made by the school and to challenge those decisions legally (Cohen, 2009).

Kirk, Gallagher, and Coleman summarized it slightly differently. They said that the law provided six key provisions that are still followed today. These provisions are zero reject, nondiscriminatory evaluations, IEPs, least restrictive environment, due process, and parental participation. IEPs stand out in relationship to the subject of this text. IEPs must be provided, and they must contain goals for the child and other information (Kirk, Gallagher, & Coleman, 2015). Thus, it should be abundantly clear that writing goals is part of federal law.

It was not that long ago that children who had learning problems, whether in communication or academics, were not receiving the services that they needed. Prior to the enactment of PL 94-142, educationally handicapped children across the country were still being denied access to an appropriate education (Giuliani, 2012).

Individuals with Disabilities Education Improvement Act (IDEIA)

In 1990, PL 94-142 was reauthorized and became known as the **Individuals with Disabilities Education Act (IDEA)**. It was reauthorized in 1997 and 2004 and is now known as the **Individuals with Disabilities Education Improvement Act (IDEIA)**. "IDEIA is the federal law in the United States that governs how states must provide special education to children with disabilities" (Giuliani, 2012, p. 23).

Cohen went on to say that IDEIA is "a statute that provides states and local school districts with federal funding on the condition that the states adhere to the special education requirements established by the U.S. Congress" and that "IDEIA, in short, provides sweeping and detailed requirements for the provision of appropriate educational services to children with disabilities as well as broad mandates for parental involvement in decision making" (Cohen, 2009, pp. 29–30, 33). It was here, on the federal level, that the need for goal writing was clarified and deemed essential. Certainly states interpret IDEIA in their own way, but the need for goals is consistent throughout the United States.

At **Committee on Special Education** meetings, writing goals is part of the proceedings. School personnel, parents and guardians, and sometimes students determine what will be taught over a predetermined period of time. An analogy for a goal is a highway for a journey. Goals should clearly state what will be taught, where it will be taught, who will teach it, how it will be measured, and when this will be achieved. Clinicians would be remiss if they viewed goals as just more paperwork. On the contrary, goals have evolved because of federal laws and regulations, state laws, and judicial rulings that were enacted to protect the educational rights of students. Goals are not designed to be complex annoyances. They are a legally necessary part of an educational plan designed to help students to be the very best they can be, no matter what that means or where they start from.

The Rowley Case

PL 94-142 spawned a number of judicial challenges. One of the most important of these was *Board of Education of the Hendrick Hudson Central School District v. Rowley,* also known as the Rowley case, which set legal precedents throughout the country. The case centered on a first-grade student named Amy Rowley. When the case began, Amy was in a general education kindergarten class. Her parents were deaf, and Amy herself had been diagnosed with a significant hearing loss at approximately 15 months of age. Her parents believed that if Amy were provided with the supportive services of a speech-language pathologist and a teacher for hearing-impaired individuals, in addition to an FM assistive technology unit, she could succeed in a regular classroom, and indeed she did. An important note is that Amy was described as an excellent speech reader. She was originally provided with a sign language interpreter, but after 2 weeks it was determined that Amy did not need this service, so it was discontinued.

Amy was scheduled to go into a fully mainstream first-grade class the following year. The school district agreed to provide her with the same services she had received in kindergarten. Her parents asked for a sign language interpreter to be reassigned to her as well. The district declined the request based on her success in kindergarten. Her parents ultimately took legal action.

This case eventually reached the Supreme Court. (It is interesting to note that the Rowleys' attorney, Michael Chatoff, was also deaf and became the first deaf lawyer to argue before the Supreme Court [Walker, 1982]). The question before the court was to define the term *free and appropriate education.* In 1982, the court ruled in favor of the school district by a six to three margin. In the majority decision, written by Justice William Rehnquist, it was clarified that *appropriate education* "does not mean a potential-maximizing education" (Turnbull, 1990, p. 318). The federal court ruling asserted that every child, regardless of his or her ability, is entitled to a free and suitable education, but the education does not have to be the very best. It merely has to meet the child's needs. The term *appropriate, not optimal* has been utilized for many years to explain to families why their children do not always receive services as often or as intensively as they feel are necessary. Turnbull further explains by stating that "the best education available does not have to be offered" and that "the child's maximum development is not the goal of his or her education" (Turnbull, 1990, p. 131). This basic premise of our public education system is often referred to as **free appropriate public education (FAPE)**. Clinicians must write their goals with this in mind.

Other Noteworthy Laws and Regulations

Numerous other laws, statutes, and judicial rulings have been made since the Rowley case was decided. Many of them, however, do not focus on special education, but rather on improving the education system in general. In 1986, the law was amended to include children from birth to age 5 years. It became known as Education of the Handicapped Amendments or **Public Law (PL) 99-457**.

The **No Child Left Behind (NCLB) Act** was enacted in 2002. It was designed to "hold states, school districts, and schools accountable for measurably improving student achievement" (Yell, 2012, p. 57). This includes students with disabilities.

NCLB was then succeeded by the **Every Student Succeeds Act (ESSA)**, which was signed by President Barack Obama on

December 10, 2015. This law was supported by both major political parties. It reauthorized "the nation's national education law and longstanding commitment to equal opportunity for all students" (U.S. Department of Education, n.d., para. 1). The ESSA reaffirms the American ideal that all children, regardless of their race, income, background, or place of residence, deserve the chance to make of their life what they choose. The act addresses both the needs of children who learn in typical ways and the needs of those who learn in different ways.

Another federal regulation that is often referred to is **Section 504 of the Rehabilitation Act of 1973**. This act was originally conceived as a civil rights protection, but, as in other instances, it has been used to aid children who are having difficulties in school. In this case, a handicapped person was defined as "any person who has a physical or mental impairment that substantially limits one or more of that person's major life activities" (Yell, 2012, p. 52). Section 504 differs from IDEIA and ESSA in that it is more lenient and open, whereas IDEIA and ESSA are more structured and have more stringent standards. Section 504 recognizes that there are circumstances when a child's learning is hampered due to an impairment of a life function, not academic, emotional, or cognitive issues. Consider, for example, a boy who is diagnosed with diabetes. He may miss some academic work because he has to take time out of class to test his glucose levels and receive insulin. Another example is a girl with asthma who might have to miss class time to receive nebulizer treatments. With small accommodations that a school can easily provide, these two children can be taught in a typical setting. Section 504 says these types of accommodations should be made to allow students with these type of problems to attend school in typical settings.

Section 504 mandates accommodations and modifications rather than direct special education services or speech-language therapy. If services are provided under Section 504, the clinician should develop goals in the same manner as for pupils who receive services under the IDEA umbrella.

Summary

As stated in the beginning of this chapter, history needs to be shared because its impact on the present and the future is immeasurable. It is crucial to understand how the history of special education services, including speech-language therapy, impacts goal writing. By having a complete understanding of the information gleaned from ongoing unbiased assessments, courses of action, or goals, are developed. Goals must be fair, measurable, and evidence based. Goals drive habilitation and rehabilitation. Goals must stand up to the scrutiny of an educational hearing and court of law. Goals are the heart, brain, and soul that enable individuals to reach their full potential, and they strongly influence how educational services are provided today.

REVIEW QUESTIONS

1. What principle did the Rowley case bring to the forefront?
   a. All members of the deaf community are entitled to the communication system of their choosing.
   b. Children should be educated in the least restrictive environment.
   c. Professionals must be trained and certified.
   d. Appropriate does not mean optimal.

2. What principle did the PARC case address for the first time?
   a. The importance of writing goals
   b. Zero reject
   c. IEPs
   d. Assessment and identification methods

3. The Brown case was originally about
   a. segregation.
   b. establishing parental rights.
   c. ensuring that special education is available to all students.
   d. mandating IEPs.

4. What does Section 504 cover?
   a. Providing services for children who need maximum support
   b. The rules and regulations needed to be followed during Committee on Special Education meetings
   c. Issues that are not considered educationally handicapped
   d. Factors that are faced by children ages 3 to 5 years

5. The regulation known as NCLB
   a. clearly takes into account students with disabilities.
   b. establishes due process procedures.
   c. confidently mandates that all children, even those with educational, physical, and emotional issues, will learn at high levels.
   d. does not address any of the above.

REFERENCES

Cohen, M. (2009). *A guide to special education advocacy: What parents, clinicians and advocates need to know.* Philadelphia, PA: Jessica Kingsley.
Education for All Handicapped Children Act of 1975, Pub. L. No. 94-142, § 6, 89 Stat. 773 (1977).
Giuliani, G. (2012). *The comprehensive guide to special education law: Over 400 frequently asked questions and answers every educator needs to know about the legal rights of exceptional children.* Philadelphia, PA: Jessica Kingsley.

Kirk, S., Gallagher, J., & Coleman, M. (2015). *Educating exceptional children* (14th ed.). Stamford, CT: Cengage Learning.

Northern Arizona University. (n.d.). PARC v the Commonwealth of Pennsylvania (1971). Retrieved from http://jan.ucc.nau.edu/~ldg/ese424/class/understanding/roots/parc.html

Turnbull, H. R. (1990). *Free appropriate public education: The law and children with disabilities* (3rd ed.). Denver, CO: Love.

U.S. Department of Education. (n.d.). Every Student Succeeds Act (ESSA). Retrieved from http://www.ed.gov/essa?src=policy

Walker, L. (1982, July 19). Though deaf, Amy Rowley is a good student—too good, says the Supreme Court. *People.* Retrieved from http://people.com/archive/though-deaf-amy-rowley-is-a-good-student-too-good-says-the-supreme-court-vol-18-no-3/

Walker, N., Brooks, C., & Wrightsman, L. (1999). *Children's rights in the United States: In search of a national policy.* Thousand Oaks, CA: Sage.

Yell, M. (2012). *The law and special education* (3rd ed.). Boston, MA: Pearson.

Unit B

Writing Goals in Speech-Language Pathology, Aural Rehabilitation and Habilitation, and Special Education

Language Disorders in Children

Margaret M. Laskowski
Terry H. Gozdziewski

Key Terms

Authentic assessment	Phonology
Content	Phonotactics
Criterion-referenced tests	Polysemous words
Dialects	Pragmatics
Dynamic assessment	Receptive language
Expressive language	Scaffolding
Form	Semantics
Language	Syntax
Morphology	Use
Norm-referenced tests	Vocabulary

Introduction: What Is Language?

The word *language*, when used in a school setting, is one of the most misinterpreted words. Many general education teachers and parents assume it refers to language arts or English as a second language. Clinicians, however, know it is far more complex than that.

Crystal defines **language** as "the systematic and conventional use of sounds (or signs or written symbols) for the purpose of communication or self-expression. This definition is short and straightforward and, although true, it is misleading in its simplicity. Language is (far more) complex and multifaceted" (Crystal, 1987). Owens defines language as a "socially shared code or conventional system for representing concepts through the use of arbitrary symbols and rule-governed combinations of those symbols" (2016, p. 4). Kennison (2014) says there are between 6,000 and 7,000 different languages spoken in the world today and that English is the third most popular spoken language; Chinese is first and Spanish is second. Owens (2016) further explains that no matter the language or the place where it is spoken, all languages share certain characteristics.

One of the shared characteristics of languages is that to sustain themselves, they must evolve and grow. If they do not, they will die; many languages have met this unfortunate fate. Many languages no longer exist because they did not generate words and phrases that accommodate more modern concepts, newer philosophies, or world happenings. Because language is socially based, society has to agree on the organization of arbitrary sounds representing specific words, phrases, and sentences. This organization must also include the rules that will be followed.

On the other hand, thousands of words and phrases have been added to English. Many of these words are from science, and many others are from technology, politics, and social media. For example, from medicine we now have the term *Zika virus*, which is new within the past few years. From politics we have new words like *ISIS* and *ground zero*. Technology is growing so fast it is hard to keep up with nouns like *tablet* and verbs like *scroll* (both were originally terms pertaining to religious history). There are new meanings for the words *mouse*, *laptop*, and *desktop*, and we have other new words like *blog* and *vlog*. And social media platforms spawned the terms *selfie* and *hashtag*.

Another characteristic of many languages, including English, is that they are spoken differently in different places. There may be slight pronunciation differences or even different words to represent the same concept. Think of how many different ways you can express the idea of a sandwich. Words such as *sub*, *submarine*, *hoagie*, *hero*, and *po'boy* are all used, depending on the geographic location. These differences are referred to as **dialects**, which are defined as "subcategories of the parent language that use similar but not identical rules" (Owens, 2016, p. 4). In light of the changing demographics in the public school population (National Center for Education Statistics, 2017), it is important to note that dialects are different from disorders. Dialects are not wrong or disordered.

The Components of Language

Language, as stated previously, is exceptionally complicated and multidimensional. The fact that *Homo sapiens* is the only species on Earth to use language at a highly sophisticated level makes us unique on this planet. Language should not be seen as one giant concept; rather, it should be broken into smaller, understandable components.

The easiest way to break down language is to view it as having receptive and expressive components. **Receptive language** refers to the understanding of arbitrary symbols, while **expressive language** is the use of these symbols. An attempt to pigeonhole language into just two divisions is no simple task. The divisions do not refer to just single words but rather intertwined, inseparable cognitive abilities involving words, phrases, sentences, paragraphs, and whole narratives. Each component strongly relies on and supports the other so we can reach our highest language potential.

Content, Form, and Use

Bloom and Lahey (1978) provided a better understanding of what language is. Knowledge of their model can significantly help clinicians when they begin to formulate goals. These researchers did not see language as just two simple interrelated elements; in their view, there are three primary components that are even more intertwined than originally thought. They named these three components content, form, and use (Lahey, 1988).

Content refers to **semantics**, which in turn refers to meaning. It is not as straightforward as just viewing one word at a time. That would be closer to the concept of **vocabulary**. Content involves the meaning of one or more words that are put together, such as in a phrase, sentence, or story. Content requires understanding objects, the relationships among objects, and relationships among events (Lahey, 1988). Equally important, semantic ability can be further divided into receptive and expressive skills.

The second dimension is **form**, which imparts rules to a language. To help describe the term, Bloom and Lahey (1978) divided it into three smaller elements: syntax, morphology, and phonology.

Syntax can be described as the external organization of words. "These rules specify word, phrase and clause order; sentence organization; and the relationships among words, word classes, and other sentence elements" (Owens, 2016, p. 18). Why is it that in English we say *red house* (with the adjective first and the noun second), while in

French we say *maison rouge* and in Spanish we say *casa rojo* (which literally translates to *house red*, with the noun first and the adjective second)? The syntax of the English language dictates that adjectives precede nouns.

Form also includes the concept of **morphology**. Morphology can be defined as the rules of language governing the internal organization of words (Owens, 2016; Turnbull & Justice, 2017). As toddlers, children begin combining words and acquire two types of morphemes (the smallest unit of meaning) that allow them to expand their vocabulary and add more specificity to their message. The addition of grammatical or inflectional morphemes, such as the present progressive *-ing* and the plural *-s*, increases the precision of the child's communication. Derivational morphemes, such as prefixes and suffixes, are another strategy to increase vocabulary and change a word's syntactic class (e.g., *friend* is a noun, whereas *friendless* is an adjective) and semantic meaning (e.g., *like* versus *dislike*) (Apel & Werfel, 2014).

The third component of form is known as **phonology**. Phonology is defined as the "rules governing the structure, distribution, and sequencing of speech sounds" (Owens, 2016, p. 19). An example of this is the hypothetical word *blib*. There is no such word as *blib* in English, but we know there could be because *blib* follows all the specific rules about how we can put speech sounds together (**phonotactics**). On the other hand, we know that *pghxxi* could never be a word in English because it does not follow the phonological rules of our language.

The third dimension of language is known as **use** or **pragmatics** (Bloom & Lahey, 1978). According to Turnbull and Justice, pragmatics "involves acquiring the rules of language that govern how language is used as a social tool" (2017, p. 57). Pragmatics also encompasses understanding the rules of discourse, such as when to take turns during conversations; when to ask a conversation partner to clarify his or her message; when to change language according to who is listening and the social situation; and how to communicate a sufficiently organized and detailed narrative (Paul & Norbury, 2012).

Complex cognitive skills like language cannot be viewed as simply black and white. The three components of content, form, and use, and the three smaller elements of syntax, morphology, and phonology, are by no means independent of one another. There are frequent, complex interactions and integrations of all these components (Lahey, 1988). In short, language is one of the most difficult, complicated, and multifaceted of all human capabilities.

Without a complete understanding of what language is and its complexity, clinicians will not understand normal development. Without the understanding of normal development, one cannot understand what atypical development is and, therefore, cannot transpose the analysis and results of assessments and observations into written goals. Lahey wrote, "Normal developmental sequences provide the best hypotheses about the sequence in which the language disordered child will learn language" (1988, p. vii). A clinician will be able to write appropriate goals only when he or she understands the scope of language and its sequence of development.

Disorders in Children's Language

Children exhibit numerous types of language disorders, and there may be issues related to any of the areas specified by Bloom and Lahey (1978). Language deficits can be associated with other disorders such as intellectual disability, learning disabilities, autism spectrum disorder, sensory impairments (such as hearing loss and visual impairment), acquired neurologic disorders (such as traumatic brain injury and focal brain lesions), or genetic syndromes (such as Down syndrome, Williams syndrome, fragile X syndrome, and Prader-Willi syndrome (Kaderavek, 2015; Paul & Norbury, 2012). Language deficits are also associated with extreme neglect and substance abuse, such as fetal alcohol spectrum disorders (Paul & Norbury, 2012; Rogers-Adkinson & Stuart, 2007). Specific language impairment, typically diagnosed during a child's school years, refers to an impairment in which a language deficit is the only impairment, and it has no readily apparent cause, such as hearing loss or neurological damage (Betz, Eickhoff, & Sullivan, 2013; Hegde & Pomaville, 2013; Kaderavek, 2015; Tomblin et al., 1997).

Pinzola, Plexico, and Haynes (2016) state that certain groups of children, besides those previously mentioned, should be considered at high risk for language disabilities. They say that children who have a history of language impairments; those with learning or reading difficulties; those who display social, emotional, and behavioral problems; and those who are beginning to struggle academically have a higher probability of having a language disability than the general population.

Regardless of whether a child is suspected of having a specific language impairment or having a language disorder due to comorbid conditions, a comprehensive speech-language evaluation must take place.

Speech-Language Evaluation: A Summary

If a child is suspected of having one or more language deficit areas, a speech-language assessment is usually recommended. This assessment may also be recommended following a screening, which typically occurs at entry into a preschool or kindergarten and may be a norm-referenced list or a checklist that is accompanied by a parent or caregiver questionnaire. The failure of a screening does not necessarily indicate the presence of a language delay or disorder. A comprehensive speech-language evaluation is necessary to diagnose a speech or language disorder, formulate goals, and design an intervention plan (Kaderavek, 2015). All areas of speech and language should be examined when conducting a comprehensive assessment, even if the primary concern is a language disorder due to the interplay of language content, form, and use (Kaderavek, 2015; Shipley & McAfee, 2016).

The therapist conducting the evaluation should gather and review as much information as possible before the start of testing. If the student is in school, a review of his or her general file can provide valuable data, such as attendance and tardy information, results of the home language survey, previous report cards, results of prior assessments or responses to interventions, and disciplinary actions. The evaluator can gain valuable insights from interviewing the student to gain firsthand information about how the student perceives his or her difficulties. Whenever possible, the evaluator should also collaborate with other professionals who interact with the student to gain their perspectives on the presenting difficulty; examples of such professionals include the classroom teacher, special area teachers, school nurse, and related service providers, such as school psychologist, physical and occupational therapists, reading teacher, and learning disability specialist. Meeting with the parents or caregivers and conducting a case history will provide additional understanding of the student's developmental and medical history and the family's perspective on the problem. At this point in the assessment process, the evaluator has gained information about the child and family's cultural and linguistic background and can take this into consideration when planning the rest of the assessment process. Useful reproducible forms for gathering case history information can be found in *Assessment in Speech-Language Pathology: A Resource Manual*, 5th edition (Shipley & McAfee, 2016).

Many components should be provided in a comprehensive speech-language evaluation, including but not limited to the following: hearing screening; oral structure and function examination;

assessment of articulation; assessment of phonology and phonological awareness; assessment of fluency, voice quality, and prosodic elements (stress, intonation, and pitch); assessment of language content, form, and use; and assessment of written language (Paul & Norbury, 2012; Shipley & McAfee, 2016). Additional assessments may be administered at the discretion of the evaluator.

Each assessment should be individually tailored to meet the needs of the student; several methods may be used in combination to accomplish this task. Skills can be assessed using **norm-referenced tests**, which allow a comparison of the child's performance to same-aged peers; **criterion-referenced tests**, which compare the child's performance to expected performance; and **authentic assessment**, which identifies what a child can and cannot do in a variety of realistic and natural contexts (e.g., language sampling in a variety of communicative contexts, sample of written work, anecdotal notes, etc.) (Kaderavek, 2015; Paul & Norbury, 2012). **Dynamic assessment** is considered an authentic assessment approach and is extremely useful when assessing children who have linguistically and culturally diverse backgrounds (Gutiérrez-Clellen & Peña, 2001).

Numerous norm-referenced and criterion-referenced tests are available that can be used to evaluate a child's language abilities. Some only evaluate one area, such as receptive vocabulary, while others focus on a child's abilities in various language domains, such as syntax, morphology, and phonological awareness. Examples include the Peabody Picture Vocabulary Test, Fourth Edition, which looks only at a child's one-word receptive vocabulary ability, and the Clinical Evaluation of Language Fundamentals, Fifth Edition (CELF-5), which evaluates many subareas of children's language. The selection of a test is based on many factors, including but not limited to client needs, clinician preferences, and availability of assessment material. The process of analyzing the results is usually the same regardless of the assessment tool used.

In summary, as in every communication area when an evaluation is administered, an evaluation must be both formal and informal in nature, and it must be dynamic as opposed to static. Evaluating a child's language skills is complicated. His or her language abilities in all areas must be considered and compared to other children (of the same gender, if possible) who are the same age and have the same cultural and linguistic background. These areas should be examined using formal tests and during informal conversations held in natural settings. Conclusions should never be drawn after only one encounter but rather should be formulated over time using multiple sources of data (Individuals with Disabilities Education Act of 2004 [IDEA], 2004).

Elements to Consider When Writing Children's Language Goals

The purpose of this chapter is to establish what a clinician should do if a child is diagnosed with a language disorder. The assessment results must be carefully and thoughtfully analyzed in a qualitative manner, not just calculated. Prior to the start of the goal writing process, the clinician should assess the student's strengths and weaknesses; analyze patterns of errors; determine the level of function in each area of language content, form, and use; consult with the family; and collaborate with educational professionals to prioritize the skills needed for social and academic functioning (Paul & Norbury, 2012).

Selecting Target Behaviors: Strengths and Weaknesses

It is obvious to novice clinicians that one has to look at the difficulties a child may display. After all, that is why we are here. However, far too often, clinicians look only at weaknesses and ignore a child's strengths, which can prove to be detrimental. When a clinician views a child as half empty, there are considerable negative connotations. The self-fulfilling prophecy becomes real; if children view themselves as incapable, they will more likely perform that way.

Knowing a child's strengths must be kept in mind when determining therapy targets and writing goals. For children to learn, they must build on previously acquired knowledge. This is known as **scaffolding** (Beed, Hawkins, & Roller, 1991; Paul & Norbury, 2012). By using a child's strengths, concepts and ideas can be taught more easily and better retention can be expected. Faster, long-lasting, positive results can be expected when this approach is used.

It is also imperative for clinicians to look for patterns of errors so that strategies to address the patterns, rather than individual errors, can be formulated. This approach is more efficient and facilitates both carryover and generalization of target skills. Again, this type of approach should be reflected in how the goals are written.

Selecting Target Behaviors: Consistent versus Inconsistent Errors

It essential to consider the consistency of errors, discovered during both formal and informal assessments, when choosing target behaviors to remediate and when writing goals (Bernthal, Bankson, & Flipsen, 2013). The errors and error patterns that students display can often be categorized as either consistent or inconsistent. Consistent errors are those that occur all the time, no matter the environment (e.g., both at school and at home, when the child is either relaxed or feels stressed, whether the child is working with a teacher or playing with friends, etc.). Inconsistent errors are those that are sometimes performed correctly and sometimes performed incorrectly. Inconsistency can be attributed to many factors, including emotional and physical states. On a more positive note, because inconsistency demonstrates that the student has the capability, it most often reflects an emerging skill. Regardless of age, an individual does not automatically move from unskilled behavior to mastery without practice and intervention. Understanding errors and patterns of errors must be considered when writing goals.

This attention to consistency is not only an important factor when working with children who have language difficulties, but also is important in all disciplines of speech-language pathology and education. Very often, inconsistency in a particular skill indicates that a child is outgrowing the skill or incorporating new, more sophisticated components into an existing skill set. The question is whether the clinician should remediate a skill that may be in progress or initiate work on skills that are not yet evident. Like so many things, there are pros and cons to both approaches.

When addressing skills that are already emerging, the targets can be achieved more quickly. The child will make more rapid progress in therapy, and that, in turn, will boost the child's self-esteem, increase his or her motivation, and may help alleviate the parents' concerns. Feelings of success and pride in accomplishments typically translate to increased motivation and better self-image. This makes future instruction easier because the child knows that he or she can succeed. Also, when families and educators begin to see success, they have a more positive attitude, which transfers to the child.

Some might argue that working on emerging skills is a waste of both the clinician's and the student's time because the skill may ultimately improve without direct intervention. These individuals believe that clinicians should work on areas that have not emerged or are not showing signs of improvement, which is often referred to as the greatest area of need. This philosophy dictates that goals should target deficit areas that do not show any signs of development and follow the typical developmental sequence (Paul & Norbury, 2012).

Level of Function: Language Content, Form, and Use

The findings of the assessment will provide a starting point for the direction of intervention and the formulation of goals. The clinician should carefully compare the child's skills in the areas of syntax, morphology, phonology, semantics, and pragmatics against typical age level expectations. The clinician can make a determination of the student's strengths and weaknesses in all areas and use this information to determine the target behaviors. More detailed information regarding the typical developmental sequences for language content, form, and use can be found at the end of this chapter in the "Additional Resources" section.

Prioritizing Target Areas: Collaboration with Family and Professionals

Developing effective goals requires collaboration on the part of the professionals, family, and child, if appropriate. The team members may change based on the age or needs of the child, but the collaborative process involved in developing goals should remain the same. Family members, along with educational professionals, should be actively engaged in prioritizing potential target areas that will facilitate the social and academic success of the child (Paul & Norbury, 2012).

When working with children from birth through age 3 years, intervention is both family and child focused, as mandated by Part C of the Individuals with Disabilities Education Improvement Act (Individuals with Disabilities Education Act of 2004). An IFSP is developed with this focus in mind. For that reason, the therapeutic team should collaborate with the family to identify what target areas they see as a priority, and they should develop goals accordingly (American Speech-Language-Hearing Association, 2008a, 2008b). Additionally, the cultural and linguistic background of the child and family must receive thoughtful consideration in this process when writing goals (Owens, 2014). Thorough coverage of this topic, as well as sample forms to assist in gathering data from the family to write goals, is presented by Roth and Worthington (2016) and Paul and Norbury (2012).

For school-aged children, it is imperative for clinicians to familiarize themselves with the CCSS (Common Core State Standards Initiative, 2010) when goals are being developed as part of the IEP. The CCSS should be reviewed in terms of syntax, semantics, pragmatics, phonology, and morphology when considering speech-language intervention and writing goals (Rudebusch, 2012). In addition to the assessment data, the clinician and the educational professional can gain information about student performance across subject matter by collaborating with classroom teachers, reading specialists, special educators, and other educational professionals. The general educator can provide additional information about the student's abilities and needs in the area of syntax, morphology, phonology, semantics, and pragmatics relative to grade level standards and also can draw comparisons against the performance of peers (Ehren, 2000; Power-deFur & Flynn, 2012).

Goal Writing: Components of a Goal

After current assessment data have been carefully and thoughtfully analyzed, areas of strength and weakness have been identified, and target behaviors have been determined, the clinician can begin the goal writing process. The educational professionals and therapists should carefully consider the needs of the whole child: academic skills, home and independent living needs, and future college or career skills. An increasingly popular framework that is useful for writing effective goals is the specific, measurable, attainable, realistic, timely (SMART) criteria, which come from an approach to the management by objectives concept developed by Peter Drucker (Greenwood, 1981; Jung, 2007; Swigert, 2014). The SMART IEP goal is as follows:

- Specific: Make the goal clear and easy to understand.
- Measurable: Measure progress at specified milestones.
- Achievable: Realistically relate the target to the most critical needs.
- Realistic: Develop the goal with a standards-based outcome in mind.
- Timely: Define clear beginning and end points.

Rudebusch (2012), Power-deFur and Flynn (2012), and Flynn (2015) all provide excellent presentations on how to write effective goals that are aligned with the CCSS. Roth and Worthington (2016) and Jung (2007) offer detailed information about the components of a goal and developing an intervention plan.

Language Content, Form, and Use: Developing Goals

If the results of an assessment provide evidence that a child displays deficits in the areas of language content (semantics), form (syntax, morphology, and phonology), and use (pragmatics), clinicians must develop goals to target these skills. But a clinician may wonder where to begin to tackle such a complex area. The answer is easy: begin at the beginning.

A solid knowledge of language development is required for formulating goals, and an abundance of information is readily available on this topic. Owens (2016) presents a detailed review of language development from birth through adolescence and adulthood. Nippold (2007) offers detailed information about language development in school-aged children (6–12 years), adolescents (13–19 years), and young adults (20 years and older). Roth and Worthington (2016) provide basic information, protocols, and developmental milestones that may be useful when developing goals. See the "Additional Resources" section of this chapter for more information.

The following sections provide an overview of areas that typically pose the greatest challenge to students presenting with language disorders. Understanding the types of challenges these students face should assist clinicians in refining and targeting specific goal areas.

Language Content: Semantic Goals

Children with language disorders may present deficits in one or more of the following areas of semantic language: vocabulary; multiple-meaning words; relational terms; semantic ambiguities; and figurative language (Owens, 2014; Paul & Norbury, 2012; Turnbull & Justice, 2017). These students have difficulty comprehending and using figurative language. When writing goals, the content information for each area should be specified, as well as the conditions or where the child will demonstrate use of the target behavior (Jung, 2007; Rudebusch, 2012).

In the school setting, vocabulary is typically introduced and learned within thematic units as part of a larger curriculum. Younger children may be introduced to thematic units, such as holidays, whereas older students will learn specific words from the math, social studies, and science curricula. As students progress through their school experience, their academic success depends on mastery of increasingly specific and abstract vocabulary. Effective goals specify the academic vocabulary that will be targeted within the thematic unit. This information can be obtained through review of the CCSS and texts used by the students.

Polysemous words, or multiple-meaning words, pose difficulties to children with language disorders, and these problems reflect their lack of word knowledge and restricted semantic categories.

Comprehension and use are difficult for students with language disorders because polysemous words are not concrete and typically change with the referent being used. Relational terms include comparative, spatial, and temporal terms. Familial terms, such as *aunt* and *sister*, and age terms, such as *younger* and *older*, can be very challenging for students to make sense of and to use in oral and written language.

Semantic ambiguities, or statements with more than one meaning, are also challenging for students because they may be inaccurately interpreted when used out of context. Semantic ambiguities include the following types: phonological, lexical, syntactic or surface structure, and deep structure. Phonological ambiguities are words that sound the same (homophones) but have different meanings (Turnbull & Justice, 2017); for example, "I ate two *pears*" (versus *pairs*). Lexical ambiguity is a word that has two or more possible meanings; for example, "I picked up the hammer and *saw*." The comprehension of lexical ambiguity is a prerequisite for understanding newspaper headlines, jokes, and riddles. Syntactic or surface structure ambiguity occurs when words in a sentence can be used in another sentence that conveys a different meaning; for example, "I told her *baby* stories" versus "I told her baby *stories*." Deep structure ambiguity occurs when a noun serves as an agent in one meaning but as an object in a different meaning; for example, "The duck is ready to eat" (Nippold, 1998, p. 140).

Figurative language has both literal and figurative meanings and covers similes, metaphors, idioms, and proverbs. Metalinguistic ability is required for the comprehension and use of figurative language. Humor is a type of figurative language that can cause difficulty for students with language disorders.

Language Form: Syntax, Morphology, and Phonology Goals

The analysis results from a language sample obtained during the assessment will yield invaluable information regarding the student's syntactic, morphological, and phonological abilities. Numerous language sample analysis methods can be used, such as Developmental Sentence Analysis (Lee, 1974), Brown's Stages of Language Development (Brown, 1973), Content, Form, and Use (Bloom & Lahey, 1978), Terminal Unit or T-Unit (Hunt, 1965), and Communication Unit or C-Unit (Loban, 1966). Owens (2014), Nelson (2010), and Paul & Norbury (2012) thoroughly cover the process of obtaining a language sample and provide in-depth explanations of each of these language sample analyses and their applications. The Systematic Analysis of Language Transcripts (SALT) software provides a computerized language sample analysis and allows a client's transcript to be compared to a database of normative language measures (Miller, 2012).

It is important to remember the linguistic and dialectal backgrounds of clients when performing a language sample analysis. Owens (2014) states that the Developmental Sentence Scoring process used in the Developmental Sentence Analysis (Lee, 1974) is not an appropriate tool for assessing the language abilities of children with culturally and linguistically diverse backgrounds. Nelson (2010) offers another option, the Black English Sentence Scoring, as a bias-free scoring measure. During the school year, continued development in the areas of complex syntax, morphology, and phonology is crucial for academic success, and students who have language disorders usually experience difficulties with one or more areas of language form. Ongoing assessments in these areas are required for developing goals.

Students who have language disorders may not present with speech sound production errors, but they may present with problems in phonological memory and awareness (Pennington & Bishop, 2009). Phonological awareness is highly correlated with success in reading (Schuele & Boudreau, 2008). Producing phonologically complex multisyllabic words and sentences may be problematic for these children. These difficulties may reflect problems in establishing accurate phonological representations (Paul & Norbury, 2012). This information should be kept in mind when considering target behaviors and writing goals.

Although it is well known that phonological awareness skills are linked to literacy success, morphological awareness is also a key component for literacy development (Apel & Werfel, 2014; Turnbull & Justice, 2017). Students with morphological deficits may have difficulties with morphemes that are hard to hear, such as past-tense endings; regular present tense; singular -s, plural -s, and possessive -s; and comparatives and superlatives (Scott, 2004).

Children with language disorders may present with difficulties understanding and producing a variety of complex syntactic structures (Nelson, 2010; Paul & Norbury, 2012). Oral and written expression can be characterized as short and sweet. These students use few complex syntactic structures with less elaboration of noun and verb phrases in their verbal and written language (Nelson, 2010). They tend to use simple sentences and have difficulty producing sentences that violate the subject–verb–object order, such as interrogative reversals, negatives, and passives (Paul & Norbury, 2012).

Language Use: Pragmatic Goals

Children who have language disorders often present with difficulties learning and mastering the rules for using language as a social tool. Difficulties are observed in using language for a variety of communicative functions, using different discourse styles, and understanding the social conventions of language (Paul & Norbury, 2012).

The most significant area of deficit for students with language disorders may be in the area of conversational pragmatics. This should be taken into consideration when developing goals (Hart, Fujiki, Brinton, & Hart, 2004). Difficulties are observed with providing sufficient elaboration and adjusting language to the age or social status of the listener. When challenges are seen in this area, goals should be written to address conversational turn-taking, topic management, and conversational repair strategies (Owens, 2014).

As might be expected, these students also have difficulties with comprehending and using other discourse genres, such as narrative, expository, and persuasive. Narrative skills have been suggested as a means of bridging conversational discourse and expository discourse (Westby, 2005). Narrative skills have been shown to be related to academic success; this should be taken into consideration when developing goals for school-age students presenting with difficulties in pragmatics (Paul & Norbury, 2012).

Summary

The components and dimensions of language are numerous and complex. It is miraculous that we can master such a complicated skill. When a child has difficulty learning this multidimensional ability, the professionals who can help must have a complete understanding of the subject, the normal developmental sequence, typical peer performance, and the specific areas that challenge the child. Only then can appropriate goals be developed that will be most effective to remediate areas of challenge.

Case Scenarios

Case Scenario 1

Josie is a fourth-grade student who is aged 9 years and 2 months. She is attending a public school and is currently in a general education class. Josie was diagnosed with significant rheumatoid arthritis at age 5 years, and she takes medication that can make her drowsy. All of her other physical abilities, including her hearing, are considered typical for her age. Her social skills are excellent, and she is even considered mature for her age. She is loved by the school personnel and her peers.

Josie presents with significant learning issues. She struggles in all academic areas; she is 2 years behind in reading and writing, 1 year behind in math computation, and 2 years behind in word problems (due to her poor reading). Her social studies and science skills are poor, but when information is read to her aloud, she does much better.

Formal testing by the school psychologist places her intelligence in the low average range, and her emotional testing shows average to above average abilities. Special education evaluations reveal that she has language-based learning disabilities. A complete speech and language evaluation was conducted. Josie's articulation, fluency, and voice skills were found to be within typical ranges.

The CELF-5 was administered to Josie, and her scores were as follows:

Core	Standard Score	Percentile Rank
Core language score	76	5
Receptive language score	73	4
Expressive language score	80	9
Subtests	**Scaled Score**	**Percentile Rank**
Concepts/following directions	4	2
Recalling sentences	6	9
Formulated sentences	9	37
Word classes—receptive	6	9
Word classes—expressive	5	5
Word classes—total	5	5
Expressive vocabulary	7	16

Case Scenarios *(continued)*

In addition to the CELF-5, the Test of Auditory Processing Skills, Third Edition (TAPS-3) was administered to Josie. The results were as follows:

Subtest	Scaled Score	Percentile Rank
Word discrimination	7	16
Phonological segmentation	6	9
Phonological blending	9	37
Number memory forward	5	5
Number memory reversed	11	63
Word memory	4	2
Sentence memory	8	25
Auditory comprehension	14	91
Auditory reasoning	10	50

When these subtests were compiled, they yielded a phonologic standard score of 87, a memory standard score of 85, a cohesion standard score of 110, and an overall index standard score of 91.

The clinician administered the Test for Auditory Comprehension of Language, Third Edition (TACL-3) as the last part of the battery. Josie's scores were as follows:

Category	Standard Score	Percentile
Vocabulary	9	37
Grammatical morphemes	12	75
Elaborated sentences	9	37
Total test	100	50

What goals would you write and then execute for Josie? Justify your choices.

Case Scenarios *(continued)*

Case Scenario 2

Paul entered the school district in September and, according to his age, was placed in a general education first-grade class. Physically he was appropriate in all areas, including hearing. Academic records were unavailable from his kindergarten year.

Paul presented as a loving child who tended to play by himself. He often appeared immature, which made it difficult for him to establish relationships with his peers.

Paul's experienced classroom teacher described his academic skills as exceptionally low in all areas. He had to receive individual instruction in all subjects, including basic prereading skills and premath skills.

Testing by the school psychologist showed Paul's cognitive skills to be within the low average range. Special education assessments placed his skills at the preschool and kindergarten levels. A full speech and language evaluation was conducted. Paul's fluency and voice skills were found to be within typical ranges. His articulation revealed that he had an interdental lisp, but all his other sounds were pronounced correctly, so the lisp was considered age appropriate.

The CELF-5 was administered, and Paul's scores were as follows:

Core	Standard Score	Percentile Rank
Core language score	82	12
Receptive language score	84	14
Expressive language score	83	13
Subtests	**Scaled Score**	**Percentile Rank**
Concepts/following directions	7	16
Word structure	7	16
Recalling sentences	7	16
Formulated sentences	7	16
Word classes—receptive	11	63
Word classes—expressive	7	16
Word classes—total	9	37
Sentence structure	4	2
Expressive vocabulary	9	37

Case Scenarios *(continued)*

The Boehm Test of Basic Concepts was administered to Paul. His scores were in the below average range, and the results showed he had gaps in his knowledge of spatial, temporal, and quantitative concepts.

What goals would you write and then execute for Paul? Justify your choices.

REVIEW QUESTIONS

1. A definition of language must include which of the following factors?
   a. It is rule governed.
   b. It is a code for the representation of both tangible and intangible thoughts.
   c. The arbitrary symbols a language uses must be agreed upon by the society that uses it.
   d. All of the above are correct.
   e. A and B are correct.
   f. B and C are correct.
   g. A and C are correct.
   h. None of the above are correct.

2. In Bloom and Lahey's model of what language is,
   a. semantics is under the domain known as *use*.
   b. pragmatics is under the domain known as *form*.
   c. morphology is under the domain known as *content*.
   d. syntax is under the domain known as *form*.

3. Receptive semantic ability and expressive semantic ability
   a. are always about the same.
   b. are always at very different levels.
   c. vary; some children are better in one than the other, and other children display roughly equal levels.
   d. have no relationship.

4. In the area of language, what are some of the factors that must be taken into account when developing goals? Choose all that apply.
   a. Cognitive abilities
   b. Inconsistent errors
   c. Consistent errors
   d. Family goals
   e. Test reliability
   f. Social abilities
   g. Physical issues
   h. Financial concerns

5. Knowledge of typical language development work will prove invaluable when a clinician is writing goals in the areas of
   a. semantics.
   b. syntax.
   c. morphology.
   d. phonology.
   e. pragmatics.

REFERENCES

American Speech-Language-Hearing Association. (2008a). Core knowledge and skills in early intervention speech-language pathology practice. Retrieved from http://www.asha.org/policy/KS2008-00292.htm

American Speech-Language-Hearing Association. (2008b). Roles and responsibilities of speech-language pathologists in early intervention: Guidelines. Retrieved from http://www.asha.org/policy/GL2008-00293.htm

Apel, K., & Werfel, K. (2014). Using morphological awareness instruction to improve written language skills. *Language, Speech, and Hearing Services in Schools, 45*, 251–260.

Beed, P. L., Hawkins, E. M., & Roller, C. M. (1991). Moving learners toward independence: The power of scaffolded instruction. *The Reading Teacher, 44*, 648–655.

Bernthal, J., Bankson, N., & Flipsen P. (2013). *Articulation and phonological disorders: Speech sound disorders in children* (7th ed.). Boston, MA: Pearson Education.

Betz, S. K., Eickhoff, J. R., & Sullivan, S. F. (2013). Factors influencing the selection of standardized tests for the diagnosis of specific language impairment. *Language, Speech, and Hearing Services in Schools, 44*, 133–146.

Bloom, L., & Lahey, M. (1978). *Language development and language disorders.* New York, NY: Wiley.

Brown, R. (1973). *A first language: The early stages.* Boston, MA: Harvard University Press.

Common Core State Standards Initiative. (2010). *Common core state standards for English, language arts and literacy in history/social studies, science and technical subjects.* Retrieved from http://www.corestandards.org/assets/CCSSI_ELA%20Standards.pdf

Crystal, D. (1987). *The Cambridge encyclopedia of language.* Cambridge, England: Cambridge University Press.

Ehren, B. J. (2000). Maintaining a therapeutic focus and sharing responsibility for student success: Keys to in-classroom speech-language services. *Language, Speech, and Hearing Services in Schools, 31*, 219–229.

Flynn, P. (2015). Speech-language goals that reflect the common core state standards (and extended standards). Case Studies by ASHA Professional Development. Retrieved from https://www.asha.org/eWeb/OLSDynamicPage.aspx?Webcode=olsdetails&title=Speech-Language+Goals+that+Reflect+the+Common+Core+State+Standards+(and+Extended+Standards)

Greenwood, R. G. (1981). Management by objectives: As developed by Peter Drucker, assisted by Harold Smiddy. *Academy of Management Review, 6*, 225–230.

Gutiérrez-Clellen, V. F., & Peña, E. (2001). Dynamic assessment of diverse children: A tutorial. *Language, Speech and Hearing Services in Schools, 32*, 212–224.

Hart, K., Fujiki, M., Brinton, B., & Hart, C. (2004). The relationship between social behavior and severity of language impairment. *Journal of Speech, Language, and Hearing Research, 47*, 647–662.

Hegde, M., & Pomaville, F. (2013). *Assessment of communication disorders in children: Resources and protocols* (2nd ed.). San Diego, CA: Plural.

Hunt, K. (1965). *Grammatical structures written at three grade levels.* Champaign, IL: National Council of Teachers of English. Individuals with Disabilities Education Act of 2004, 20 U.S.C. § 1400 et seq.

Jung, L. A. (2007). Writing SMART objectives and strategies that fit into the ROUTINE. *TEACHING Exceptional Children, 39,* 54–58.

Kaderavek, J. (2015). *Language disorder in children: Fundamental concepts of assessment and intervention* (2nd ed.). New York, NY: Pearson.

Kennison, S. (2014). *Introduction to language development.* Los Angeles, CA: Sage.

Lahey, M. (1988). *Language disorders and language development.* New York, NY: Macmillan.

Lee, L. L. (1974). *Developmental sentence analysis.* Evanston, IL: Northwestern University Press.

Loban, W. (1966). *Language ability: Grades seven, eight and nine.* Washington, DC: U.S. Government Printing Office.

Miller, J. F. (2012). *Systematic analysis of language transcripts (SALT).* Madison, WI: SALT Software.

National Center for Education Statistics. (2017). The condition of education: English language learners in public schools. Retrieved from https://nces.ed.gov/programs/coe/indicator_cgf .asp

Nelson, N. W. (2010). *Language and literacy disorders: Infancy through adolescence.* Boston, MA: Allyn & Bacon.

Nippold, M. A. (1998). *Later language development: The school-age and adolescent year and adolescent years* (2nd ed.). Austin, TX: PRO-ED.

Nippold, M. A. (2007). *Later language development: School-age children, adolescents, and young adults* (3rd ed.). Austin, TX: PRO-ED.

Owens, R. (2014). *Language disorders: A functional approach to assessment and intervention* (6th ed.). New York, NY: Pearson.

Owens, R. (2016). *Language development: An introduction* (9th ed.). Boston, MA: Pearson.

Paul, R., & Norbury, C. (2012). *Language disorders from infancy through adolescence: Listening, speaking, reading, writing, and communicating* (4th ed.). Saint Louis, MO: Elsevier Mosby.

Pennington, B., & Bishop, D. (2009). Relations among speech, language, and reading disorders. *Annual Review of Psychology, 60,* 283–306.

Pinzola, R., Plexico, L., & Haynes, W. (2016). *Diagnosis and evaluation in speech pathology* (9th ed.). Boston, MA: Pearson.

Power-deFur, L., & Flynn, P. (2012). Unpacking the standards for intervention. *SIG 16 Perspectives on School-Based Issues, 13,* 11–16. doi:10.1044/sbi13.11

Rogers-Adkinson, D. L., & Stuart, S. K. (2007). Collaborative services: Children experiencing neglect and the side effects of prenatal alcohol exposure. *Language, Speech, and Hearing Services in Schools, 38,* 149–156.

Roth, F., & Worthington, C. (2016). *Treatment resource manual for speech-language pathology* (5th ed.). Clifton Park, NY: Cengage Learning.

Rudebusch, J. (2012). From common core state standards to standards-based IEPs: A brief tutorial. *Perspectives on School-Based Issues, 13,* 17–24. doi:10.1044/sbi13.1.17

Schuele, C., & Boudreau, D. (2008). Phonological awareness intervention: Beyond the basics. *Language, Speech, and Hearing Services in Schools, 39,* 3–20.

Scott, C. (2004). Syntactic ability in children and adolescents with language and learning disabilities. In R. Berman (Ed.), *Language development across childhood and adolescence* (pp. 111–134). Philadelphia, PA: John Benjamins.

Shipley, K. G., & McAfee, J. G. (2016). *Assessment in speech-language pathology: A resource manual* (5th ed.). Boston, MA: Cengage Learning.

Swigert, N. (2014). Patient outcomes, NOMS, and goal writing for pediatrics and adults. *SIG 13 Perspectives on Swallowing and Swallowing Disorders (Dysphagia), 23,* 65–71. doi:10.1044 /sasd23.2.65

Tomblin, J., Records, N., Buckwalter, P., Zhang, X., Smith, E., & O'Brien, M. (1997). Prevalence of specific language impairment in kindergarten children. *Journal of Speech, Language, and Hearing Research, 40,* 1245–1260.

Turnbull, K. L. P., & Justice, L. M. (2017). *Language development from theory to practice* (3rd ed.). New York, NY: Pearson.

ADDITIONAL RESOURCES

Developmental sequences for language content, form, and use can be found on the American Speech-Language-Hearing Association website:

- Developmental Norms for Speech and Language. http://www.asha.org/SLP/schools/prof-consult/norms/
- Social Language Use (Pragmatics). http://www.asha.org/public/speech/development/Pragmatics/
- Speech Sound Disorders: Articulation and Phonological Processes. Phonology and articulation. http://www.asha.org/public/speech/disorders/SpeechSoundDisorders/

Detailed information regarding typical language development can be found in the following books:

McLeod, S., & Baker, E. (2017). *Children's speech: An evidence-based approach to assessment and intervention.* Boston, MA: Pearson.

Nippold, M. A. (2016). *Later language development: School-age children, adolescents, and young adults* (4th ed.). Austin, TX: PRO-ED.

Owens, R. (2016). *Language development: An introduction* (9th ed.). Boston, MA: Pearson.

Paul, R., & Norbury, C. (2012). *Language disorders from infancy through adolescence: Listening, speaking, reading, writing, and communicating* (4th ed.). Saint Louis, MO: Elsevier Mosby.

Roth, F., & Worthington, C. (2016). *Treatment resource manual for speech-language pathology* (5th ed.). Clifton Park, NY: Cengage Learning.

Turnbull, K. L. P., & Justice, L. M. (2017). *Language development from theory to practice* (3rd ed.). New York, NY: Pearson.

Westby, C. (2005). Assessing and facilitating text comprehension problems. In H. Catts & A. Kahmi (Eds.) *Contextualized language intervention* (pp. 157–232). Boston, MA: Allyn & Bacon.

CHAPTER 4

Speech Disorders in Children

Renee Fabus
Terry H. Gozdziewski

Key Terms

Articulation disorder
Assessment
Diagnosis
Phonological contrast approaches
Phonological disorders

Speech sound disorders
Stimulability
Traditional (motor or phonetic)
  approach

Introduction

This chapter is geared for novice clinicians who are learning how to analyze data from the speech sound assessment and develop an intervention plan. The chapter cannot possibly include information about all the elements of the assessment and intervention process; please refer to the "Additional Resources" section in this chapter for more information.

According to the ASHA, **speech sound disorders** "is an umbrella term referring to any combination of difficulties with perception, motor production, and/or the phonological representation of speech sounds and speech segments (including phonotactic rules that govern syllable shape, structure, and stress, as well as prosody) that impact speech intelligibility" (2016, Overview section, para. 3). Originally, speech sound disorders were simply regarded as articulation impairments, but over time it was realized that the production of sounds in words and connected speech is an extremely complex and multifaceted process.

Currently, the term **articulation disorder** refers to impairments in the motor processes that are involved in the production of speech sounds (Bauman-Waengler, 2012; Bernthal et al., 2013). Articulation disorders are "speech sound disorders (that) can impact the form of speech sounds" (Bauman-Waengler, 2012, p. 410). A child may be diagnosed with an articulation disorder if he or she has difficulty executing these speech movements or difficulty producing speech sounds. Articulation disorders can result from functional impairments (e.g., an interdental lisp) or organic impairments (e.g., cleft palate) (Roth & Worthington, 2016). Articulation disorders are usually the result of a child substituting, omitting, or distorting one or a few speech sounds.

Speech sound disorders that impact the way speech sounds function within a language are referred to as **phonological disorders** (Bauman-Waengler, 2012). Bleile states that "persons with articulation disorders are presumed to experience difficulty either producing or perceiving speech" (Bleile, 2014, p. 46). Therefore, a child who exhibits a phonological disorder has difficulty understanding the rules underlying the language. A child may be diagnosed with a phonological delay or disorder if he or she still exhibits phonological patterns beyond the age those patterns should be eliminated, or if he or she exhibits unusual phonological patterns in speech production.

It is important for clinicians to be knowledgeable about the classification of consonants and vowels in English. For information about the place and manner of consonants and vowels in English, refer to the following references: American Speech-Language-Hearing Association, 2016; and University of Arizona, n.d. The following references are additional sources: Bauman-Waengler, 2012; Bernthal, Bankson, & Flipsen, 2013; McLeod & Baker, 2017; Pena-Brooks & Hegde, 2015; Shipley & McAfee, 2015; and Stein-Rubin & Fabus, 2018.

Phonological processes (more recently referred to as *patterns* in the literature) are what children use when learning to speak in order to simplify modeled adult productions. There are three types of phonological patterns: syllable structure, assimilation, and substitution (Fabus & Gironda, 2018; Lowe 2009; Pena-Brooks & Hegde, 2015). For a listing of the different types of phonological patterns that exist in a typical child's speech production, please refer to the following references: American Speech-Language-Hearing Association, 2016; Fabus & Gironda, 2018; and Pena-Brooks & Hegde, 2015. When a child exhibits a typical phonological pattern past the age that the process or pattern should be eliminated, the child may exhibit a phonological error pattern or a phonological delay. If a child is exhibiting additional unusual or idiosyncratic processes or patterns, he or she may be diagnosed with a phonological disorder. For a listing of idiosyncratic or unusual processes, please refer to the following references: Lowe, 2009; and Pena-Brooks & Hegde, 2015.

Comprehensive Assessment

Prior to discussing the purpose and components of an overall assessment, it is important to define the terms *assessment, evaluation,* and *diagnosis.* Hegde and Pomaville describe **assessment** as "inclusive of several kinds of clinical activities that result in naming the communication disorder of a child, making statements about prognosis for improvement with or without treatment, and offering recommendations for communication treatment (and) additional assessment of other kinds of specialized services" (2013, p. 4). Those authors also say the terms *evaluation* and *assessment* tend to be synonymous, whereas **diagnosis** refers to the actual naming of the communication disorder (Hegde & Pomaville, 2013). According to the ASHA (2016), the clinical indications for a speech sound assessment are initiated by a referral from a healthcare or education professional, the child's medical status, or the failure of a speech-language screening. For a comprehensive list of speech screening measures, refer to the following references: Bleile, 2014; and Hegde & Pomaville, 2013.

Although a child may fail a screening measure, that does not necessarily mean the child has a speech sound disorder. The clinician may choose to educate the parents or guardian about typical speech-language development or monitor the child's speech-language skills (American Speech-Language-Hearing Association [ASHA], 2016). A screening is designed to be a simple, fast, and efficient measure with a pass–fail option that may indicate the need for a more in-depth evaluation or assessment.

Bauman-Waengler (2012) says there are two components in the assessment process: appraisal and diagnosis. The appraisal is when the clinician is choosing the tests and materials for the evaluation. The decision to use particular measures and materials during the assessment may directly impact the results of the evaluation. The diagnosis is determined when the clinician identifies the presence or absence and severity of a disorder after analyzing the data from the testing situation.

Components of a Comprehensive Assessment

There are important aspects to consider when designing the assessment protocol for a child. Some of these include the child's cultural experience, linguistic background and dialect, cognitive skills, social abilities, physical capabilities, interests, the family's perceptions of the speech sound delay or disorder, and other possible communication or concomitant disorders. It is also imperative to take into account the child's likes and dislikes when developing stimuli for testing measures.

A comprehensive assessment should include the following components (ASHA, 2016, 2017c; Fabus & Gironda, 2018):

- A case history or intake should be obtained from the child's parent or guardian. It should include the child's medical history, birth and developmental milestones (including speech-language and motor), languages spoken in the home, social and academic history, previous therapy (including speech-language therapy, occupational or physical therapy, psychological services, and special education), and additional concerns.
- An oral–peripheral mechanism should be performed, including articulatory diadochokinetic rates.
- A pure-tone hearing screening should be conducted.
- A speech sound assessment should be performed (including both single words and connected speech; an assessment of intelligibility, stimulability, and severity in different contexts; and evaluations of stimulability and severity).
- Additional measures may be indicated, such as a language screening or evaluation, an auditory discrimination and phonological awareness assessment, and an assessment of voice quality and fluency measures.

The first component is gathering the case history of the child. There are many sample case history forms available in the literature (Hegde & Pomaville, 2013; Shipley & McAfee, 2015). The case history form should include, but is not limited to, information about the family's perception of the child's speech-language difficulties, developmental milestones (in all areas including speech-language, motor, social, and cognitive), family history of speech-language and hearing difficulties, the family's perception of the child's intelligibility, the child's educational history and performance, the child's social interaction skills, the child's native language, and information regarding any other specialized services received. If applicable, the clinician should obtain information from the child's teacher and note if the child is aware of his or her speech production patterns in the classroom. The clinician may want to ascertain if the child participates in classroom activities.

Another important component in the assessment process is the oral–peripheral examination. The clinician must examine the structures and functions of the articulators that are necessary for speech production. Fabus and Gironda (2018) provide a description and instructions about how to conduct an oral–peripheral examination.

A third component of the assessment process is the pure-tone hearing screening. This screening is a pass–fail measure. If the child fails the screening, he or she should be referred for a complete audiological evaluation by a certified audiologist. The child's ability to hear the difference in sounds, often known as auditory discrimination, must be taken into account, but it is not part of a pure-tone screening. The clinician may choose to examine a child's auditory discrimination skills when determining if the child can be stimulated to produce the error sound.

The speech sound assessment itself, of course, is the heart of the evaluation. The speech sound evaluation includes the formal testing, eliciting, transcribing, and analyzing the conversational speech sample; stimulability testing; and intelligibility and severity measures. Published measures that are used to assess speech sound disorders in children and adults are available in the following references: Fabus, Yudes-Kuznetsov, & Gozdziewski, 2015; Hegde & Pomaville, 2013; Pena-Brooks & Hegde, 2015; Shipley & McAfee, 2015; and Stein-Rubin & Fabus, 2018. In addition, refer to **TABLE 4-1** for a selection of published tests for speech sound disorders in children; also refer to **TABLE 4-2** for a list of phonological awareness tests.

TABLE 4-1 Selected Tests for Speech Sound Disorders

Name of Test	Age Range	Publisher
Arizona Articulation Proficiency Scale, Third Revision (Arizona-3)	1–18 years	LinguiSystems
Bankson-Bernthal Test of Phonology (BBTOP)	3–9 years	PRO-ED
Clinical Assessment of Articulation and Phonology, Second Edition (CAAP-2)	2 years, 6 months–11 years, 11 months	Super Duper
Diagnostic Evaluation of Articulation and Phonology (DEAP)	3–8 years	Pearson
Fisher-Logemann Test of Articulation Competence (FLTOAC)	Children–adult	PRO-ED Australia

TABLE 4-1 Selected Tests for Speech Sound Disorders *(Continued)*

Name of Test	Age Range	Publisher
Goldman-Fristoe Test of Articulation, Third Edition (GFTA-3)	2 years–21 years, 11 months	Pearson
Hodson Assessment of Phonological Patterns, Third Edition (HAPP-3)	3–8 years	PRO-ED
Khan-Lewis Phonological Analysis, Third Edition (KLPA-3) used with GFTA-3	2 years–21 years, 11 months	Pearson
LinguiSystems Articulation Test (LAT)	3–21 years	LinguiSystems
Photo Articulation Test, Third Edition (PAT-3)	3 years–8 years, 11 months	PRO-ED
Secord Contextual Articulation Test (S-CAT)	4 years–adult	Super Duper
Slosson Articulation Language Test with Phonology (SALT-P)	3 years–5 years, 11 months	Slosson

TABLE 4-2 Select Phonological Awareness Tests

Name of Test	Age Range	Publisher
Comprehensive Test of Phonological Processing (CTOPP)	4 years–24 years, 11 months	PRO-ED
Phonological Awareness Literacy Screening (PALS)	Prekindergarten–grade 3	University of Virginia
Phonological Awareness and Reading Profile—Intermediate	8–14 years	LinguiSystems
Test of Phonological Awareness Skills (TOPAS)	5–10 years	PRO-ED Australia
Test of Phonological Awareness, Second Edition: PLUS (TOPA-2+)	5–8 years	PRO-ED

Tests may be standardized or nonstandardized. Standardized tests have procedures for administration and scoring that are the same for all participants (Epstein, 2018). Standardized tests provide an objective, reliable method for quantifying an individual's scores. Standardized tests can be norm-referenced tests; they allow the clinician to compare an individual's scores to the scores of other individuals who are the same age, and sometimes the same gender (Epstein, 2018).

All types of test measures have advantages and disadvantages. The clinician needs to consider certain factors when choosing a test for a speech sound assessment. These factors include the child's age and culture; the population the test was normalized for; if the test examines only speech in single words or if it includes an analysis of connected speech; the child's cognitive skills, including attention; the child's linguistic skills; and if the test examines articulation, phonology, or both (Fabus & Gironda, 2018).

In addition to formal testing measures, the clinician should obtain a conversational speech sample (connected speech). Depending on the factors previously listed, the clinician should choose different activities to elicit the speech sample. Additionally, the child's likes and interests should be important factors when determining the activity. After the clinician elicits the speech sample, it is essential to transcribe a representative number of utterances using the International Phonetic Alphabet (IPA). For further information about choosing activities and eliciting and transcribing the speech sample, please refer to the following references: Bauman-Waengler, 2012; Bleile, 2014; and Hegde & Pomaville, 2013.

After the conversational speech sample has been obtained and transcribed, the child's phonetic and phonemic systems should be analyzed, including the following elements:

- Sounds
- Sound combinations
- Syllable shapes produced accurately, including sounds in various word positions (e.g., initial, medial, and final word position; or prevocalic, intervocalic, and postvocalic, respectively) and in different phonetic contexts
- Phoneme sequences (e.g., vowel combinations, consonant clusters, and blends)
- Speech sound errors, including the type of errors (e.g., deletions, omissions, substitutions, distortions, and additions)

- Position of targeted sounds within words
- Phonological processes (e.g., syllable structure, assimilation, and substitution processes)

In addition, the clinician should be aware that there are vowel processes, such as vowel backing, which are thoroughly described in Lowe (2009).

After the formal testing has been completed, the clinician needs to determine if the child is stimulable for producing the error sound. The severity of the disorder or delay, and the intelligibility of the child's speech, should also be determined. Stimulability is an important prognostic factor in the intervention process. **Stimulability** refers to the "child's correct or improved production of an erred speech sound following the clinician's model" (Hegde & Pomaville, 2013, p. 173). It is usually assessed in isolation, syllable, word, and phrase levels (ASHA, 2016). Some test measures have a stimulability section in the formal measure. For tests that do not include that section, the clinician can create a stimulability assessment measure after the child's errors are known.

The clinician also needs to examine the child's speech intelligibility in words, phrases, and connected speech (i.e., reading, if applicable, and conversational speech). Intelligibility is usually documented on a perceptual rating scale; the intelligibility is usually rated as good, fair, or poor (ASHA, 2016) in known or unknown contexts. Percentages of intelligible speech are used to express typical conversational abilities of children (Coplan & Gleason, 1988; Flipsen, 2006):

- 1 year: 25 percent intelligible
- 2 years: 50 percent intelligible
- 3 years: 75 percent intelligible
- 4 years: 100 percent intelligible

Hegde and Pomaville (2013) also suggested that a percentage of intelligibility should be determined. To do so, the clinician can divide the number of intelligible words by the total number of words in the sample, then multiply that number by 100. The resulting intelligibility rating can be used as a baseline when the clinician initiates speech-language therapy. In terms of severity, the clinician makes a qualitative judgment of the child's speech sound disorder after analyzing the results of the speech evaluation.

It is of great importance to properly assess ethnoculturally diverse children. Procedures for assessing these populations are provided in the following references: American Speech-Language-Hearing

Association, 2016 (see the "Special Considerations: Bilingual/Multilingual Populations" section); American Speech-Language-Hearing Association, 2017b; Hegde & Pomaville, 2013; and Shipley & McAfee, 2015.

In addition to speech sound testing, it is important to evaluate the child's language skills, (including receptive and expressive semantics, receptive and expressive syntax, and pragmatics), fluency, and voice quality. Additionally, the clinician should assess the child's phonological awareness and speech discrimination skills. Even if the child's skills are typical, this information must be documented in the diagnostic or evaluation report. Information about assessing these skills are provided in the following reference: American Speech-Language-Hearing Association, 2016.

Analysis and Interpretation of Assessment Data

The analysis of all assessment data (including the case history, intake, and interview; oral–peripheral examination; hearing screening; speech sound assessment; and other communication testing measures, such as receptive and expressive language, fluency, voice, auditory discrimination, and phonological awareness skills) is necessary to determine the diagnosis, if any. If a diagnosis is indicated, the clinician can then design an appropriate intervention plan with functional goals.

The clinician can begin interpreting the results by analyzing the statistical data obtained from the formal testing measures. This should include scoring the speech sound assessment measures and any additional formal testing measures. However, the data analysis is not complete when the test measure is scored. The score simply provides information about how the child's speech sound system compares to that of other children who are the same age or gender, depending on the test. The score itself does not provide all the necessary data to design an intervention plan with measurable goals.

The clinician should analyze the data from the formal measures and compare it to the results of the informal measures (e.g., conversational speech sample or reading passage). The clinician will look for a possible articulation or phonological delay or disorder; some tests report this specific information. The clinician should document the following information for both the formal and informal measures:

- The nature of the errors (the type of consonants in error according to place, manner, and voicing)
- The number of consonants in error (the number of consonants in error and how many times each consonant is in error)
- The nature of vowel errors (determining the vowel errors based on the vowel quadrangle)
- The number of vowels in error (the number of vowels in error and how many times each vowel is in error) and if there are patterns of errors
- The position of sounds in error (initial, medial, or final position; or prevocalic, intervocalic, or postvocalic, respectively) and the context of the errors (the sounds prior to or after the sound in error)
- The number of phonological patterns that should have been eliminated by the child's current chronological age
- The type of phonological patterns (both typical and unusual)
- The number of sounds affected in a class of sounds for each phonological pattern
- The consistency of phonological patterns that are present (the number of opportunities for a pattern to occur and the number of occurrences of the pattern)

The clinician should then review the norms for speech sound acquisition and phonological patterns. The following references document the approximate age when English phonemes are acquired and phonological patterns are eliminated: American Speech-Language-Hearing Association, 2016; Fabus & Gironda, 2018; Pena-Brooks & Hegde, 2015; and Shipley & McAfee 2015.

With clear knowledge of the expected sequence of sound acquisition, the clinician can determine the sounds that are not mastered and the phonological patterns that are not eliminated.

For additional information about the frequency of consonant occurrence in English and the norms for speech and language skills, please refer to the following references:

- American Speech-Language-Hearing Association, 2017a: Information about developmental norms for speech and language skills is presented.
- Lof, 2004: This presentation provides background information that is helpful prior to a review of developmental norms.
- Pena-Brooks & Hedge, 2015; and Shipley & McAfee, 2015: These sources provide tables indicating the frequency of occurrence of

individual consonants in the English language and the variability of age norms in the development of speech and language skills.

The variability of age norms in the development of speech and language skills can be related to the manner in which data from the speech sound acquisition tables are interpreted (Bankson & Bernthal, 1990; Bernthal et al., 2013; Lof, 2004). For example, the data from the Sander's norms are based on when 50 percent of children produced the sound, which is called customary production, and when 90 percent of children produced the sound, which is called mastery production. The clinician should keep this variability in mind when interpreting results based on age norms.

Phonetic development and acquisition data have customarily been derived from initial position, single-word testing. The resulting average age estimates range from the median age of correct articulation to the older age level at which 90 percent of the children tested accurately produced the target (Pena-Brooks & Hegde, 2015). Pena-Brooks and Hegde (2015) review various research studies, including the types of studies, the norms reported in the studies, and the criteria in the studies for mastering the production of consonant sounds.

An important factor to consider is whether the clinician will use a traditional (motor or phonetic) approach or a phonological contrast approach (described in the "Types of Intervention Approaches" section later in this chapter). If the clinician uses a traditional approach, he or she should decide which sounds to target first in the therapy session. The clinician may choose to take either a developmental or nondevelopmental approach (Roth & Worthington, 2016). With a developmental approach, the clinician would examine the sounds in error and compare them to the developmental acquisition of phonemes. Afterwards, the clinician would choose the sounds that should have been acquired first, according to the developmental norms to target in the treatment sessions.

A nondevelopmental approach is best described with an example. It is important to consider the family's values during treatment. Parents may believe that certain sounds are more important for their child to learn than others. The child may also have strong preferences. For example, if a child has difficulty pronouncing the unvoiced fricative sound *s* and the child's name starts with that sound, it may be important to work on that sound even though that phoneme is usually developed later. Respecting these preferences may enhance the rate of success in speech-language therapy. This approach is called the non-developmental approach.

Forming Specific Goals

As mentioned previously in this chapter, many elements must be considered before choosing what to target in the area of speech sound disorders. When sounds or patterns are targeted for remediation, the general rules of goal writing must always apply. Some general considerations include, but are not limited to, the child's age and cognitive and linguistic skills; the child's likes and dislikes for the selection of treatment stimuli; the implementation of teaching strategies (e.g., phonetic placement, shaping, modeling, instructions, prompts, and corrective feedback [Bauman-Waengler, 2012; Bleile, 2014; Pena-Brooks and Hegde, 2015]); cultural factors; and the family's perception of the speech sound disorder and their involvement in the intervention process.

After analyzing the results of the speech sound assessment, the clinician should consider which incorrect sounds the child should have already acquired and which phonological patterns should have already been eliminated, based on developmental norms. The clinician may want to consider which sounds are easier to remediate because of their visibility or place of articulation. Sounds that contribute to increasing speech intelligibility may be important to target first. If a clinician chooses to address a phonological pattern, he or she may target a phonological pattern that has fewer sounds in an affected class or more sounds in an affected class, based on the phonological contrast method used in the therapy session (minimal contrast method compared to maximal contrast method).

Prior to beginning the therapy sessions, the clinician must obtain baseline, quantitative data from the child. Baseline data are different from a probe. A probe is a procedure to determine if the targeted speech sound was generalized. Baseline procedures can assist in the evaluation of the child's progress over time. The therapy sessions and goals can be modified, as necessary, based on the baseline data and the child's progress.

Many data recording sheets are available (e.g., Roth & Worthington, 2016), but the clinician can create data sheets as well. The clinician also needs to decide whether to use evoked trials or modeled trials. With evoked trials, the clinician does not provide a model for the child;

with modeled trials, the clinician does provide a model. Modeled trials can provide valuable information. If the child produces a sound by following a model, the clinician can evaluate if that sound is a good target to address in the therapy session.

When the clinician determines what target sounds and/or phonological patterns will be addressed in the therapy session, the clinician should formulate the long-term and short-term goals. The short-term goals should contain the following elements (Hedge, 1998; Pena-Brooks & Hedge, 2015): the response topography; the quantitative criterion for performance (e.g., 80 percent accuracy); the response mode and level (e.g., production training and in words); the response setting (e.g., in the clinic); and the number of sessions. Roth and Worthington (2016) provide a detailed description for writing goals using appropriate verbs, which are measurable. The clinician needs to write detailed goals because many insurance companies and agencies limit the number of sessions based on the child's progress and other prognostic indicators. The clinician should indicate estimated completion times for short-term goals.

The clinician must take into account how often the child will receive therapy services. An approval for a certain number of therapy sessions is sometimes dictated by the insurance company, the team meeting at the school, the IEP, or the family's financial resources to pay for services. For example, state regulations and school district policies may stipulate the frequency of service in public schools, whereas a medical insurance policy may dictate the number of sessions provided at a medical facility.

When writing goals, it is crucial to identify whether speech-language therapy should be administered individually or in a group. Although many speech-language pathologists strongly prefer one model over the other, some children perform better when they are seen individually, and others perform better in a group. Therefore, the circumstances should dictate the delivery model. In either case, the delivery model must be considered during the goal writing process.

Types of Intervention Approaches

The clinician must choose an intervention approach based on evidence-based practice, regardless of what sounds or phonological patterns are chosen to be targeted in the therapy session (Baker &

McLeod, 2011a, 2011b). The following approaches could be implemented for children diagnosed with speech sound disorders:

- Traditional approach (Van Riper, 1978)
- Distinctive feature approach
- Phonological contrast approaches (including minimal contrast, maximal contrast, multiple contrasts, and empty set)
- Cycles approach (Prezas & Hodson, 2010)
- Core vocabulary approach (Dodd, Holm, Crosbie, & McIntosh, 2006)
- Naturalistic speech intervention approach
- Metaphon therapy (Dean, Howell, Waters, & Reid, 1995)

Refer to the following references for information about the listed evidence-based treatment approaches for speech sound disorders: American Speech-Language-Hearing Association, 2016; Baker & McLeod, 2011a, 2011b; Bauman-Waengler, 2012; Bernthal, Bankson, & Flipsen, 2013; Hegde & Pomaville, 2013; Pena-Brooks & Hegde, 2015; and Ruscello, 2008. Additionally, refer to the following reference for information about evidence-based treatment for children who are bilingual: Fabiano, 2007.

Each approach has limitations, and the clinician must choose which approach best suits the child. The clinician may modify the approach as therapy progresses and as the child improves or does not improve. Note that some approaches require the clinician to obtain a certification. Computer technology support, including electropalatography (EPG) and ultrasound, is available for children diagnosed with speech sound disorders as a result of functional and organic speech disorders (Dagenais, 1995; Preston, Brick, & Landi, 2013). The traditional approach and some of the phonological approaches are described in the following paragraphs.

Traditional Approach

The **traditional (motor or phonetic) approach** contains the elements of sensory–perceptual training, production training, transfer, and carry-over of the sound or targeted behavior (ASHA, 2016; Pena-Brooks & Hegde, 2015). The clinician uses auditory discrimination tasks to help the child increase his or her awareness of the error sounds. Afterwards, the clinician instructs the child to produce the sound in isolation, nonsense syllables, words, phrases, sentences, and conversation. The clinician incorporates transfer and carry-over activities into the session after the child is able to produce the sound correctly prior to conversation.

Phonological Contrast Approaches

Phonological contrast approaches are used to eliminate phonological patterns in a child's speech. The clinician will employ contrast therapy, in which the child has to produce contrastive pairs of words. This approach emphasizes sound contrasts that are different from each other and includes the following approaches: minimal opposition contrasts (minimal pairs), maximal opposition contrasts, treatment of the empty set, and multiple oppositions (ASHA, 2016). The clinician will choose the approach depending on the number and type of phonological patterns that are not eliminated.

Summary

The clinician must take many different factors and variables into account prior to writing goals for children diagnosed with speech sound disorders. A careful understanding and analysis of assessment results begins the process, along with complete knowledge of the child's physical, social, emotional, cognitive, and cultural factors, as well as input from family members. The best therapy approach for the individual child must then be taken into consideration. After consideration of all these factors, goals can be contemplated then formulated.

 Case Scenarios

Case Scenario 1

Andrea, aged 4 years, 6 months, was referred to the ABC Speech and Language Clinic by her mother, Mrs. Smith, because she was concerned about her daughter's speech. Andrea was described as an attentive and cooperative girl who was performing well in preschool, according to her teachers. Her medical history was unremarkable with no ear infections, major illnesses, or hospitalizations. Mrs. Smith reported that her daughter's speech-language and motor milestones occurred at the appropriate ages. Andrea was learning all of the prereading and premath skills, demonstrated good play skills, and had many friends. Her gross motor skills were age appropriate, but her fine motor skills were weak (i.e., she had difficulty coloring and holding a pencil). It was also noted that the Audiology Van from the local university had visited Andrea's preschool at the beginning of the school year, and Andrea's hearing was found to be within normal limits. Andrea was not frustrated or bothered by her

Case Scenarios (continued)

speech. An informal speech screening revealed that Andrea had many mispronunciations, so a complete speech-language evaluation was recommended.

The results of the evaluation indicated that Andrea was cooperative and motivated during the evaluation. She easily engaged in conversation with the clinician. The oral–peripheral examination revealed that all structures and functions of the articulators were within normal limits. Her receptive and expressive vocabulary skills appeared to be age appropriate, as were her fluency, speech discrimination, and phonological awareness skills. The speech sound assessment revealed numerous speech sound errors, and Andrea was intelligible approximately 75 percent of the time when the context was not known by the clinician.

Andrea exhibited many errors on the Sounds-in-Words subtest of the GFTA-3. They included the following: [/θ/ → /s/; /ð/→ /z/; /w/ → /r/]. In total, Andrea earned a raw score of 36 on the test, which gave her a percentile rank of 5, an age-equivalency score of 2–9, and a standard score of 76 with a 90 percent confidence level of 72–83.

Questions

1. What questions would you ask Mrs. Smith during the interview for the evaluation?

2. Which error sounds would you possibly address first? Which factors would influence your decision?

3. With the information gleaned from the formal and informal sections of the diagnostic evaluation, write one long-term goal and two short-term goals that could be addressed in a therapy section.

4. Which six factors would you consider prior to developing short-term goals for Andrea?

Case Scenario 2

Christopher, aged 7 years, 4 months, attends his neighborhood school and is in a self-contained special education class with a 12:1–2 student to teacher ratio. His math skills are appropriate, but his reading skills are approximately 1.5 years behind where they should be. Christopher has particular difficulty with sound–symbol relationships, and he has overall auditory comprehension deficits.

Mr. Jones, Christopher's father, reported that his son's medical history includes numerous bouts of middle ear infections between the ages of 2 and 5 years. Christopher had a bilateral myringotomy when

📋 Case Scenarios *(continued)*

he was 5, and his ear infections ceased. Mr. Jones indicated that Christopher's speech-language and motor milestones were delayed, but he did not provide details. The oral–motor examination was unremarkable, but Christopher's diadochokinetic production was slow and labored. He recently received a comprehensive audiological evaluation, and the results were within normal limits. Christopher is aware of his speech sound deficits and sometimes becomes frustrated when people do not understand his speech.

Christopher was administered the DEAP test. On the Articulation Single Word Production subtest, he displayed nine errors. On the phonological assessment, Christopher displayed several phonological processes, including 11 fronting errors (/k/ and /g/ → /t/ and /d/, respectively), 7 consonant reduction errors all involving the *s* sound (for example, he produced *paidδ* for *spaidδ*) and 6 final consonant deletions (he omitted all final /p/, /t/ and /k/ phonemes at the end of words).

The results of the articulation assessment are as follows:

Raw score = 9

Scaled score = 1

Standard score = 55

Percentile rank = 0.1

Stanine = 1

The results of the phonological assessment are as follows:

Raw score = 24

Fronting errors = 11

Final consonant deletion = 6

Consonant reduction = 7

Scaled score = 1

Standard score = 55

Percentile rank = 0.1

Stanine = 1

Formal testing that was previously completed revealed that Christopher's overall cognitive skills were within normal range for his age, with the exception of his verbal intelligence, which was slightly below average. Academic testing revealed that his math calculation and reasoning skills were within the average range, but his English language skills, including phonics, reading comprehension, listening

📋 **Case Scenarios** *(continued)*

comprehension, writing, and spelling, were all at least 1.5 standard deviations below the mean. The results from the CELF-5 revealed that Christopher's receptive and expressive language abilities were all below his age level.

Questions

1. What questions would you ask Mr. Jones during the interview for the evaluation?

2. With the information gleaned from the formal and informal sections of the diagnostic evaluation, write one long-term goal and two short-term goals that could be addressed in a therapy section.

3. Which six factors would you consider prior to developing short-term goals for Christopher?

4. Which phonological patterns would you possibly address first? Which factors would influence your decision?

REVIEW QUESTIONS

1. How can a speech sound disorder be defined?
   a. A disorder involving the misperception of sounds
   b. A disorder involving difficulty with motor production
   c. A disorder involving poor phonotactic rules of speech
   d. All of the above
   e. None of the above

2. The clinician should take into account which of the following factors to determine goals for a child diagnosed with a speech sound disorder?
   a. The child's social, medical, and academic history
   b. Stimulability for error sounds
   c. Typical sound development
   d. A and B
   e. All of the above

3. What are the components of a speech sound evaluation?
   a. Case intake or history only
   b. Case intake or history, oral–peripheral examination, and hearing screen
   c. Case intake or history, oral–peripheral examination, hearing screen, speech sound assessment (including intelligibility, stimulability, and severity), and additional measures
   d. Speech sound assessment (including intelligibility, stimulability, and severity) only
   e. None of the above

4. The phonological contrast approaches include which of the following?
   a. Isolation, syllable, phrase, sentence, and connected speech
   b. Minimal opposition contrasts (minimal pairs), maximal opposition contrasts, treatment of the empty set, and multiple oppositions
   c. Core-vocabulary and metaphon therapy
   d. Cycles approach and electropalatography
   e. None of the above

5. Which class of speech sounds is acquired first?
   a. Plosives
   b. Nasals
   c. Approximants
   d. Fricatives

REFERENCES

American Speech-Language-Hearing Association. (2016). Speech sound disorders—articulation and phonology. Retrieved from http://www.asha.org/PRPSpecificTopic.aspx?folderid=8589935321&section=Assessment

American Speech-Language-Hearing Association. (2017a). Developmental norms for speech and language. Retrieved from http://www.asha.org/slp/schools/prof-consult/norms/

American Speech-Language-Hearing Association. (2017b). Phonemic inventories across languages. Retrieved from http://www.asha.org/practice/multicultural/Phono/

American Speech-Language-Hearing Association. (2017c). Speech sound disorders: Articulation and phonological processes. Retrieved from http://www.asha.org/public/speech/disorders/SpeechSoundDisorders/

Baker, E., & McLeod, S. (2011a). Evidence-based practice for children with speech sound disorders: Part 1 narrative review. *Language, Speech, and Hearing Services in Schools, 42*, 102–139. doi:10.1044/0161-1461(2010/09-0075)

Baker, E., & McLeod, S. (2011b). Evidence-based practice for children with speech sound disorders: Part 2 application to clinical practice. *Language, Speech, and Hearing Services in Schools, 42*, 140–151. doi:10.1044/0161-1461(2010/10-0023)

Bankson, N. W., & Bernthal, J. E. (1990). Bankson-Bernthal test of phonology. Austin, TX: PRO-ED.

Bauman-Waengler, J. A. (2012). *Articulatory and phonological impairments.* New York, NY: Pearson Higher Education.

Bernthal, J., Bankson, N. W., & Flipsen, P., Jr. (2013). *Articulation and phonological disorders.* New York, NY: Pearson Higher Education.

Bleile, K. (2014). *Manual of speech sound disorders: A book for students and clinicians* (3rd ed.). New York, NY: Cengage.

Coplan, J., & Gleason, J. R. (1988). Unclear speech: Recognition and significance of unintelligible speech in preschool children. *Pediatrics, 82*(3), 447–452.

Dagenais, P. A. (1995). Electropalatography in the treatment of articulation/phonological disorders. *Journal of Communication Disorders, 28*(4), 303–329.

Dean, E. C., Howell, J., Waters, D., & Reid, J. (1995). Metaphon: A metalinguistic approach to the treatment of phonological disorder in children. *Clinical Linguistics and Phonetics, 9*, 1–19.

Dodd, B., Holm, A., Crosbie, S., & McIntosh, B. (2006). A core vocabulary approach for management of inconsistent speech disorder. *Advances in Speech-Language Pathology, 8*(3), 220–230.

Epstein, B. (2018). Psychometrics of assessment. In C. Stein-Rubin & R. Fabus (Eds.), *A guide to clinical assessment and professional report writing in speech-language pathology.* Thorofare, NJ: Slack.

Fabiano, L. (2007). Evidence-based phonological assessment of bilingual children. *Perspectives on Communication Disorders and Sciences in Culturally and Linguistically Diverse Populations, SIG -14, 14,* 21–23. doi:10.1044/cds14.2.21

Fabus, R., & Gironda, F. (2018). Speech sound disorders in children. In C. Stein-Rubin & R. Fabus (Eds.), *A guide to clinical assessment and professional report writing in speech-language pathology.* Thorofare, NJ: Slack.

Fabus, R., Yudes-Kuznetsov, J., & Gozdziewski, T. (2015). *Clinical case studies of children with articulation and phonological disorders.* San Diego, CA: Plural.

Flipsen, P., Jr. (2006). Measuring the intelligibility of conversational speech in children. *Clinical Linguistics & Phonetics, 20*(4), 202–312.

Hegde, M. N. (1998). *Treatment procedures in communicative disorders.* Austin, TX: PRO-ED.

Hegde, M. N., & Pomaville, F. (2013). *Assessment of communication disorders in children.* San Diego, CA: Plural.

Lof, G. L. (2004). *Confusion about speech sound norms and their use.* Retrieved from https://myspeechteacher.wikispaces.com/file/view/confusion+about+speech+-sound+norms+and+their+use.pdf

Lowe, R. (2009). *Workbook for the identification of phonological processes and distinctive features* (4th ed.). Austin, TX: PRO-ED.

McLeod, S., & Baker, E. (2017). *Children's speech: An evidence based approach to assessment and intervention.* New York, NY: Pearson.

Miccio, A. W., & Elbert, M. (1996). Enhancing stimulability: A treatment program. *Journal of Communication Disorders, 29,* 335–352.

Miccio, A. W., & Williams, A. L. (2010). Stimulability treatment. In A. L. Williams, S. McLeod, & R. J. McCauley (Eds.), *Interventions for speech sound disorders in children* (pp. 179–202). Baltimore, MD: Paul H. Brookes.

Owens, R. (2014). *Language development: An introduction* (8th ed.). Boston, MA: Pearson.

Pena-Brooks, A., & Hegde, M. N. (2015). *Assessment and treatment of speech sound disorders in children: A dual-level text* (3rd ed.). Austin, TX: PRO-ED.

Preston, J. L., Brick, N., & Landi, N. (2013). Ultrasound biofeedback treatment for persisting childhood apraxia of speech. *American Journal of Speech-Language Pathology, 22*(4), 627–643.

Prezas, R. F., & Hodson, B. W. (2010). The cycles phonological remediation approach. In A. L. Williams, S. McLeod, & R. J. McCauley (Eds.), *Interventions for speech sound disorders in children* (pp. 137–157). Baltimore, MD: Paul H. Brookes.

Roth, F. P., & Worthington, C. K. (2016). *Treatment resource manual in speech-language pathology* (5th ed.). New York, NY: Delmar Cengage Learning.

Ruscello, D. (2008). *Treating articulation and phonological disorders in children.* St. Louis, MO: Mosby Elsevier.

Shipley, K. G., & McAfee, J. G. (2015). *Assessment in speech-language pathology: A resource manual* (5th ed.). Clifton Park, NY: Delmar Cengage Learning.

Stein-Rubin, C., & Fabus, R. (2018). *A guide to clinical assessment and professional report writing in speech-language pathology.* Thorofare, NJ: Slack.

University of Arizona. (n.d.). *Consonant chart (English).* Retrieved from http://www.u.arizona.edu/~ohalad/Phonetics/docs/Cvchart.pdf

Van Riper, C. (1978). *Speech correction: Principles and methods* (6th ed.). Englewood Cliffs, NJ: Prentice-Hall.

ADDITIONAL RESOURCES

American Speech-Language-Hearing Association. For Speech-Language Pathologists. Clinical topics and professional issues for speech-language pathologists. http://www.asha.org/Practice-Portal/Speech-Language-Pathologists/

American Speech-Language-Hearing Association. The Practice Portal. http://www.asha.org/practice-portal/

Bowen, Caroline. Speech-Language-Therapy Dot Com. http://speech-language-therapy.com/index.php?option=com_content&view=featured&Itemid=101

Childhood Apraxia of Speech Association of North America. Apraxia-KIDS. http://www.apraxia-kids.org/

Fisher, Hilda, and Jeri A. Logemann. (1971). *The Fisher-Logemann Test of Articulation Competence.* Boston, MA: Houghton Mifflin, 1971.

George Mason University. The Speech Accent Archive. http://accent.gmu.edu

Goldman, Ronald, and Macalyne Fristoe. *GFTA-3: Goldman Fristoe 3 Test of Articulation.* Bloomington, MN: PsychCorp, 2015.

Hodson, Barbara Williams. *HAPP-3: Hodson Assessment of Phonological Patterns.* Austin, TX: PRO-ED, 2004.

International Phonetic Association. https://www.internationalphoneticassociation.org/

Khan, Linda M., and Nancy Lewis. *KLPA 3: Khan-Lewis Phonological Analysis.* Bloomington, MN: PsychCorp, 2015.

Kuster, Judith Maginnis. Net Connections for Communication Disorders and Sciences: An Internet Guide. Examples of materials that can be adapted for therapy. http://www.mnsu.edu/comdis/kuster2/welcome.html

TypeIt. Type IPA Phonetic Symbols. http://ipa.typeit.org

CHAPTER 5

Pediatric Feeding and Swallowing Disorders

Cindy G. Arroyo

Key Terms

Failure to thrive
Feeding disorder
Neonatal intensive care unit
(NICU)
Nonnutritive sucking

Nutritive sucking
Pediatric dysphagia
Sensory integration intervention
Swallowing disorder

Introduction

Infants and children may experience a feeding or **swallowing disorder** at various ages and stages in their development. Consequently, feeding, which is generally perceived as a pleasurable and natural process, can suddenly create stress for the family and health concerns for the child. Infants and children with a feeding disorder may have a history of poor weight gain or **failure to thrive**. The American Psychiatric Association (2000) describes a **feeding disorder** of infancy or early childhood as including children who fail to eat sufficient quantities or varieties of foods, which may result in chronic malnutrition, poor weight gain, or weight loss before 6 years of age, in the absence of an organic component. Children may exhibit refusal behaviors toward feeding and have rigid, restricted food preferences. A feeding disorder may or may not be associated with a swallowing disorder (**pediatric dysphagia**). A swallowing disorder is characterized by difficulties in one or more of the swallowing phases; that is, oral, pharyngeal, and esophageal (Arvedson, 2008).

The Centers for Disease Control and Prevention (2015) characterizes feeding difficulties as a heterogeneous group. They identify a variety of possible etiologies, including metabolic abnormalities or absorption defects, such as cystic fibrosis or short bowel syndrome; gastrointestinal difficulties, such as reflux; structural or anatomical defects, such as cleft palate; oral–motor deficits, such as dysphagia; and sensory-related hypersensitivity to new foods and textures (Sharp, Jaquess, Morton, & Herzinger, 2010).

The incidence of feeding and swallowing disorders has been estimated from 25–45 percent in typically developing children. This may include developmental issues, such as difficulties progressing to textured foods at the appropriate age, or behavioral issues, such as food refusal, in the absence of a developmental disability diagnosis. Children with mild feeding concerns may be considered picky eaters. The incidence of feeding and swallowing disorders increases to up to 80 percent in children with some type of developmental disability, such as cerebral palsy (Arvedson, 2008; Lefton-Greif & Arvedson, 2008; Linscheid, Budd, & Rasnake, 2003). Children with a diagnosis of cerebral palsy have the highest prevalence of feeding and swallowing difficulties, with an estimated incidence of 85–90 percent (Lefton-Greif & Arvedson, 2008). The prevalence of feeding problems in children with autism spectrum disorders has been reported as 70–90 percent, with the primary concern being food selectivity that leads to a significantly restricted food repertoire and a high occurrence of behavioral difficulties (Kodak & Piazza, 2008; Ledford & Gast, 2006; Twachtman-Reilly, Amaral, & Zebrowski, 2008).

The speech-language pathologist is the professional who should have the prominent role in the assessment, diagnosis, and treatment of feeding or swallowing disorders in infants and children (American Speech-Language-Hearing Association [ASHA], 2016b). Therefore, it is imperative for speech-language pathologists to be adequately educated and trained in the knowledge and skills necessary to work with the pediatric population (Arvedson, 2008; ASHA, 2017). Training and experience in adult dysphagia is not sufficient to qualify speech-language pathologists to provide assessment and intervention to infants and children with feeding or swallowing problems (ASHA, 2017).

Comprehensive Assessment

A referral for a feeding or swallowing assessment may be initiated by a professional, such as a pediatrician, or a parent or caregiver who expresses concerns about a child's feeding or swallowing skills. An infant who is born prematurely or with medical complications may be assessed while he or she is in the **neonatal intensive care unit (NICU)**. In all cases, it is imperative to use developmental milestones as a framework or baseline for identifying differences in feeding behaviors. It is also important to consider that the course of typical development is made up of a sequence of connected elements and transitions, rather than isolated skills (Morris & Klein, 2000). A child's oral–motor functioning for feeding and swallowing must be evaluated in relation to the entire body. Any difficulties or differences in postural tone or stability and movement in the pelvis, trunk, shoulder girdle, or neck may influence jaw stability (Alexander, Boeheme & Cupps, 1993; Morris & Klein, 2000). Because the jaw is the proximal structure for distal movements of the lips, tongue, and cheeks, stability is necessary for more controlled and diverse oral–motor movements.

An interdisciplinary team approach is best practice for both assessment and treatment. The speech–language pathologist addresses oral–motor concerns, swallowing disorders, and food presentation. A physical therapist may contribute information regarding positioning and any need for adaptive seating. An occupational therapist may address sensory issues, self-feeding skills, and the need for adaptive equipment. Additional team members may include a dietician or nutritionist, behavior specialist, and medical pediatric specialists (e.g., pediatric gastroenterologist, cardiologist, etc.). It is imperative for parents and caregivers to be involved in all assessments, team decisions, and interventions (Bruns & Thompson, 2010; Owen et al., 2012).

As part of the assessment, it may be helpful to categorize feeding or swallowing disorders by the types of limitations affecting the child's abilities. It is important, however, to recognize that many children may demonstrate characteristics across more than one category (Morris & Klein, 2000). The types of limitations are as follows:

- Structural limitations: Differences in structures or anatomy may interfere with feeding and swallowing skills, such as cleft lip, cleft palate, or tracheoesophageal atresia or fistula.
- Motor-based or physiological limitations: Motor-based diagnoses, such as cerebral palsy, result in differences in postural muscle tone

and movement. Examples of physiological limitations may be seen in children with cardiac, respiratory, or other medical conditions.

- Experientially based limitations: This may include children who have had invasive or extensive medical interventions or conditions, such as gastroesophageal reflux, which may result in behavioral reactions such as food refusal.
- Sensory-based limitations: These children may have difficulty modulating and integrating sensory input (visual, auditory, smell, taste, and touch). Many children with autism spectrum disorder exhibit these characteristics.
- Environmental limitations: This may include socioeconomic factors or personal limitations of parents or caregivers. It may also include the influence of the feeding environment (Morris & Klein, 2000).

A comprehensive assessment should identify the child's strengths and needs, incorporate observations and concerns from parents or caregivers, and explore the child's skills or behaviors in a variety of environments. This should provide information that can be used to develop goals and an effective intervention plan (Morris & Klein, 2000; Silverman, 2010). The initial step should therefore be to gather a thorough medical, developmental, and feeding history. Some information may be available from medical records, but it is important to ask more detailed questions of the parent or caregiver (Arvedson, 2008; Wolf & Glass, 1992). Recounting a difficult medical or feeding history may be a very emotional experience for a parent or caregiver; therefore, the evaluator must gather information in a supportive, empathetic manner. It may be helpful to send a questionnaire prior to the assessment to allow parents or caregivers time and privacy to respond to delicate questions. Evaluation and assessment checklists are available that may be helpful in organizing and guiding assessments. Examples of questionnaires and assessment checklists are provided in the "Additional Resources" section in this chapter.

An oral–peripheral examination should be administered to observe the symmetry and appearance of the oral structures. Oral reflexes (e.g., suck, swallow, gag, rooting, and phasic bite) should be evaluated and compared to developmental norms (Arvedson, 2008). It is also important to conduct clinical observations of posture, movement, and muscle tone; respiratory patterns; affect and alertness levels; and responses to sensory stimulation (e.g., visual, tactile, and auditory) because they can influence a child's readiness and participation for feeding (Arvedson, 2008; Morris & Klein, 2000).

There will be differences in the assessment process depending on the age or functional level of the child. For example, the assessment of feeding skills for an infant younger than 4–6 months would evaluate only **nutritive sucking** (breast or bottle) and **nonnutritive sucking** (pacifier or finger) because those skills are expected in that developmental age range. A child aged 4–6 months should be evaluated for oral–motor skills related to sucking purees from a spoon. From 6 months to 1 year of age there are developmental norms related to chewing and biting various food textures and tastes. Cup and straw drinking are expected and assessed at other age ranges. This requires the clinician to have a base of knowledge regarding the typical developmental milestones in the acquisition of feeding skills (Arvedson, 2008; Morris & Klein, 2000; Wolf & Glass, 1992).

In all assessments there should be an emphasis on the whole child, including medical status, neurologic status, neuromotor function, behavioral profile, and general developmental abilities (Redstone, 2014; Wolf & Glass, 1992). It is also imperative to consider the family, cultural practices, and communication during the feeding process (Bruns & Thompson, 2010; Davis-McFarland, 2008; Morris & Klein, 2000). Feeding practices and food preferences differ across cultures and are also impacted by socioeconomic status and religious background (Davis-McFarland, 2008).

The assessment should include observation of a typical meal or feeding in a familiar environment, with the parent or caregiver feeding the child. The child should be fed in the typical position or seating system, and the child's ability to maintain postural stability should be noted. When seated, the child's ability to maintain postural stability or upright positioning depends on 90° flexion at the hips, knees, and ankles (Arvedson, 2008; Redstone, 2014). The evaluator should then try feeding the child to get a closer perspective of the child's skills or needs and to implement some techniques or strategies that may assist the child in more effective feeding patterns. This dynamic process may indicate the potential for change and assist in the development of appropriate goals and interventions (Redstone, 2014).

There are no standardized assessments of pediatric feeding or swallowing skills. Feeding behaviors are generally compared to typical patterns of development using a reference such as the Developmental Pre-Feeding Checklist (Morris & Klein, 2000). There are some scales and checklists for specialized populations; an example is the Neonatal Oral–Motor Assessment Scale (NOMAS), which was designed for infants who are being evaluated in the NICU due to premature birth or medical complications. The NOMAS is a checklist of feeding behaviors categorized by normal, disorganized, or dysfunctional movements of the tongue and jaw during nutritive sucking from a breast or bottle and nonnutritive sucking from a pacifier or finger (Palmer, 2014; Palmer, Crawley & Blanco, 1993).

The Child's Eating Behavior Inventory-Revised (CEBI-R) and the Brief Autism Mealtime Behavior Inventory (BAMBI) are reliable and valid measures in terms of psychometric properties. In both inventories, the parent or caregiver is asked to indicate how often a child engages in a specific feeding behavior (Archer, Rosenbaum, & Streiner, 1991; Lukens & Linscheid, 2008).

Data Analysis and Additional Tests

According to ASHA (2017), the purpose of a pediatric feeding and swallowing assessment is to determine the presence and possible etiologies of a disorder and to determine the need for additional referrals. Additionally, the results of the assessment should first and foremost determine whether the child can eat and drink in a safe manner. If there are any concerns with regard to safe feeding or swallowing, particularly if there are signs of possible aspiration, a referral for additional testing is warranted (Arvedson, 2008; Lefton-Greif & Arvedson, 2008). This should be discussed with the child's pediatrician and any other relevant members of the medical team. The team, along with the parents, will then pursue appropriate diagnostic tests, which may include the following:

- Videofluoroscopic swallow study (VFSS), also known as modified barium swallow study: This study may provide information on the swallowing phases, presence of aspiration, risk factors, and consistencies of food that the child can safely swallow.
- Fiberoptic endoscopic evaluation of swallowing (FEES): This study may provide information regarding the laryngopharynx or upper aerodigestive tract in a dynamic fashion.
- Upper gastrointestinal (GI) series: This test may identify structural abnormalities and provide information about the function and motility of the GI tract.
- pH probe: This test is used over a specified time period to quantify the frequency and duration of gastroesophageal reflux.
- Bronchoscopy and laryngoscopy: These tests may identify structural abnormalities in the upper airway structures (Arvedson, 2008; Morris & Klein, 2000).

Based on the results of the diagnostic tests, medical management or additional referrals may be necessary, such as to a pediatric gastroenterologist for treatment of reflux. The results may also indicate the need for alternate feeding methods, such as tube feedings, if oral feedings are not medically possible (as in the case of aspiration). Another outcome from the diagnostic tests may be a recommendation for the use of a particular consistency of food or liquid to ensure safe and effective swallowing. These recommendations must always be implemented with medical guidance and consultation.

The frequency and duration of therapy should be determined on an individual basis, and the environment may influence the recommendations. For example, an infant may be receiving services in the NICU. A child between the ages of birth and 3 years may be seen in the home environment through an early intervention program. Older children may be seen in the school. Individual therapy sessions allow for the implementation of specific techniques and training for families. Group sessions may benefit children through peer modeling, social interaction, and engagement in food preparation activities.

Swallowing and feeding services associated with complex medical needs may be reimbursed by Medicaid under the categories of speech-language pathology or nursing services. Note that Medicaid eligibility requirements and coverage vary from state to state (Power-deFur & Alley, 2008).

Children with medically complex conditions are increasingly being integrated into school settings, and the number of these cases are expected to rise (ASHA, 2016a). An ASHA schools survey (2016a) reported that 14 percent of school-based speech-language pathologists in the United States serve students with feeding or swallowing problems. Although medical issues were historically considered separate from educational goals, the need for adequate nutrition and a child's ability to participate in mealtimes with peers has been recognized as part of academic and social development (ASHA, 2000; Lefton-Greif & Arvedson, 2008). The safety and nutritional needs of children in schools are also supported by the Individuals with Disabilities Education Act (U.S. Department of Education, 2004), which mandates that school systems provide health-related services, including feeding (Lefton-Greif & Arvedson, 2008; Mabry-Price, 2014).

Forming Specific Goals

Morris and Klein say that short-term goals should contain the following related components: "What will the child do?; Under what circumstances will the child do it?; With what degree of proficiency will the child do it?" (2000, p. 216). An example of a goal that uses these components is as follows: John will exhibit a controlled, sustained bite on a cracker placed on lateral chewing surfaces, four out of six times, when seated upright during snack time.

When forming goals and treatment plans, Morris and Klein (2000) discuss important considerations in the use of terminology. The term *feeding program* may focus too narrowly on improving a child's eating and drinking skills. This narrow focus may not address the child's physical, sensory, and oral–motor needs, which are crucial for successful feeding and swallowing. It is important to recognize that the term *oral–motor treatment* is often used while developing goals that emphasize specific stimulation and movements of the jaw, tongue, and lips. Clinicians often develop goals using oral stimulation or exercises, such as blowing or tongue resistance, because they believe these techniques may assist in feeding and swallowing issues. However, these goals and strategies become things we do to children; they do not engage children as active participants in a functional feeding activity (Morris & Klein, 2000). There is limited evidence supporting the use of oral–motor exercises for children with feeding and swallowing difficulties (Arvedson, Clark, Lazarus, Schooling, & Frymark, 2010; Lof & Watson, 2008; McCauley, Strand, Lof, Schooling, & Frymark, 2009), and the total needs of the child will not be addressed in this narrow scope of treatment.

The term *mealtime program* has been suggested to include the treatment of the child's feeding and oral–motor issues in a larger context. This includes the influence of cultural, health, and socioeconomic factors, which may impact the child in the context of the family or the community (Morris & Klein, 2000). In all facets of goal development and treatment programs, it is crucial to directly train the individuals who are involved with feeding the child, including parents, teachers, and classroom aides. Such training may include a written description of goals and intervention techniques, modeling techniques, the provision of feedback while observing the parent or caregiver feeding the child, and review of a video-recorded feeding session in a natural environment (Silverman, 2010). The therapy goals and feeding skills must also be integrated into all relevant settings (e.g., home, school, and day care) for the outcomes to be successful, functional, and generalized.

Evidence-based practice is the gold standard for developing goals and interventions, but there are often limited resources in pediatric feeding and swallowing. Therefore, adequate knowledge and skills and clinical judgment must also be used in goal formulation (Arvedson et al., 2010).

Although a discussion of appropriate goals and interventions for specific diagnoses and populations is beyond the scope of this chapter, some important considerations should be noted. When working with premature or young infants, feeding goals and interventions must be infant-driven and focused on quality, rather than quantity or volume (Shaker, 2012). Modifications to the feeding process are based on the infant's stress cues, such as cardiac and respiratory rates, oxygen saturation levels, and suck–swallow–breathe coordination (Shaker, 2012; Wolf & Glass, 1992). With this in mind, an example of an inappropriate goal is as follows: The infant will suck 4 ounces of formula in 20 minutes. A more appropriate goal is the following: The infant will exhibit a coordinated suck–swallow–breathe pattern during bottle feeding in a side-lying position when provided with external pacing for 15 minutes. Measurable feeding goals may often be difficult to establish or irrelevant to the situation. It is more important to establish age-appropriate patterns, safe and efficient feeding, and a pleasurable, stress-free experience for the infant and the parent or caregiver. Again, quality is more important than quantity. "Successful oral feeding must be measured in quality of mealtime experiences with best possible skills, while not jeopardizing a child's functional health status or the parent-child relationship" (Arvedson, 2008, p. 125).

The transition from tube feeding to oral feeding is a process that requires medical guidance and consideration of readiness factors, which may include the overall health of the child, the results of a swallow study, oral–motor skills, and the potential to develop hunger–satiation cycles. The child's interest and cooperation in eating, and the parent's readiness, must also be considered. The critical question may be whether the child is ready to and wants to eat orally, or if this is the goal of the clinician or parents (ASHA, 2000; Lefton-Greif & Arvedson, 2008; Morris & Klein, 2000).

The goals for children with sensory-based feeding difficulties may focus on behavioral issues, such as decreasing behavioral resistance, increasing positive interactions between the child and the parent or caregiver, and improving the structure and routine of meals. The goals may also target increasing the quantity and variety of foods that the child eats and increasing the textures of foods according to developmental norms (Fischer & Silverman, 2007; Silverman, 2010).

Intervention Approaches

Feeding and swallowing difficulties will rarely be remediated with just one technique or method. The selection of intervention techniques and strategies must be a dynamic process that meets the child's changing needs (Wolf & Glass, 1992). Furthermore, pediatric feeding and swallowing problems are not homogeneous in nature, and they require individualized treatment plans (Linscheid, 2006). The best practice employs a case-based approach, founded in ethics, that focuses on developing strategies to allow for a range of options that apply to the individual child (Brady-Wagner, 2001).

Due to the heterogeneous nature of pediatric feeding and swallowing issues, problem solving is an effective way to integrate assessment and treatment. Problem solving may involve organizing information gathered from the assessment and clinical observations, prioritizing goals and skills to be targeted, and determining the appropriate strategies and techniques for intervention (Morris & Klein, 2000). The assessment and treatment should be intertwined when working with children who have feeding and swallowing problems. Children will present differently from session to session, influenced by physical, sensory, maturational, and environmental factors. The clinician must be able to assess the situation, adapt goals as needed, and explore treatment options to address the needs of the child in that particular session (Morris & Klein, 2000).

As mentioned earlier, it is critical to address the whole child in interventions. There must be considerations for the components of physical status and postural stability; sensory input, such as taste, smell, and texture; nutritional factors; and communication, including nonverbal and verbal signals and interactions (Arvedson et al., 2010; Morris & Klein, 2000).

It is essential to be sensitive to cultural and linguistic differences when developing goals and treatment protocols. Families should be encouraged to attend meetings, or bring an advocate, and they should be informed that they are entitled to a translator. There may be distinct variations in feeding practices, preferred foods, and communication styles across cultures. There may be financial constraints and religious or cultural prohibitions against eating certain foods (Davis-McFarland, 2008). These factors must be considered when developing goals or making recommendations regarding the food types and textures that will be used in treatment.

While goals typically address specific skills, treatment should also include procedures to support and enhance the feeding session. The procedures may include the following (Morris & Klein, 2000):

1. Preparing the feeding environment, including minimizing auditory and visual distractions
2. Seating and positioning for postural stability (a physical therapy or occupational therapy consultation should be considered)

3. Determining the communication methods (verbal, nonverbal, or augmentative and alternative communication [AAC] so the child can indicate choices, emotions, pain, etc.)
4. Training and counseling the parent or caregiver, with appropriate referrals as necessary

It is particularly important to identify and prioritize treatment needs and goals for children with feeding or swallowing difficulties; this approach is called *therapeutic balance* (Twachtman-Reilly et al., 2008). For example, a child with a diagnosis of autism spectrum disorder may exhibit extreme food selectivity, a strong preference for specific rituals, and high-risk choking behaviors. The first priority should be to facilitate safe feeding behaviors with foods that are already in the child's repertoire. If too many issues are targeted at one time, the child may show resistance and negative behaviors (Twachtman-Reilly et al., 2008). Other strategies may include combining new foods with familiar foods, choosing foods based on attributes such as color and texture, peer modeling, and minimizing distractions in the environment (Ernsperger & Stegen-Hanson, 2004). There are also programs that address sensory behaviors related to feeding, such as acceptance, toleration, touch, smell, taste, and eating. This may allow the child's sensory system to shift slowly into acceptance, reducing negative and aversive behaviors (Toomey & Ross, 2011; Twachtman-Reilly et al., 2008). Intervention approaches that incorporate the principles of operant conditioning and systematic desensitization are frequently used with children who have autism spectrum disorder and sensory-based feeding problems. Operant conditioning may be considered a top-down approach in which a specific behavior is expected, often elicited through shaping or chaining. Systematic desensitization is more of a bottom-up approach in which the child is exposed to a stimulus he or she perceives as negative, such as a particular food. Reinforcement activities are generally paired with this process. More evidence is needed to support the efficacy of these approaches (Marshall, Ware, Ziviani, Hill, & Dodrill, 2015).

Behavioral approaches, such as contingency management, appetite manipulation, and reinforcement strategies, are often cited in the literature as part of a feeding program, particularly for children with autism spectrum disorder or sensory-based feeding disorders (Linscheid, 2006). An example of a strategy in appetite manipulation is reducing liquid intake while increasing food intake. Meals are generally restricted to 25–30 minutes, and there should be adequate intervals between feedings, perhaps 3–4 hours, to create an appetite. Contingencies may include the use of positive reinforcement, including praise and access to preferred toys or preferred foods (Linscheid, 2006).

Sensory integration intervention is often implemented by an occupational therapist; however, recommendations for a sensory diet may be provided to parents and other team members to support the achievement of feeding goals. Sensory integration activities may include vibration, therapeutic brushing, rhythm or music activities, and proprioceptive activities, such as joint compression and crawling through a tunnel (Addison et al., 2012).

Interventions may also target the development or refinement of specific feeding skills or processes, including sucking, lip closure for spoon feeding, cup and straw drinking, and a controlled, sustained bite. Chewing should progress from a vertical munching pattern to a diagonal rotary movement of the jaw. Separation of movement should result in tongue lateralization in chewing, which aids in forming a bolus and channeling the food for safe, efficient swallowing (Morris & Klein, 2000).

It is of paramount importance to ask permission, instead of tricking the child, and to follow the child's lead (Morris & Klein, 2000). Feeding and oral treatment interventions should never be stressful for the child, and under no circumstances should a child be force fed (Lefton-Greif & Arvedson, 2008). Intervention plans for children of all ages should stress safe feeding that supports and maintains the child's health and nutrition. The plans should also be farsighted and consider future implications for the child (Wolf & Glass, 1992). Additionally, mealtimes should be pleasurable and as stress-free as possible for the child and family.

Summary

Infants and children may experience a feeding and/or swallowing disorder at various ages and stages in their development. Speech-language pathologists should have the prominent role in the assessment, diagnosis, and treatment of feeding and/or swallowing disorders in infants and children; however, team/family collaboration is essential.

Evidence-based practice should be the foundation for developing goals and interventions, along with adequate knowledge and skills and clinical judgment. In all cases, goals and interventions should support safe feeding, maintenance of the child's health and nutrition, and a pleasurable experience for both the child and the family.

Case Scenarios

Case Scenario 1

Billy is 4 years, 3 months old. At 18 months he was diagnosed with autism spectrum disorder and sensory integration disorder. He is very sensitive to loud noises, and he gets overstimulated in loud, bright environments. He resists touch in the oral–facial area, and he does not cooperate for tooth brushing. Billy does not like his hands to be dirty, and he refuses to touch foods and substances that are wet or sticky. He is receiving occupational therapy to address his sensory issues. His occupational therapist has designed a sensory diet for Billy, which includes therapeutic brushing; the use of calming, rhythmic music; and proprioceptive activities, such as bouncing on a therapy ball.

Billy exhibits muscle tone within normal limits, and he has achieved all of the typical fine and gross motor milestones for his age. An oral–peripheral examination revealed all structures to be symmetrical with normal range of motion. Billy's oral reflexes are age appropriate, although a hyperactive behavioral gag has been observed when he is presented with new foods or foods that are wet or sticky.

Billy has no history of significant medical concerns. His hearing and vision evaluations were within normal limits. His weight gain has been poor, and he is below the 10th percentile for his age.

Billy exhibits extreme food selectivity. He primarily eats dry, crunchy snack foods, such as pretzels and crackers. He grazes on these foods throughout the day and does not have an established feeding schedule. His chewing pattern is age appropriate, characterized by diagonal and rotary jaw movement and adequate tongue lateralization. There are no swallowing difficulties. If a new food is presented on Billy's tray or table, he gags and screams. He drinks water throughout the day from a bottle, and his pediatrician thinks this is restricting Billy's appetite for food. Billy attends a preschool program 5 days a week, and he refuses to sit at the table to eat snacks with the other children.

Billy's receptive language is slightly delayed for his chronological age (1 standard deviation below the mean) based on the Auditory Comprehension section of the Preschool Language Scale, Fifth Edition (PLS-5). Billy scored more than 2 standard deviations below the mean on the Expressive Communication section of the PLS-5, which is a significant delay. He communicates with a few manual signs, and he is beginning to point to pictures on a communication board to indicate choices and emotions. Billy's vocalizations are limited to vowel sounds and grunts, and he does not engage in vocal imitation. He becomes frustrated very easily when he cannot communicate effectively, then he engages in behaviors such as crying and throwing objects.

📋 **Case Scenarios** *(continued)*

Billy's parents are extremely concerned with his limited diet, slow weight gain, and nutrition. The observation of a typical feeding session at home revealed stressful interactions between Billy and his parents.

In developing goals and interventions for Billy, the whole child must be considered and his parents must be involved. The feeding environment should be as distraction-free as possible, and Billy should be seated in a chair that facilitates 90° flexion at the hips, knees, and ankles. This position will improve his postural stability and help him remain calm and organized. Following a consultation with Billy's occupational therapist, it may be helpful to incorporate some activities from his sensory diet, such as therapeutic brushing and proprioceptive activities, prior to the feeding session. Rhythmic music may help calm his sensory system during the meal.

A consultation with Billy's parents revealed that their primary concerns are his limited diet, extreme behavioral reactions, and dependence on bottle drinking. When comparing Billy's feeding skills to developmental norms, he should be drinking from a cup or straw rather than from a bottle. Because his limited weight gain and nutrition are also concerns, a more nutritious drink should be introduced. A consultation with a nutritionist may assist in this recommendation.

Long-Term Goal 1

Billy will develop the ability to drink liquid from a straw.

Short-Term Goals 1

1. Billy will smell a novel liquid without a negative response in three out of five trials.
2. Billy will touch and taste a novel liquid, given verbal reinforcement and modeling, in three out of five trials.
3. Billy will use an efficient suck–swallow pattern when presented with a novel liquid in a cup with a straw in 8 out of 10 trials.

The short-term goals use the desensitization approach, allowing the sensory system to slowly shift into acceptance. If new liquids or foods are presented too quickly without allowing the gradual accommodation of the senses (sight, smell, and touch), there is often a negative reaction. The same approach should be used to introduce new foods into Billy's repertoire. New foods should be chosen based on nutritional value (consult with a nutritionist) and should share properties with Billy's preferred foods.

Long-Term Goal 2

Billy will increase his repertoire of accepted foods.

📋 Case Scenarios *(continued)*

Short-Term Goals 2

1. Billy will visually accept a new food on his plate, without a negative reaction, four times per session.
2. Billy will smell a new food, given verbal reinforcement and modeling, four times per session.
3. Billy will touch a new food, given verbal reinforcement and modeling, four times per session.
4. Billy will taste a new food, given verbal reinforcement and modeling, four times per session.

The clinician and parents will model the behaviors, such as tasting and smelling, and model positive language. It is important to recognize that mealtimes are opportunities for communication. Billy's communication board should be available with appropriate pictures to label the foods, indicate choices and emotions, and describe the qualities of the foods. These strategies should be shared with the teachers at Billy's preschool so they can encourage participation in snack time at school with his peers.

Case Scenario 2

Chase was born prematurely, and he suffered a cerebral hemorrhage related to his prematurity. He was diagnosed with spastic cerebral palsy at 2 months of age. Chase is presently 2 years old. He exhibits extreme spastic muscle tone (hypertonia) throughout his body. He is unable to sit or walk independently, and he is fed in an adaptive seating system that supports his head and trunk. The adaptive chair also maintains his hips, ankles, and knees at 90° flexion. Chase's arms are often in a retracted position, and he is unable to grasp and hold objects because of the flexed position of his fingers due to spasticity. Chase exhibits upper lip retraction and therefore has difficulty with lip closure. He uses atypical tongue movements, particularly strong thrusting, in his attempts to form and swallow a bolus of food. Chase eats only pureed foods or smooth foods such as yogurt or applesauce. His mother has tried to introduce textured table foods, with limited success. Chase does not demonstrate vertical jaw movement for chewing; rather, he uses a sucking pattern when textured foods are introduced, either pushing the food out with his tongue or gagging when it moves toward the back of his tongue. His mother is now reluctant to introduce table foods, even though her pediatrician has emphasized that it is developmentally and socially appropriate.

Chase has demonstrated responses to receptive identification tasks (objects and pictures) and verbal commands via eye gaze and head shakes (for yes and no), and his skills have informally been judged to be close to age appropriate. His expressive language is significantly delayed,

📋 **Case Scenarios** *(continued)*

with a score more than 3 standard deviations below the mean on the PLS-5. Chase has not been able to use sign language as a communication mode because of his fine motor limitations. His speech-language pathologist has designed a no-tech, partner-assisted scanning AAC system so Chase can nod his head when the speech-language pathologist reads his desired choice from a communication board that displays relevant symbols and messages for feeding. This communication system will be used during feeding sessions.

Chase's parents would like him to eat regular table foods with the family at mealtimes. Chase had a VFSS, which revealed normal results in the oral and pharyngeal phases of swallowing and no evidence of aspiration. Some delays in formation and transit of the bolus were noted, but no premature spillage or misdirection of the bolus were observed. These delays were attributed to immature chewing skills, limited tongue lateralization, and lack of experience with textured foods.

Long-Term Goal

Chase will develop age-appropriate feeding skills.

Short-Term Goals

1. Chase will demonstrate a vertical chewing pattern with textured foods that are placed on lateral chewing surfaces, when provided with jaw support by the feeder, in six out of eight trials.
2. Chase will demonstrate tongue lateralization during chewing with textured foods that are placed on lateral chewing surfaces, when provided with jaw support by the feeder, in six out of eight trials.
3. Chase will demonstrate improved lip closure and reduced loss of food during chewing and swallowing activities, when provided with jaw support by the feeder, in six out of eight trials.

Chase's parents will be trained in the techniques of jaw support, choosing appropriate textured foods that dissolve easily, and food placement on the lateral chewing surfaces. Upright positioning and postural stability must be monitored and maintained throughout the feeding session to ensure safe swallowing and optimal oral–motor stability and mobility.

REVIEW QUESTIONS

1. Which is true of a feeding disorder in infancy or childhood?
   a. May result in malnutrition or poor weight gain
   b. May or may not be associated with a swallowing disorder (pediatric dysphagia)
   c. May cause stress for the family
   d. All of the above

2. What should a comprehensive assessment do?
   a. Utilize an interdisciplinary team approach
   b. Incorporate observations and concerns from parents and caregivers
   c. Focus only on feeding and oral–motor skills
   d. Both A and B are correct

3. Which method is an effective way to integrate assessment and treatment?
   a. Standardized tests
   b. An oral–peripheral examination
   c. Problem solving and prioritizing goals
   d. VFSS

4. Which of the following is *not* important and lacks evidence for feeding or swallowing interventions?
   a. Seating and positioning for postural stability
   b. Sensitivity to families' cultural and linguistic differences
   c. Oral–motor exercises
   d. Parent training and appropriate referrals

5. When working with premature or young infants, goals and interventions
   a. must be infant-driven.
   b. should focus on quantity of intake.
   c. will always be measurable.
   d. should be developed without input from the parents or caregiver.

REFERENCES

Addison, L., Piazza, C., Patel, M., Bachmeyer, M., Rivas, K., Milnes, S., & Oddo, J. (2012). A comparison of sensory integrative and behavioral therapies as treatment for pediatric feeding disorders. *Journal of Applied Behavior Analysis, 45*(3), 455–471.

Alexander, R., Boehme, R., & Cupps, B. (1993). *Normal development of functional motor skills.* Tuscon, AZ: Therapy Skill Builders.

American Psychiatric Association. (2000). *Diagnostic and statistical manual of mental disorders* (4th ed.). Washington, DC: Author.

American Speech-Language-Hearing Association. (2000). *Guidelines for the roles and responsibilities of the school-based speech-language pathologist.* Rockville, MD: Author.

American Speech-Language-Hearing Association. (2016a). *Schools survey report: SLP caseload characteristics trends 1995–2016.* Retrieved from http://www.asha.org/uploadedFiles/2016-Schools-Survey-SLP-Caseload-Characteristics-Trends.pdf

American Speech-Language-Hearing Association. (2016b). Scope of practice in speech-language pathology. Retrieved from http://www.asha.org/policy/SP2016-00343/

American Speech-Language-Hearing Association. (2017). Pediatric dysphagia practice portal. Retrieved from http://www.asha.org/Practice-Portal/Clinical-Topics/Pediatric-Dysphagia

Archer, L. A., Rosenbaum, P., & Streiner, D. (1991). The children's eating behavior inventory: Reliability and validity results. *Journal of Pediatric Psychology, 16*, 629–642.

Arvedson, J. C. (2008). Assessment of pediatric dysphagia and feeding disorders: Clinical and instrumental approaches. *Developmental Disabilities Research Reviews, 14*, 118–127.

Arvedson, J., Clark, H., Lazarus, C., Schooling, T., & Frymark, T. (2010). Evidence-based systematic review: Effects of oral motor interventions on feeding and swallowing in pre-term infants. *American Journal of Speech-Language Pathology, 19*, 321–340.

Brady-Wagner, L. C. (2001). Dysphagia management for school children: Dealing with ethical dilemmas. *ASHA Division 16 Newsletter, 2*, 18–20.

Bruns, D. A., & Thompson, S. D. (2010). Feeding challenges in young children: Towards a best practices model. *Infants & Young Children, 23*(2), 93–102.

Centers for Disease Control and Prevention. (2015). *International Classification of Diseases, Ninth Revision, Clinical Modification (ICD-9-CM)*. Retrieved from http://www.cdc.gov/nchs/icd/icd9cm.htm

Davis-McFarland, E. (2008). Family and cultural issues in a school swallowing and feeding program. *Language, Speech, and Hearing in Schools, 39*, 199–213.

Ernsperger, L., & Stegen-Hanson, T. (2004). *Just take a bite: Easy, effective answers to food aversions and eating challenges*. Arlington, TX: Future Horizons.

Fischer, E., & Silverman, A. (2007). Behavioral conceptualization, assessment and treatment of pediatric feeding disorders. *Seminars in Speech and Language, 28*, 160–165.

Kodak, T., & Piazza, C. (2008). Assessment and behavioral treatment of feeding and sleeping disorders in children with autism spectrum disorders. *Child and Adolescent Psychiatric Clinics of North America, 17*(4), 887–905.

Ledford, J. R., & Gast, D. L. (2006). Feeding problems in children with autism spectrum disorders: A review. *Focus on Autism and Other Developmental Disabilities, 21*, 153–166.

Lefton-Greif, M. A., & Arvedson, J. C. (2008). Schoolchildren with dysphagia associated with medically complex conditions. *Language, Speech, and Hearing in Schools, 39*, 237–248.

Linscheid, T. R. (2006). Behavioral treatment for pediatric feeding disorders. *Behavior Modification, 30*(1), 6–23.

Linscheid, T. R., Budd, K. S., & Rasnake, L. K. (2003). Pediatric feeding problems. In M.C. Roberts (Ed.), *Handbook of pediatric psychology* (pp. 481–498). New York, NY: Guilford Press.

Lof, G. L., & Watson, M. M. (2008). A nationwide survey of nonspeech oral motor exercise use: Implications for evidence-based practice. *Language, Speech, and Hearing Services in Schools, 39*, 392–417.

Lukens, C. T., & Linscheid, T. R. (2008). Development and validation of an inventory to assess mealtime behavior problems in children with autism. *Journal of Autism and Developmental Disabilities, 38*, 342–352.

Mabry-Price, L. (2014). Dysphagia services in the school setting: Challenges and opportunities. *SIG 13, Perspectives on Swallowing and Swallowing Disorders, American Speech-Language-Hearing Association, 23*, 152–156.

Marshall, J., Ware, R., Ziviani, J., Hill, R. J., & Dodrill, P. (2015). Efficacy of interventions to improve feeding difficulties in children with autism spectrum disorders: A systematic review and meta-analysis. *Child: Care, Health and Development, 41*(2), 278–302.

McCauley, R. J., Strand, E., Lof, G. L., Schooling, T., & Frymark, T. (2009). Evidence-based systematic review: Effects of nonspeech oral–motor exercises on speech. *American Journal of Speech-Language Pathology, 18*, 343–360.

Morris, S. E., & Klein, M. D. (2000). *Pre-feeding skills: A Comprehensive Resource for Mealtime Development* (2nd ed.). Tucson, AZ: Therapy Skill Builders.

Owen, C., Ziebell, L., Lessard, C., Churcher, E., Bourget, V., & Villeneuve, H. (2012). Interprofessional group intervention for parents of children age 3 and younger with feeding difficulties: Pilot program evaluation. *Nutrition in Clinical Practice, 27*(1), 129–135.

Palmer, M. M. (2014). Feeding in the NICU. In F. Redstone (Ed.), *Effective SLP interventions for children with cerebral palsy* (pp. 131–163). San Diego, CA: Plural.

Palmer, M., Crawley, K., & Blanco, I. (1993). Neonatal oral–motor assessment scale: A reliability study. *Journal of Perinatology, 13*, 28–35.

Power-deFur, L., & Alley, N. S. (2008). Legal and financial issues associated with providing services in schools to children with swallowing and feeding disorders. *Language, Speech & Hearing Services in Schools, 39*, 160–166.

Redstone, F. (2014). Feeding the whole child using NDT. In R. Redstone (Ed.), *Effective SLP interventions for children with cerebral palsy* (pp. 93–130). San Diego, CA: Plural.

Shaker, C. S. (2012). Feed me only when I'm cueing: Moving away from a volume-driven culture in the NICU. *Neonatal Intensive Care, 25*(3), 27–32.

Sharp, W. G., Jaquess, D. L., Morton, J. F., & Herzinger, C. V. (2010). Pediatric feeding disorders: A quantitative synthesis of treatment outcomes. *Clinical Child Family Psychological Review, 13*, 348–365.

Silverman, A. H. (2010). Interdisciplinary care for feeding problems in children. *Nutrition in Clinical Practice, 25*, 160–165.

Toomey, K. A., & Ross, E. S. (2011). SOS approach to feeding. *Perspectives on swallowing and swallowing disorders, 20*, 82–87.

Twachtman-Reilly, J., Amaral, S. C., & Zebrowski, P. (2008). Addressing feeding disorders in children on the autism spectrum in school-based settings: Physiological and behavioral issues. *Language, Speech, and Hearing Services in Schools, 39*(2), 261–272.

U.S. Department of Education. (2004). Building the legacy: IDEA 2004. Retrieved from http://idea.ed.gov/

Wolf, L. S., & Glass, R. P. (1992). *Feeding and swallowing disorders in infancy.* Tucson, AZ: Therapy Skill Builders.

ADDITIONAL RESOURCES

The following resources contain questionnaires and evaluation forms for pediatric feeding and swallowing:

Arvedson, Joan, and Linda Brodsky. *Pediatric Swallowing and Feeding.* San Diego, CA: Singular, 1993. Oral–Motor and Feeding Evaluation, pp. 283–293.

Morris, Suzanne Evans, and Marsha Dunn Klein. *Pre-Feeding Skills: A Comprehensive Resource for Mealtime Development* (2nd ed.). Tucson, AZ: Therapy Skill Builders, 2000. Sample Mealtime Questionnaires, pp. 175–183. Developmental Pre-Feeding Checklist: A Sequential Approach, pp. 712–726. Spanish Translations of Parent Questionnaires, pp. 727–740.

Wolf, Lynn S., and Robin P. Glass. *Feeding and Swallowing Disorders in Infancy.* Tucson, AZ: Therapy Skill Builders, 1992. Feeding History/Clinical Feeding Evaluation of Infants, pp. 150–158.

CHAPTER 6

Adult Dysphagia

Laurie Wenerholm
Renee Fabus

Key Terms

Clinical swallow evaluation
Dysphagia
Electrical stimulation (e-stim)
Fiberoptic endoscopic
   evaluation of swallowing
   (FEES)
Functional communication
   measures (FCMs)
Levels of evidence

Modified barium swallow
   study (MBSS)
Nil per os (NPO, nothing by
   mouth)
Palliative care
Patient's goals
Percutaneous endoscopic
   gastrostomy (PEG)
Per os (PO, by mouth)

Introduction

Dysphagia (swallowing disorders) can manifest in many adult populations as a result of numerous disease processes. Dysphagia can be defined as "problems involving the oral cavity, pharynx, esophagus, or gastroesophageal junction" (American Speech-Language-Hearing Association [ASHA], 2017). Logemann defined dysphagia as "behavioral, sensory, and preliminary motor acts in preparation for the swallow, including cognitive awareness of the upcoming eating situation, visual recognition of food, and all of the physiological responses . . . such as increased salivation" (Logemann, 1998, p. 1).

The incidence of dysphagia in the stroke population ranges between 26 and 60 percent, depending on the author's research (Groher & Crary, 2010). Dysphagia in patients with head and neck cancer can range between 20 and 50 percent prior to treatment and as high as 80 percent after treatment (Raber-Durlacher et al., 2012). A high incidence and prevalence of patients who are tracheostomized or ventilator dependent present with dysphagia (Dikeman & Kazandjian, 2002). "Dysphagia cuts across so many diseases and age groups, its true prevalence in adult populations is not fully known and is often underestimated" (ASHA, 2017, Incidence and Prevalence section).

According to ASHA, dysphagia signs and symptoms include drooling and poor oral management; food or liquid remaining in the oral cavity after the swallow; complaints of food "sticking"; globus sensation or complaints of fullness in the neck; complaints of pain when swallowing; wet or gurgling sounding voice during or after eating or drinking; coughing during or right after eating or drinking; difficulty coordinating breathing and swallowing; recurring aspiration pneumonia, respiratory infection, or fever; and weight loss or dehydration from not being able to eat enough. Some people ignore their symptoms until their dysphagia affects their mental health or lifestyle. One of the most common complaints is that food gets stuck or the patient notices a sticking sensation in the throat.

Regardless of dysphagia etiology, the consequences of swallowing impairment include significant health risks, including malnutrition, dehydration, pulmonary infection, and, in severe cases, death (Mann, 2000). Conservative estimates of the annual heath costs associated with dysphagia and its complications are as high as $550 million (Cichero & Altman, 2012). The cost of treating one episode of aspiration pneumonia, which is the result of a patient's oropharyngeal dysphagia, is as high as $17,000. Other factors, such as the impact dysphagia may have on a patient's social function, family interaction, economic state, and quality of life, are much more difficult to quantify.

Beginning in the 1980s, speech-language pathologists took the lead in evaluating and treating oropharyngeal dysphagia (Langmore, 2001). In 2001, ASHA created a policy document that outlines the knowledge and skills speech-language pathologists need to provide services to people with swallowing and feeding disorders (ASHA, 2001a). In addition, by 2005, standards for certification by ASHA required competency in dysphagia. In 2004, the first submission for specialty recognition in swallowing and swallowing disorders was received by the American Board of Swallowing and Swallowing Disorders. The creation of these standards of practice and specialty recognitions confirmed that clinicians who work with this population require a solid understanding of normal and abnormal anatomy and physiology of the swallowing process. These standards established that clinicians must remain current with the literature in a fairly new and growing domain of practice. They must be competent to perform evaluations and design intervention plans with appropriate management strategies. For clinical dysphagia practice, goal setting is paramount for managing this complex condition to address swallowing deficits, reduce their potential consequences, and maximize the quality of life for individuals with dysphagia. This chapter is designed to help clinicians use diagnostic and patient-specific information to create goals and deliver evidence-based practice interventions.

Comprehensive Assessment

In some institutions, dysphagia screening is the first step in the evaluation process. Several screening measures are available in the literature. A swallow screen does not diagnose dysphagia; it indicates whether further evaluation is warranted. Some examples of swallow screens include the Eating Assessment Tool (EAT-10), Gugging Swallowing Screen (GUSS), Toronto Bedside Swallowing Screening Test, and Yale Swallow Protocol. Refer to the "Additional Resources" section of this chapter for additional information about these and other dysphagia screening and assessment measures.

To understand the nature of dysphagia in adults, a comprehensive and thorough evaluation must be performed. According to ASHA, the speech-language pathologist is the primary team member responsible for the assessment and intervention of dysphagia. Depending on the diagnosis contributing to the dysphagia, other team members may include otolaryngologist, gastroenterologist, radiologist, neurologist, dentist, nurse, dietitian, occupational therapist, pulmonologist, or respiratory therapist.

A speech-language pathologist who is working with patients diagnosed with dysphagia must be able to perform a clinical examination of swallowing (ASHA, 2001b). There is controversy among experts in the field regarding the utility of a **clinical swallow evaluation** (McCullough, Leder, & Coyle, 2015). Although this method of assessment is criticized for its inability to detect silent aspiration, it remains a valuable tool for gaining information about the history of the patient, the patient as an individual, and the gross status of the swallow (Fabus & Dondorf, 2014). If a speech-language pathologist were to perform a

modified barium swallow study (MBSS) or a **fiberoptic endoscopic evaluation of swallowing (FEES)** without having seen the patient, it would be a difficult task. The clinical swallow evaluation is the method of assessment during which the clinician becomes familiar with the patient's swallowing function, including his or her positioning, affect, cognitive function, motivation, and compliance. An SLP performing an MBSS/FEES without conducting the clinical swallow exam is akin to a neurologist ordering a CT scan or MRI without performing a physical examination. The clinical swallow evaluation includes several components: the case history, the cranial nerve (CN) examination, and an assessment of swallowing different liquids and consistencies (if the patient is a candidate for oral intake or bolus trials).

The first of these components is an in-depth review of any medical records or pertinent medical history (including medical history; current medications; previous hospitalizations; allergies; physicians' findings; oral, enteral, or parenteral intake; previous pneumonia; artificial airway ventilator or tracheostomy; patient's perception of the problem; course of complaint; the impact of dysphagia on the activities of daily living; and previous treatment) that can assist in formulating a hypothesis for the etiology of the swallowing impairment. The speech-language pathologist will obtain relevant medical history from the patient, the patient's family members, or other healthcare providers. The importance of interprofessional collaboration among clinicians is essential during the assessment and intervention process (Dondorf, Fabus, & Ghassemi, 2016) to obtain pertinent information regarding the patient's medical status and possibly the reason for the referral. For example, if a 73-year-old male who has dysphagia and Parkinson disease were admitted with a respiratory infection, this may indicate possible progression of dysphagia or an inability to tolerate current diet consistencies. At times, the medical chart may have paucity of information that can be obtained only during the patient–family interview. A family member may say, "Oh yes, my father had a stroke in 2005 that affected his right side," but this information might not be documented in the patient's history and physical report or admission data. However, the information is critical for understanding the nature of the patient's swallowing function. Sometimes the family reveals pertinent information during an interview at the bedside.

The second component of a clinical swallow evaluation includes an oral peripheral or CN examination, which includes a sensory and motor examination of the cranial nerves for speech and swallowing. Speech-language pathologists must have a proficient knowledge of CN function for swallowing: trigeminal (CN V); facial (CN VII);

glossopharyngeal (CN IX); vagal (CN X); accessory (CN XI); and hypoglossal (CN XII). In graduate settings, speech-language pathology students are often taught a series of CNs and are required to memorize them. They are also taught how to perform an oral–peripheral examination (Fabus, Gironda, & Museyeva, 2018). However, there is often a disconnect when they are asked how to assess CNs and how this relates to sensory and motor swallowing activity. Students need to apply their knowledge about CN function when working with patients. For example, in practice, a patient who presents with a severe pharyngeal dysphagia after cardiac valve replacement may have permanent or temporary damage to CN X, resulting in asymmetric velar movement and changes in vocal function (for example, loudness or quality). The same patient may not be able to trigger a pharyngeal swallow response and may have reduced sensation of the pharynx due to an embolic CVA within the brainstem. A speech-language pathologist with advanced understanding of CN function can assist a puzzled surgeon in defining the possible etiology of the patient's dysphagia and guide the team toward appropriate assessment and intervention. In practice, understanding the neurology behind the swallow is critical and essential. It is important to incorporate evidence-based practice into dysphagia assessment and intervention. Two procedures are used today, but the level of support is controversial. One is cervical auscultation, and the other is the modified Evans blue dye test for patients with tracheostomy tubes. Fiorelli and colleagues published a paper that says a new modified Evans blue due test could be more accurate for screening tracheostomized patients (Fiorelli et al., 2016).

After a thorough CN exam, and if it is appropriate and the patient is medically stable, the clinician can administer bolus trials in calibrated amounts to identify if there are overt swallowing deficits, such as anterior spillage from the oral cavity, or overt signs of aspiration after the swallow, like coughing or a change in vocal quality to wet or gurgling sounds. Anterior spillage may indicate incompetent valving at the lips, and aspiration may indicate poor airway closure or delayed swallow response with airway invasion. Because the anatomy and physiology of the pharynx and esophagus cannot be visualized during a clinical swallow evaluation, specific goals to address changes in physiology or appropriateness of postures or maneuvers cannot be determined only with a clinical swallow evaluation. The clinician can write goals, based on the results of the clinical exam, about certain elements of the swallow. If oral care is considered poor, as judged by the oral–peripheral examination, a goal that addresses oral hygiene may be written. Goals addressing swallowing physiology components cannot be determined based upon the results of the clinical swallow exam alone, because physiology cannot be viewed, only inferred.

A clinician is not required to use a published clinical swallow evaluation measure. Novice clinicians or students may choose to use a published measure because they do not have to reflect about the components that must be assessed. More experienced clinicians can create their own clinical swallow evaluation measures to ascertain information about the patient's CN for speech and swallowing function. An example of a psychometrically sound clinical swallow evaluation is the Mann Assessment of Swallowing Ability (MASA) (refer to the "Additional Resources" section in this chapter). This examination was originally standardized with an acute stroke population. It contains a series of clinical observations that are evaluated to derive a total score; a higher score indicates a greater impairment. The components of the assessment are typically evaluated during a nonstandardized examination (general clinical swallow evaluation) and include cognition, secretion management, breathing, and presence of coughing. The MASA assessment was created to provide statistically valid clinical scores for patients with head and neck cancer. Although there are several standardized clinical examinations, many times the questions about the patient's swallowing function cannot be answered at the bedside or in the office setting without a more detailed physiologic delineation.

If the clinician cannot determine an appropriate and safe plan for the patient's alimentation from the clinical swallow evaluation, instrumentation is warranted (Murry & Carrau, 2001). Currently, the two main methods of visualizing swallow physiology are the MBSS (also referred to as a videofluoroscopic swallow study, or VFSS) and the FEES. The MBSS is a dynamic assessment method; during the study, a clinician can view the oral phase, pharyngeal phase, and aspects of the esophageal phase of the swallow in real time (Logemann, 1983). It was first performed by Jeri Logemann in the 1980s, and for many years it was considered the gold standard in dysphagia assessment. The efficiency of the swallow can be identified based on bolus flow characteristics and patterns of residue. Any airway compromise, namely penetration and aspiration, can be viewed before, during, or after the swallow. From this examination, specific physiologic deficits can be identified and goals can be written. For example, if there is postswallow residue in the valleculae and there is visualized impaired base of tongue to posterior pharyngeal wall movement, strengthening exercises can be prescribed to target this deficit. Similarly, if an effortful swallow helps clear this residue, a goal can be written to use this technique. The MBSS requires the patient to be transported to radiology and be exposed to low doses of radiation. Patients are required to consume barium products, which has been criticized as potentially reducing the naturalness of the swallowing task. In addition, there is poor resolution for viewing the anatomical structures (i.e., shadow, bone, and black bolus), which is sometimes a criticism.

Training to become competent in performing and analyzing a MBSS varies extensively. There are no specific guidelines for the number of supervised MBSS exams before a clinician can independently conduct this procedure. In addition, interrater reliability is very low for specific physiologic components of the swallow. For example, one rater might judge base of tongue retraction as impaired, and another rater might report it as grossly intact. To improve interrater reliability, Martin-Harris created the Modified Barium Swallow Impairment Profile (MBSImP), which is a standardized protocol that guides the administration and scoring of the MBSS (Martin-Harris et al., 2008). The MBSImP allows a clinician to provide more concrete information about the safety and efficiency of the swallow mechanism after examining 17 components in the four stages of the swallow. Clinicians must be specifically trained and certified to use the MBSImP. From the MBSImP, patients receive an impairment score (the higher the score, the more impaired the function). The administration and scoring of the MBSImP will allow the clinician to develop treatment goals that are more accurate and in line with the patient's swallowing physiological impairments.

Langmore developed the FEES in the 1980s to enhance the portability of dysphagia assessment and to provide a superior view of anatomy and secretions during the swallow. In this examination, a nasoendoscope is passed through the naris (nostril) and positioned above the endolarynx while the patient swallows secretions and calibrated volumes of liquids, purees, and solids (Langmore, Schatz, & Olsen, 1988). The foodstuffs are often dyed with blue or green food coloring to enhance the visualization of the mucosa in the pharynx and larynx. Postures and maneuvers can be implemented during a FEES exam, and they can also be used as biofeedback while the patient is swallowing. FEES provides a superior view of anatomy and excellent information regarding airway edema, vocal fold movement, and symmetry, as well as secretions management. FEES is inferior to MBSS in that the oral phase, the moment of swallow and anything inferior to the esophageal inlet cannot be viewed because there is a period of whiteout during the swallow. This whiteout period occurs as the epiglottis flaps down to cover the laryngeal vestibule and obscures the view at the moment of the swallow.

Because of its minimally invasive nature, the training for FEES has been well outlined in different states (Hiss & Postma, 2003). Generally, it is recommended that a clinician in training should pass an endoscope and analyze the examination under the supervision of a trained endoscopist at least 25 times. These 25 passes should include a variety of patients both with and without dysphagia. The risks of FEES include laryngospasm, epistaxis, discomfort, and inability to tolerate the endoscope. Some authors recommend the use of a nasal anesthetic prior to the FEES exam to enhance the patient's ability to tolerate the endoscope (Johnson, Belafsky, & Postma, 2003; Leder, Ross, Brinskin, & Sasaki, 1997). Initially, the use of a nasal anesthetic was thought to desensitize the mucosa of the pharynx and larynx and that this change in sensation could alter the swallowing physiology. Recently, Lester and colleagues reported no such change in swallowing physiology; they agreed with others that the use of an anesthetic could improve patient comfort during FEES (Lester et al., 2013).

The Penetration–Aspiration Scale (Rosenbek, Robbins, Roecker, Coyle, & Wood, 1996) is commonly used because numerical scores are typically not obtained from MBSS and FEES instrumentation, with the exception of the MBSImP. The Penetration–Aspiration Scale has 8 points for determining the depth of the airway invasion and the patient's response to that invasion. It is validated for use during MBSS and FEES exams. The difference between a score of 1 (material does not enter the airway) and a score of 8 (material enters the airway, passes below the vocal folds, and no effort is made to eject it) provides information to the dysphagia clinician and other healthcare providers about the patient's ability to clear the airway, which is a predictor of swallowing safety. These data can guide the clinician in determining recommendations, and they serve as a comparison from one procedure to the next to help measure swallowing outcomes. This information is helpful for clinicians to determine the benefits of treatment, and it is imperative for reimbursement. Additional dysphagia scales and outcome tracking tools are provided in the "Additional Resources" section of this chapter.

It is critical to understand that viewing penetration and aspiration are only one observed outcome of using swallowing instrumentation. It is well documented that determining the presence of penetration and aspiration should not be the only important outcome of instrumentation (Crary, 2000; Martin-Harris et al., 2008). It is critical for clinicians (particularly novice clinicians) to value the efficiency of the swallow as a possible predictor of malnutrition and dehydration, not solely the risk of aspiration.

It is imperative for clinicians to view dysphagia instrumentation as a means to understand the complex physiology and pathophysiology that results in impaired safety or efficiency of the swallow. Logemann referred to the MBSS as a rehabilitative study (2013) in which the role of the speech-language pathologist is to note any change in the swallow using postures, maneuvers, or swallow strategies. She spoke out against the idea of an MBSS being viewed as a pass–fail exam that defines *only* if the patient is aspirating. Logemann also urged clinicians to stop restricting patients from intake of certain liquids and consistencies if they present with solely laryngeal penetration. She challenged us to *make them aspirate* (2013), meaning that clinicians should assess the swallowing mechanism with different volumes and viscosities. If a patient is determined to have a compromised airway, Logemann challenges us to determine the pathophysiology behind the swallowing deficits (2013).

The interpretation of data obtained from swallowing assessment measures should allow the clinician to determine whether the symptoms that are observed during **per os (PO, by mouth)** trials truly represent impairment. Did the clinician's judgment translate into actual physiologic impairment? Many times a patient will demonstrate overt signs of aspiration at the bedside but not have any airway compromise or significant physiologic deficits as demonstrated by the results of the MBSS or FEES. This is particularly common in patients who are diagnosed with chronic obstructive pulmonary disease (COPD) or active pneumonia. These patients cough at baseline after every swallow, but they may not show any evidence of a delayed pharyngeal swallow response, or airway closure compromise, during instrumentation.

In addition to accepting or rejecting the null hypothesis (whether the instrumentation confirmed or refuted the presence of a dysphagia), the clinician should be able to identify the physiologic deficits that contribute to the dysphagia and any compensatory strategies or maneuvers that enhance efficiency and safety of the swallow. PO or **nil per os (NPO, nothing by mouth)** status should be determined, and recommendations should be made for the consistencies that are best tolerated. Most importantly, targeted outcomes and goals should be formulated for patients who will be seen for clinical swallow management or treatment. It is common in clinical practice that many patients will not and cannot participate in an exercise program due to cognitive impairments, physical limitations, or compliance; however, the clinician must formulate goals that are appropriate for the client. For example, if Mrs. Jones is not able to improve her tongue motion for bolus transport with targeted exercises due to her inability to follow commands, goals may be formulated to address the placement of a bolus within the oral cavity to facilitate transit.

Assessing the Data and Treatment Options

The MBSS and the FEES illustrate the stages of swallowing at one moment in time. Therefore, it is critical that recommendations and goals be developed based on a combination of the clinical and instrumental data that have been acquired after the assessment is done. Only then can the clinician gain an understanding about the general condition and medical status of the patient, the swallowing motivation, and the positioning and feeding environment. In addition, the patient's prognosis, age, advance directives, and goals for care must be well understood. The **patient's goals** and the goals of the family must be paramount. If the goals are unattainable, there should be a discussion with the patient and family to create goals that have functional outcomes.

For example, suppose that Mr. Smith has an uncoordinated swallow for liquids and aspirates on all consistencies of liquids, as evidenced by using instrumentation. Mr. Smith has a remarkable medical history consisting of several strokes, one in the cerebellum, and multiple aspiration pneumonias requiring inpatient hospitalizations. After an MBSS, the speech-language pathologist may choose the following goal: The patient will swallow nectar-thick liquids using a supersupraglottic swallow maneuver in 10 trials without overt signs of aspiration after a volitional cough. Mr. Smith may be seen in his home, and he may decide to consume thin liquids, contrary to the speech-language pathologist's recommendations. Another goal for this patient might be the following: The patient will swallow small sips of thin liquids three times per day and remain free from pneumonia and avoid hospital admissions for 1 month. What should the speech-language pathologist do in this situation? Perhaps the clinician could focus on Mr. Smith's ability to effectively cough using expiratory muscle strength training (EMST) instead of asking him to eliminate thin liquids and consume only thick liquids. Mr. Smith might opt out of treatment if his expectations were different compared to the speech-language pathologist.

According to Groher and Crary, the "selection of any treatment for the patient with dysphagia should be based on the best available evidence from the published literature, the patient's wishes, and the clinician's experience with similar problems" (Groher & Crary, 2010, p. 232). The authors indicate that the combination of these variables is referred to as EBP. It is best to evaluate published literature by using **levels of evidence** (Robey, 2004). The levels are assigned numbers 1 through 4. The highest level of evidence for efficacy or effectiveness of treatment is level 1a, systematic review of randomized controlled trials (RCTs). In research, RCTs are considered paramount to indicate that the treatment is effective to treat the disorder.

For example, Langmore and colleagues (2015) published data from their RCT on the effects of neuromuscular **electrical stimulation (e-stim)** on swallowing in patients who were treated for head and neck cancer. This study involved a large number of grossly homogenous patients. They were required to perform 60 swallows per day. The treatment group received e-stim while performing the swallows. The sham (control) group had the same electrodes with severed wires (they were blinded to this information). The results revealed that both groups improved with regard to swallowing. However, the sham group did better than the e-stim group. This evidence helped clinicians select treatment modalities and formulate goals. For example, although e-stim is widely publicized as a successful treatment approach for patients with intractable dysphagia, this RCT suggests that the clinician might proceed with caution before selecting this modality for patients with chronic dysphagia.

On the other end of the levels of evidence spectrum is level 5, expert opinion without critical appraisal. An example of this is a clinician's review of a treatment technique. It can be loosely compared to a food critic's appraisal of a new restaurant. Because the critic expresses an opinion, it presents little valid evidence of the restaurant's quality. Although one patient or a handful or patients may benefit from a technique, that does not mean the positive outcome will generalize to the larger population. Therefore, expert opinion is the lowest level of evidence to guide treatment.

Although evidence from the literature is critical for treatment planning, the importance of the patient's wishes is a critical aspect for determining the treatment plan. Also, a clinician's experience with similar patients using a similar treatment cannot be undervalued. For example, one might prefer to see a cardiac surgeon who has performed 500 bypasses instead of a surgeon just out of fellowship who has performed only 75 of these procedures. This specialization is also present in speech-language pathology. Clinicians who treat dysphagia are often not only swallowing disorders specialists, but they focus on one select sample of the population. For example, there are speech-language pathologists with specialization in tracheostomy and ventilator related dysphagia, head and neck cancer related dysphagia, or neurogenic dysphagia.

To summarize, the clinician will formulate a series of goals based on evidence-based practice, patient wishes, and the clinician's clinical judgment. These goals will be established to address one or more of the following areas:

1. Safety and efficiency of PO consistencies as measured by overt symptomology or change in medical status
2. Specific performance in treatment sessions as measured in the patient's accuracy of skill or strength tasks or change in a physiologic parameter noted on repeat instrumentation
3. Implementation of safe feeding and swallowing strategies by the caregiver after training

Irrespective of the target goals, the patient must demonstrate measurable gains. In dysphagia intervention, many goals cannot be measured in percentage accuracy due to the nature of the disorder and how it impacts the patient's medical status. Therefore, using measurable phrases like "within 1 week" or "over the course of 5 sessions" or "without change in pulmonary status or respiratory status" may be required for measurement. Examples of measurable dysphagia goals are provided in the following hypothetical scenario.

A 93-year-old male patient with head and neck cancer completed concurrent chemotherapy and radiation (CCRT) with posttreatment dysphagia. This patient crashed at week two of CCRT due to hyponatremia and aspiration pneumonia. He received a feeding tube during his hospital admission but continued limited PO intake throughout treatment. When the treatment was completed and the patient wished to resume more PO feeds and begin weaning off **percutaneous endoscopic gastrostomy (PEG)** feeds, he was seen for a clinical swallow evaluation and an MBSS. Clinically, the patient had obvious CN X deficits related to his glottic cancer and its treatment. He had a complete paralysis of the left true vocal fold on an ear, nose, and throat (ENT) exam. His vocal quality was significantly breathy and rough, but it was dry at baseline, indicating adequate secretion management. Coughing was noted postswallow for thin liquids and nectar-thick liquids intermittently on bolus trials. No overt signs of dysphagia were observed for purees or chewable solids. An MBSS revealed a grossly intact oral phase of the swallow. The pharyngeal swallow was moderately delayed, and laryngeal elevation was reduced, as was laryngeal vestibular closure. This resulted in penetration and aspiration before the swallow for thin and nectar-thick liquids via spoon and cup feeds. A supersupraglottic swallow (SSG) maneuver improved airway protection for nectar-thick liquids in small volumes. He was able to perform the SSG swallow maneuver with accuracy but required cues.

The possible goals to address might be as follows:

1. To address safety and efficiency: The patient will tolerate PO feeds of soft solids and nectar-thick liquids using an SSG over 1 week without a change in weight or pulmonary status.
2. To address specific performance in treatment sessions: The patient will perform breath hold swallow maneuvers to improve glottic closure using nectar-thick and thin liquid boluses in 7 out of 10 trials while under endoscopy for biofeedback.
3. To address using safe swallowing techniques: The patient will complete an oral hygiene regimen with his caregiver before each meal and use upright positioning for all PO intake.

Assume the patient was able to achieve all goals except the breath hold maneuver. This goal could be targeted during the next 10 sessions. If the patient still does not achieve this goal, the clinician can modify it to include only nectar-thick liquid swallows. For example, if his glottic closure and swallow delay resulted in a significant amount of thin liquid penetration and aspiration as identified with endoscopy biofeedback, this might not be a realistic expectation and is therefore an unachievable objective. The goal may need to be revised with support from visual endoscopic data.

Based on this endoscopic observation, the patient might be recommended for consideration of medialization thyroplasty because glottic closure was not achieved using behavioral intervention. The goal could be modified to reflect a referral and evaluation by a laryngologist for consideration of laryngoplasty for glottic closure within a 2-month time frame. If the patient were to be evaluated by the laryngologist and it were determined that the risks of this procedure would outweigh the benefits, the goal of swallowing thin liquid could be omitted from the treatment plan. This patient might not be able to safely consume thin liquids despite the best efforts of multiple professionals.

These examples of goals are for a particular patient with a particular diagnosis in an outpatient setting. Depending on the length of time the patient is expected to be in treatment, the goals and their features may vary. Typically speech-language pathologists set goals for outpatients based on 10 visits because G-coding requires reevaluation after every 10 visits (discussed later in this chapter). Inpatients and patients in rehabilitation centers may have shorter or longer stays based on their level of functioning and treatment needs. Whatever the expected length of treatment, it is wise to aim low so progress can be demonstrated. The clinician should establish a baseline and create goals and projected outcomes based on these baseline data. For example, third-party payers would be more likely to cover services for a patient who has made slow and steady gains with goals set slightly above baseline than to cover services for a patient who has met no goals because the goals are beyond the expectations.

As stated previously, the clinician is responsible for formulating goals that are measurable. In fact, the Council for Clinical Certification in Audiology and Speech-Language Pathology (CFCC) Knowledge and Skills Acquisition (KASA) form specifies that the speech-language pathologist must "identify measurable short- and long-term treatment goals targeting functional outcomes" (ASHA, 2001a). Writing from experience, goals may be difficult to measure, and they may vary from one treatment session to another. To assist clinicians in establishing goals and measuring gains, ASHA created **Functional Communication Measures (FCMs)**. FCMs were established in 1998, and they mirror the Functional Independence Measures (FIM) that were created to guide reimbursement for acute rehabilitation admissions. The FCMs include seven levels of functioning that pertain to a specific skill set. To document functional gains for patients diagnosed with dysphagia, an FCM for swallowing was created.

Presently, FCMs can be applied to guide G-coding, which is the method used by the Centers for Medicare and Medicaid Services (CMS) to assess the cost effectiveness of speech-language pathology services for patients with dysphagia. For example, G-codes are scored on an initial evaluation, and the clinician is asked to provide a score that reflects a level of functioning (FCM). The clinician is then required to set a goal G-code and predict a level of functioning that the patient will achieve during 10 dysphagia treatment visits. This requires the gains to be measurable, or CMS can deny further treatment if the goal criterion is not achieved. Most insurance providers mirror the CMS process. Therefore, clinicians should have an understanding of G-coding for swallowing and recall the mantra to aim low. The use of FCMs requires participation in ASHA's National Outcomes Registry; therefore, FCMs are no longer available for general use.

There are several other swallowing measurement scales, including EAT-10 (Belafsky et al., 2008), the Functional Oral Intake Scale (FOIS) (Crary, Carnaby-Mann, & Groher, 2005), and the Functional Assessment Measure (FAM) (Allcot & Dixon, 1997). These allow the clinician to use psychometrically sound scales to establish goals and measure progress over time. For example, the FOIS consists of 7 levels. Examples of specific levels are as follows:

- Level 1: Nothing by mouth
- Level 2: Tube dependent with minimal attempts of food or liquid
- Level 6: Total oral diet with multiple consistencies without special preparation, but with specific food limitations

An example of a measurable objective is if a patient can advance from Level 1 to Level 6 in a treatment period. A clinician may incorporate goal setting using such a scale because it gives both the clinician and the patient tangible, concrete objectives.

Forming Specific Goals

When forming goals, the clinician must have a baseline of the patient's swallowing function. A baseline is the minimum or starting point, prior to the intervention, that can be used for later comparisons (New Oxford Dictionary of English, 2010). The treatment baseline may be related to a specific task or exercise, such as the amount of oral intake consumed, specific parameters for avoiding adverse outcomes, or the accuracy of a caregiver's feeding techniques. Progress can be measured only if there is a change from the baseline. This seems simple, but if goals are established far above the baseline, chances are the patient will not attain the goals. Therefore, the time frame for establishing goals must be considered. For example, if a patient can perform only one effortful swallow maneuver at baseline, he or she will not be able to perform 10 effortful swallow maneuvers in 1 week; 2 or 3 effortful swallow maneuvers in this time frame is more realistic. The speech-language pathologist should discuss the results of the evaluation, possible therapy goals, and functional outcomes with the patient. For example, a 46-year-old patient diagnosed with ALS may not be able to perform high-effort tasks, while a 63-year-old female diagnosed with posttraumatic brain injury may be capable of intense swallowing exercises.

As stated previously, patients are more likely to participate in therapy if the goals are functional and important to them. In some facilities goals stated by the patient and family are documented at the top of the interdisciplinary conference form. During team conferences the professionals discuss the patient's progress, and the treatment team is continually reminded of the goals that are important to the patient and family. For example, a patient-stated goal that is not measurable or functional is "I want to get better." The speech-language pathologist may want to help the patient develop a more functionally appropriate goal with measurable outcomes, such as "The patient will consume puree consistency at breakfast, for 2 days, without coughing."

The only way to improve swallowing function is to allow the patient to swallow something, even if only sips of water. In fact, disuse of the swallowing musculature can have a deleterious effect on the swallowing mechanism (Langmore, Krisciunas, Miloro, Evans, & Cheng, 2012). The swallowing treatment should focus on the task of swallowing. Indirect treatment (swallowing exercises with no PO intake) techniques are not being used as often because, in select populations, the benefit of improving swallowing strength or coordination is worth the risk of trace aspiration of a trial bolus. The speech-language pathologist may want to consider developing goals that target increasing lingual movement, vocal fold closure, and pharyngeal constriction during swallowing different types of bolus consistencies. During Langmore's e-stim treatment trial study (Langmore et al., 2015), patients were encouraged to take a sip of water between swallows to give them an incentive to swallow. Many of these patients were aspirating thin liquids at their baseline. No patient suffered from pneumonia as a result of the exercises.

An example of a weak goal is the following: "The patient will perform 25 tongue clicks to improve base of tongue retraction." This goal has been used for many years, and it is concerning because tongue clicks are exercises for the back of the tongue, not the base of tongue. Tongue base retraction is achieved with exercises like the effortful swallow and the tongue hold swallow or the Masako maneuver. The speech-language pathologist might suggest writing the goal as follows: "The patient will perform 10 repetitions of an effortful swallow consuming a puree bolus." This could translate into the following long-term goal: "Patient will consume 4 oz of puree using an effortful swallow in a 5 minute period without a need for a liquid wash." The amount and location of residue could be identified with the use of FEES for biofeedback, and the strength of the effortful swallow could be measured by surface electromyography (sEMG).

Another example of a weak goal is one that is created with criteria that are much higher than the baseline performance level. If a patient is consuming one meal per day of soft solids and thin liquids and is using a feeding tube for the remainder of his or her nutrition and hydration, a weak goal might be the following: "The patient will consume all nutrition, hydration via PO feeds without adverse outcomes (weight loss or respiratory issues) within 2 weeks." This goal is not realistic or attainable. The speech-language pathologist might choose to rewrite the goal as follows: "The patient will consume 1–2 meals per day and reduce tube feeding by 1–2 cans without adverse outcome over 2 weeks." Depending on the disease process, this still may not be an attainable goal for this patient.

There are some pearls of wisdom for selecting treatment modalities and setting goals for dysphagia:

- Select targeted exercises or tasks that are appropriate for the patient's deficits (no tongue clicks for tongue base deficits).
- Understand the patient's underlying disease state and prognosis.
- Understand the patient's and family's expectations when developing goals.
- Help the patient and family create realistic goals and expectations.
- Understand and respect the baseline and assessment results attained during the clinical bedside evaluation and with instrumental measures (MBSS or FEES).
- Select exercises or maneuvers that have evidence-based practice support.
- Consider the patient's quality of life and comfort.
- Refer to clinicians who specialize with a specific population.
- Do not be afraid to ask questions.
- Stay current with the literature.

If you heed these 10 pearls of wisdom, dysphagia intervention, including developing goals, will be a piece of cake—a soft solid cake with a liquid wash, of course! Most speech-language pathologists who specialize in dysphagia in adults realize it is a privilege to work with this population. It involves a degree of risk, and it requires a great deal of knowledge. This knowledge must evolve and change over time in this relatively new and growing area of practice. Knowledge about the mechanics of the oropharynx and the pulmonary system is critical; more critical is the clinician's ability to understand the patient as a whole and not just shadows and bone on a fluoroscopic image.

The speech-language pathologist will collaborate with physicians, pain and **palliative care** experts, and other professionals to make decisions for complex disease processes in which dysphagia is a symptom. Palliative care professionals are responsible for improving the quality of life for patients and families who are facing life-threatening illnesses (Jocham, Dassen, Widdershoven, & Halfens, 2009). The expertise of these professionals can be extremely important when working with patients diagnosed with terminal diseases and dysphagia.

Types of Interventions

The speech-language pathologist must be knowledgeable about evidence-based practices to formulate interventions for patients diagnosed with dysphagia (refer to **TABLE 6-1** in the appendix of this chapter).

A speech-language pathologist develops an intervention plan based on an understanding of the anatomy, neurology, and physiology of the swallow mechanism. The overall goal is safe and efficient intake of the least restrictive diet for adequate nutrition and hydration. The speech-language pathologist is required to review the results of the clinical bedside evaluation and the instrumental evaluation, consider treatment candidacy (alertness, orientation, endurance, ability to control and execute voluntary movements), and employ selection principles (least tiring, least restrictive intervention that is easiest to execute) when creating the intervention plan. Any of the mainstream treatment programs, even the ones that require specific certification like the McNeill Dysphagia Therapy Program (MDTP) (Crary, Carnaby-Mann, LaGorio, & Carvajal, 2012), typically involve instructing the patient to perform swallow maneuvers. In terms of intervention techniques, there are compensatory strategies, which include postures, sensory input, and modification of the patient's diet. There are swallow maneuvers, which include the effortful swallow, Mendelsohn maneuver, supraglottic swallow, and the super-supraglottic swallow. A speech-language pathologist may prescribe a treatment program that includes a combination of oral, pharyngeal, and laryngeal exercises. The different types of exercises are beyond the scope of this chapter. For further information, please refer to the reference list.

Postures may be used for a variety of different disorders, and they can be implemented with minimal training and practice. Postures help redirect the bolus to improve swallowing efficiency and safety (Crary, 2006). The use of instrumentation is required to determine if a specific posture or maneuver is effective in reducing penetration or aspiration.

The first posture is called the chin tuck or chin down posture. In practice, it is common for patients to be shown this posture to make the swallow safer. This positioning is commonly recommended by a nurse or physician at the bedside or in the office without instrumental assessment data to identify the effectiveness of the posture. The chin tuck position places the base of tongue closer to the posterior pharyngeal wall to cap the airway and widen the valleculae for patients who may have premature loss of material or a delayed pharyngeal swallow response and airway invasion before the swallow trigger. However, this posture also reduces the constriction forces of the pharynx and may result in increased residue that may be aspirated after the swallow (Crary, 2006). Therefore, it is critical to use MBSS or FEES to observe whether any posture is making the expected changes for a patient. The chin tuck posture may be implemented if a patient has a pharyngeal swallow delay or premature spillage of material into the pharynx. This can potentially cause airway invasion before the swallow. This posture should not be used in patients with excess residue in the pyriform because the residue may spill over into the larynx.

Another posture is called the head turn to the affected (weak) side. This posture closes off the weakened hemipharynx to divert the bolus down the stronger side (Logemann, Kahrilas, & Vakil, 1989). If the patient has a right-sided weakness, the head should be turned to the right side. A head turn can also compress the weak side and improve clearance of the residue. This should be assessed in an anterior–posterior (AP) view on a MBSS.

Another posture is called the chin up, head back. This posture may be appropriate for patients who are status postglossectomy or who have severe oral transit issues (Logemann, 1998). Gravity pulls the bolus to the posterior oral cavity and into the pharynx for initiation of the pharyngeal swallow response. Patients should be cognitively intact because it is often combined with a breath hold maneuver (supersupra-glottic swallow maneuver) to prevent laryngeal penetration and aspiration. This posture should not be used with patients who have any pharyngeal stage deficits.

One maneuver is called the Mendelsohn maneuver. This maneuver may be used to prolong hyolaryngeal elevation and thereby increase the extent and duration of the cricopharyngeus muscle opening (Bartolome & Neumann, 1993). This maneuver may be used in patients who have postswallow residue in the distal pharynx (pyriform sinuses). It is also used as an exercise regimen to improve strength and skill without any food consistencies.

Another maneuver is called effortful swallow. This maneuver may be used to enhance pharyngeal swallow constriction force, especially where the tongue base and posterior pharyngeal wall meet (Hind, Nocosia, Roecker, Carnes, & Robbins, 2001). It is often implemented when a patient presents with excessive residue in the valleculae after the swallow. It is also commonly used in treatment paradigms to build strength and skill. It is the easiest maneuver for a patient to execute.

The supraglottic swallow and supersupraglottic swallow maneuvers are used to promote preswallow airway closure at the level of the vocal folds. They are often implemented when patients demonstrate airway compromise (laryngeal penetration or aspiration) before or during the swallow (Logemann, Pauloski, Rademaker, & Colangelo, 1997). The supraglottic swallow is a breath hold, and the supersupra-glottic swallow combines a breath hold with bearing down, thereby tilting the arytenoids to the petiole of the epiglottis to promote tight airway closure. These maneuvers are often used in treatment regimens to build strength and control the airway mechanism.

Another maneuver is the head raise or Shaker exercise. This technique is not used during swallowing tasks involving foodstuff because the patient lies flat on his or her back and raises the chin to the chest. It is designed to improve the strength and contraction of the suprahyoid muscles that pull the larynx superiorly. This upward movement should then translate into an improved cricopharyngeal opening (Shaker et al., 1997). It is often used with patients who exhibit decreased laryngeal elevation and reduced cricopharyngeal distention, which commonly results in residue in the pyriform sinuses after the swallow.

For example, a patient diagnosed with dysphagia poststroke may present with significant postswallow residue in the distal pharynx (pyriform sinuses). During an instrumental examination, the clinician can decipher if an effortful swallow is most effective for that patient compared to the Mendelsohn maneuver. Given the baseline physiological deficit, the Mendelsohn maneuver would be more appropriate because it prolongs hyolaryngeal elevation, thereby increasing the cricopharyngeal opening to aid in the clearance of distal pharyngeal residue. The effortful swallow maneuver may have been appropriate for vallecular residue because it stimulates more base of tongue retraction. The Mendelsohn maneuver is typically not appropriate for patients with respiratory issues because it prolongs swallow apnea and can increase the work of breathing in certain populations, such as those with motor neuron diseases (Crary, 2006).

The effects of maneuvers can be viewed during an instrumental examination and can help the speech-language pathologist incorporate them into a patient's treatment regimen. For example, if a patient demonstrates poor airway closure due to removal of tissue above the glottis larynx (supraglottic laryngectomy) or impaired laryngeal vestibule closure, a supersupraglottic swallow maneuver is important to improve vocal fold adduction and cease respiration before the swallow. For patients exhibiting aspiration before or during the swallow, this maneuver can be an invaluable tool. Specifically, the supersupraglottic swallow maneuver improves vocal fold closure at the time of its use, and patients can learn to use it effectively; however, it has not been shown to increase vocal fold and glottic closure specifically as a strengthening task (Crary, 2006).

It is not uncommon to question whether a patient is performing an effortful swallow, a Mendelsohn maneuver, or a supersupraglottic swallow with any degree of accuracy. Biofeedback can aid the clinician and the patient in this regard. For example, sEMG can be used to provide visual feedback or numerical information on the strength of muscle contraction and the length of contraction for certain swallow maneuvers. FEES can be used to train patients on swallow maneuvers in real time, and the patients can see the effects of the maneuvers.

In addition to postures and maneuvers, many therapeutic techniques are designed to improve swallowing function. As swallowing specialists, speech-language pathologists should select techniques based on the underlying pathophysiology of the swallow deficits in each patient and ensure that treatments are based on evidence-based practice. One exercise is called expiratory muscle strength training (EMST). It is designed to achieve improved expiratory muscle strength for improved cough. As speech-language pathologists, we often ignore the last protective mechanism against aspiration—a productive cough response. This is critical for continued oral intake for at-risk patients who are diagnosed with weak musculature. Patients with an impaired cough remain at greater risk for developing pneumonia from their aspiration. It involves the use of an expiratory muscle strength training device that looks like a small blower or horn. It has progressive resistance that makes exhalation more difficult, and the force of exhalation generates a productive cough (Sapienza & Troche, 2011).

Other devices are used to increase lingual strengthening. The Iowa Oral Performance Instrument (IOPI) is a device that requires sustained oral tongue pressure on a bulb (Adams, Mathisen, Baines, Lazarus, & Callister, 2013). The appropriate use of this device can improve tongue pressure and enhance oral transit times in multiple populations. The Madison Oral Strengthening Therapeutic Device (MOST) was created by Robbins and colleagues (Robbins et al., 2007). It is a mouthpiece with multiple sensors that is molded to a patient's hard and soft palates then placed in the patient's mouth. The mouthpiece is attached to a laptop with software that reads the pressures the patient's tongue exerts against the sensors. The pressures are graduated to improve strength and thereby improve function and swallowing safety. There is well-regarded evidence regarding the efficacy of this device (Robbins et al., 2007). Another more recent device that has evidence-based support is the SwallowSTRONG, which is used to increase lingual strengthening (Swallow Solutions, 2014).

Summary

Dysphagia can be defined as an impairment in the oral, pharyngeal or esophageal stages of the swallow. Regardless of the dysphagia etiology, the consequences of swallowing impairment may include malnutrition, dehydration, pulmonary infection, and, in severe cases, death. The impact of dysphagia on a patient's social function, family interaction, economic state, and quality of life can be quite distressing. It is important for the speech-language pathologist to perform a comprehensive evaluation to determine if a dysphagia exists and to design an appropriate intervention plan.

Case Scenarios

Case Scenario 1

Mr. Budda is 72 years old and has a history of multiple CVAs diagnosed with moderate ataxic dysarthria and dysphagia. He has been admitted on multiple occasions (this is the first time to this medical center) with lower lobe pneumonia and presumed aspiration pneumonia. His hospitalizations, according to his wife, were preceded by coughing with PO intake that was severe enough to induce vomiting and respiratory distress after vomiting. He was seen after his second admission by a speech-language pathologist after a consult request was placed by the hospitalist. The clinician reviewed Mr. Budda's medical chart and labs, which were significant for dehydration, and interviewed the wife and patient at the bedside. The patient's wife indicated that according to a prior swallowing evaluation, her husband was told to consume thick liquids and regular solids. She was not certain of the assessment method (clinical or instrumental) and that he had received swallowing therapy, but he had been discharged. She indicated that her husband "coughs all the time when he is eating." She noted that the last stroke had affected his speech significantly. The patient acknowledged and confirmed his wife's reported information and noted that he could not eat without vomiting.

The speech-language pathologist's original hypothesis was that this dysphagia was possibly related to a GI issue, given the report of persistent vomiting. However, Mr. Budda's neurogenic presentation and history of dysphagia indicates that a possible oropharyngeal etiology is part of the clinical picture. During the clinical swallow evaluation, unsteadiness of movement (ataxia) was the overwhelming symptom. Labial, buccal, and lingual weakness (protrusion and elevation were reduced) was noted. There was reduced velar movement and fatigue, which progressed over time. Partial dentition was noted, and they were in fair condition. The patient's breathing was labored, and he was receiving 2 liters of oxygen via nasal cannula. His vocal quality was mildly wet and gurgling at baseline. His cough was judged to be weak, and he was not eliciting a

📋 Case Scenarios *(continued)*

cough in response to material likely at the level of the vocal folds. The volitional cough was weak and unproductive. An eventual clearance of some vocal wetness was noted after multiple cued swallows. Oral care was provided prior to PO trials. Two half teaspoons of water were presented. The patient's oral containment was adequate, and the bolus transport was delayed. After the pharyngeal swallow was triggered, as noted by laryngeal elevation on palpation, there was immediate coughing (again weak) and increased vocal wetness within the airway and during vocalizations. It was recommended that the patient remain NPO and receive an MBSS that afternoon. The physician ordered an MBSS, which was performed later that day.

The MBSS revealed impaired coordination of the oral and pharyngeal phases of the swallow. Intermittently, the pharyngeal swallow response was triggered at the level of the valleculae; at other times it was triggered when the bolus was in the laryngeal vestibule for thin liquids. The cough was not effective in clearing liquids from the airway, and aspiration occurred. The patient was not able to coordinate movement to produce a supersupraglottic swallow maneuver, and he was not able to perform a bolus hold and swallow it all at once. A chin tuck increased the degree and depth of aspiration. There was mild postswallow residue in the valleculae and in the bases of the pyriform sinuses post liquid swallow. There was no overwhelming weakness; there was rather poor coordination and timing of the swallow with reduced airway closure. There was laryngeal penetration without aspiration for nectar-thick liquids and the same physiological deficits and poor overall coordination. Puree and solid consistencies were intact with the exception of some mild postswallow residue.

The patient was discharged several days later from acute care with a regular diet consistency and nectar-thick liquids, strict oral care guidelines, mobility suggestions (stay mobile), and recommendations for swallowing therapy. He was subsequently seen for therapy, and the following goals were established based on his coordination and timing deficits:

1. The patient will perform a bolus hold and swallow it all at once to improve timing using thin and nectar-thick liquids.

2. The patient will perform EMST to improve expiratory muscle strength for cough effectiveness for 25 repetitions at level 60 (baseline was level 45).

Case Scenarios *(continued)*

3. The patient will perform effortful swallows to improve base of tongue retraction for 20 repetitions (baseline was 10).

4. The patient will consume regular solids and nectar-thick liquids without adverse outcomes, such as weight loss or respiratory sequelae, over 10 weeks.

5. The patient will report his performance of oral care prior to all PO meals for 10 weeks, and the caregiver will confirm this report.

The patient attended all therapy sessions and appeared fatigued after each session. He often required periods of rest during the therapy session. He reported that he had upgraded himself to thin liquids and was noncompliant with thick liquid recommendations. The speech-language pathologist counseled him about the importance of consuming the thick liquids due to his history of silent aspiration and multiple pneumonias. His response, despite counseling was, "I want thin liquids." The speech-language pathologist counseled him to swallow water without food and in small sips following oral care. He was noncompliant with this recommendation too. The speech-language pathologist modified the goals to include obtaining a cough-assist device to use after PO intake, given the understanding that he is at risk for silent aspiration after each meal. The speech-language pathologist also communicated with the patient's pulmonologist and general practitioner about the situation. They were in agreement that the goal should be modified to the following: "The patient will swallow thin liquid and use a cough-assist device after meals to remain free of pulmonary compromise over 10 weeks." Afterward, the patient was counseled regarding the possibility of pulmonary fibrosis, given his history of chronic aspiration. He communicated that he understood the speech-language pathologist's recommendation, but he refused to abide by it. The remaining goals regarding oral care and swallow coordination were addressed during each session.

The patient received an evaluation every 10 weeks, or sooner if needed. He remained free of pneumonia and other respiratory issues during the duration of treatment. There were mild improvements in coordination of the oral and pharyngeal phases of the swallow for thin liquids; however, he continued to demonstrate inconsistency and intermittent silent aspiration on his final MBSS exam.

Case Scenarios *(continued)*

Questions

1. Given the chronicity of the patient's dysphagia, which of the following is reasonable?

   A. Continue monthly monitoring of the patient and repeat MBSS every month.

   B. Continue monthly monitoring of the patient, take a chest X-ray every 3 months, and repeat MBSS if swallowing function appears to worsen (i.e., patient exhibits overt signs of aspiration for solids).

   C. Discharge the patient completely and refer him if his dysphagia status worsens.

   D. Continue aggressive therapy to address weakness of the musculature.

2. The patient should be discharged from service given his noncompliance with liquid recommendations.

   A. True

   A. False

3. Which of the following professionals, in addition to the speech-language pathologist, should be involved in interdisciplinary care for this complex patient? Choose all that apply.

   A. Pulmonologist

   B. Primary care physician

   C. ENT specialist

   D. Cardiologist

4. Treatment refractory dysphagia, in this case, is likely due to

   A. noncompliance.

   B. multiple bilateral CVAs.

   C. history of pneumonia.

   D. silent aspiration.

5. Which of the following additional activities might have been useful in assisting the patient during treatment?

   A. E-stim

   B. Psychological referral

   C. FEES as biofeedback during postures and maneuvers to improve swallowing safety and efficiency

   D. None of the above

Case Scenarios *(continued)*

Case Scenario 2

Mr. Schmidt is 48 years old and has a history of heroin abuse. He has no other significant medical history. He was admitted for cardiac failure and rapid atrial fibrillation, "throwing plaque/vegetation off the mitral valve." He was taken to the operating room for a valve replacement, and a porcine valve was placed. The patient was NPO with a naso-gastric tube (NGT) for 2 days postoperatively. He was referred for a clinical swallow evaluation while still in the ICU. The patient's chart was thoroughly reviewed, and the nursing notes indicated that Mr. Schmidt "has been using Yankauer consistently." He had failed the nurse's swallow screen, which was notable for coughing postintake while consuming sips of water from a cup. The patient was seated upright in a chair with his significant other at the bedside. The NGT was in place. The ICU team purported that dysphagia was likely due to postextubation edema. The patient was awake, alert, oriented times 4, and his speech was intelligible. He was using Yankauer to manage his secretions, and his vocal quality was intermittently wet and gurgling. A cough was present and very productive, and the patient was able to manage his oral secretions.

The oral–peripheral exam revealed intact labial, buccal, and lingual range of motion and strength. Slight velar asymmetry was noted, and there were no suspected laryngeal impairments. His oral care was fair, and oral hygiene was provided before PO trials. The absence of the gag reflex was observed bilaterally, and there was no palpable pharyngeal swallow response with secretions or a 3 ml water trial. The patient was encouraged to reduce his use of Yankauer and attempt to swallow secretions. A neurology consult was recommended due to suspicion of postop CVA. The ICU team was reluctant to consult neurology despite CN evidence of possible central injury. The dysphagia did not resolve over the next several days. The patient received a PEG at postop day 8, and he still was not seen by neurology. The speech-language pathologist called the chief of neurology, and the neurologic exam was completed, which revealed CN deficits. An MRI revealed possible embolic infarction of the medulla. During the patient's acute inpatient stay, the following goals were formulated:

1. The patient will swallow secretions successfully after thermal tactile, cold, or sour stimulation three times per session.
2. The patient will reduce use of the Yankauer suction device, as measured by the amount of secretions in the suction container over 2 days.

Case Scenarios *(continued)*

3. The patient will perform aggressive oral care 3–4 times per day according to the outline provided by the speech-language pathologist.

4. The patient will maintain daily mobility, ambulating three times per day with physical therapy.

5. The patient will utilize ice chips after oral care for swallow stimulation without adverse events.

Mr. Schmidt was discharged to a rehabilitation facility with PEG placement and recommendations for daily dysphagia therapy, including frequent oral care and allowance of ice chips or small sips of water to facilitate swallow recovery. The risk of trace aspiration of water boluses were judged to be outweighed by the benefits of stimulating the patient's swallowing by providing him with swallowing experience—in line with the use it or lose it principle.

The patient went to a subacute rehabilitation facility, and the speech-language pathologist there requested that he not swallow ice chips. The patient later reported that he would cheat and swallow whenever he could if his mouth was clean. The patient came for follow-up at the original acute facility as an outpatient and was reporting that he was able to swallow his secretions and no longer used a spittoon. He was also swallowing small amounts of water and other liquids. His chest X-ray was negative for pneumonia, and his respiratory and pulmonary statuses were stable. He was evaluated clinically, and his reports were accurate. There was mild throat clearing after several thin liquid swallows, but no issues were present as he had demonstrated in the past. An MBSS was recommended for the following day, 3 months after his initial inpatient evaluation.

The MBSS revealed a grossly functional oral phase of the swallow. There was some initial hesitancy (mild bolus holding) prior to oral transport. The pharyngeal swallow was mildly delayed, triggering at the pyriform sinuses, and there was trace penetration to the level of the vocal folds. There was complete retrieval of the material and no aspiration. Pharyngeal weakness was noted for purees, and it was more significant for chewable solids. There was mild to moderate residue in the valleculae and pyriform sinuses that was cleared with a secondary swallow. There was no airway compromise for puree or solid consistency. Mr. Schmidt patient was counseled regarding the findings, and he was tearful about how he had improved. He was eager to be weaned from his PEG. The PEG was removed 6 weeks after the MBSS and after 2 weeks of nonuse and adequate maintenance of his weight. He was followed for 4 years

118 Chapter 6

📋 Case Scenarios *(continued)*

and was found to not have further complications from his dysphagia. Mr. Schmidt was often seen in the hospital cafeteria eating dough-nuts and having coffee with his wife. He gained almost 70 pounds and was counseled to consult with a dietician about his food choices, but he refused.

Questions

1. This patient's dysphagia was due to postextubation trauma to the laryngeal structures.

   A. True
   B. False

2. The speech-language pathologist's understanding of which factor assisted in the proper diagnosis and management of this complex patient?

   A. Atrial fibrillation
   B. Substance abuse
   C. Neurology of the swallow and cranial nerve function
   D. Critical illness

3. This patient's outcome might have been different in which of the following situations?

   A. If the speech-language pathologist had immediately performed an MBSS
   B. If the patient were kept dry NPO, without stimulation for swallow recovery
   C. If the patient were cognitively intact
   D. None of the above

4. The patient exhibits swelling of the laryngopharyngeal structures but not absent swallow response that is persistent at postextubation.

   A. True
   B. False

5. The patient did not require an MBSS at the time of initial diagnosis because

   A. he could not even manage his secretions, and aspiration of barium was a significant risk.
   B. the dysphagia was so severe and so obvious.
   C. the oral phase was impaired.
   D. the team would not place the order for the exam.

REVIEW QUESTIONS

1. Clinicians should take which of the following into consideration when formulating goals?
   a. The patient's goals
   b. The prognosis for improvement
   c. The patient's baseline level of functioning
   d. The patient's cognitive skills
   e. All of the above

2. When establishing an intervention plan with goals, the clinician must do which of the following?
   a. Formulate goals that are measurable
   b. Make decisions about treatments with low levels of evidence
   c. Restrict patients from swallowing their saliva or small sips of water due to fears about aspirating
   d. Formulate goals that do not exceed the patient's capabilities
   e. None of the above

3. A goal for a patient diagnosed with dysphagia who cannot participate in active treatment due to advanced dementia may have which of the following possible goals? Choose all that apply.
   a. The patient will perform effortful swallows for 20 repetitions independently.
   b. The patient's caregiver will position the patient in an upright position, provide oral care prior to PO intake, and feed at a slow rate over 1 week.
   c. The patient will perform a supersupraglottic swallow maneuver with biofeedback using sEMG for 10 repetitions.
   d. The patient will consume three meals of puree with thin liquids without adverse outcomes (i.e., no pulmonary or respiratory compromise) over 1 week.
   e. None of the above apply.

4. ASHA and the American Board of Swallowing and Swallowing Disorders indicate that speech-language pathologists working with patients who have dysphagia must do which of the following? Choose all that apply.
   a. Possess the knowledge and skills to evaluate and treat patients with swallowing disorders
   b. Use evidence-based practice to guide treatment and management
   c. Be competent to perform FEES exams
   d. Refer to another speech-language pathologist if he or she is not competent or prepared to work with the patient

5. If the patient has different goals than the speech-language pathologist, the speech-language pathologist should work with the patient, the family, and the physicians to develop reasonable goals and create compromise.
   a. True
   b. False

REFERENCES

Adams, V., Mathisen, B., Baines, S., Lazarus, C., & Callister, R. (2013). A systematic review and meta-analysis of measurements of tongue and hand strength and endurance using the Iowa Oral Performance Instrument (IOPI). *Dysphagia, 28*, 350–369.

Allcot, D., & Dixon, K. (1997). The reliability of the scales of the Functional Assessment Measure (FAM): Differences in abstractness between FAM scales. *Disability Rehabilitation, 19*(9), 355–358.

American Speech-Language-Hearing Association. (2001a). *Knowledge and skills for speech- language pathologist providing services to individuals with swallowing and feeding disorders.* Rockville, MD: Author.

American Speech-Language-Hearing Association. (2001b). *Roles of speech-language pathologists in swallowing and feeding disorders* [Position paper]. Rockville, MD: Author.

American Speech-Language-Hearing Association. (2017). Adult dysphagia. Retrieved from http://www.asha.org/Practice-Portal/Clinical-Topics/Adult-Dysphagia/

Bartolome, G., & Neumann, S. (1993). Swallowing therapy in patients with neurological disorders causing cricopharyngeal dysfunction. *Dysphagia, 8*, 146–149.

Belafsky, P. C., Mouadeb, D. A., Rees, C. J., Pryor, J. C., Postma, G. N., Allen, J., & Leonard, R. J. (2008). Validity and reliability of the Eating Assessment Tool (EAT-10). *Annals of Otology, Rhinology & Laryngology,117*, 919–924.

Cichero, J., & Altman, K. (2012). Definition, prevalence, and burden of oropharyngeal dysphagia. *Nestle Nutritional Institute Workshop Service, 72*, 1–11.

Crary, M. (2000, July 19). *The Florida Dysphagia Institute* [course]. Orlando, FL.

Crary, M. (2006, September 22 & 23). *Advanced course on treatment of adult dysphagia* [course]. Boston, MA.

Crary, M., Carnaby-Mann, G., & Groher, M. (2005). Initial psychometric assessment of a functional oral intake scale for dysphagia in stroke patients. *Archives of Physical Medicine & Rehabilitation, 86*, 1516–1520.

Crary, M., Carnaby-Mann, G., LaGorio L., & Carvajal, P. (2012). Functional and physiological outcomes from an exercise-based dysphagia therapy: McNeill dysphagia therapy program. *Archives of Physical Medicine & Rehabilitation, 93*(7), 1173–1178.

Dikeman, K., & Kazandjian, M. (2002). *Communication and swallowing management of tracheostomized and ventilator-dependent adults.* San Diego, CA: Singular.

Dondorf, K., Fabus, R., & Ghassemi, A. (2016). The interprofessional collaboration between nurses and speech-language pathologists working with patients diagnosed with dysphagia in skilled nursing facilities. *Nursing Education and Practice, 6*(4), 17–20.

Fabus, R., & Dondorf, K. (2014). Training speech-language pathology students to perform the clinical swallow evaluation and a multidisciplinary approach in a skilled nursing facility. *Express, an International Journal of MultiDisciplinary Research, 1*(11), 1–24.

Fabus, R., Gironda, F., & Museyeva, S. (2018). Conducting the oral peripheral exam. In C. Stein-Rubin (Ed.), *Guide to clinical assessment and professional report writing in speech-language pathology* (2nd ed.). Thorofare, NJ: Slack.

Fiorelli, A., Ferraro, F., Nagar, F., Fusco, P., Mazzone, S., Costa, G., . . . Santini, M. (2016). A new modified Evans blue dye test as screening test for aspiration in tracheostomized patients. *Journal of Cardiothoracic and Vascular Anesthesia, 31*(2), 441–445.

Groher, M., & Crary, M. (2010). *Dysphagia: Clinical management in adults and children.* St. Louis, MO: Mosby Elsevier.

Hind, J., Nocosia, M., Roecker, E., Carnes, M., & Robbins, J. (2001). Comparison of effortful and noneffortful swallows in healthy middle-aged and older adults. *Archives of physical medicine and rehabilitation, 82*, 1661–1665.

Hiss, S., & Postma, G. (2003). Fiberoptic endoscopic evaluation of swallowing. *Laryngoscope, 113*, 1386–1393.

Jocham, H., Dassen, T., Widdershoven, G., & Halfens, R. (2009). Evaluating palliative care—a review of the literature. *Palliative Care Research and Treatment, 3*, 5–12.

Johnson, P., Belafsky, P., & Postma, G. (2003). Topical nasal anesthetic for transnasal fiberoptic laryngoscopy: A prospective, double-blind, cross over study. *Otolaryngology Head and Neck Surgery, 128*(4), 452–454.

Langmore, S. (2001). *Endoscopic evaluation and treatment of swallowing disorders.* New York, NY: Thieme.

Langmore, S., Krisciunas, G., Miloro, K., Evans, S., & Cheng, D. (2012). Does PEG use cause dysphagia in head and neck cancer patients? *Dysphagia, 27*(2), 251–259.

Langmore, S., McCullough, T., Krisciunas, G., Lazarus, C., Van Daele, D., Pauloski, B., . . . Doros, G. (2016). Efficacy of electrical stimulation and exercise for dysphagia in patients with head and neck cancer: A randomized clinical trial. *Head and Neck, 38*(Suppl. 1), E1221–E1231.

Langmore, S., Schatz, K., & Olsen, N. (1988). Fiberoptic endoscopic examination of swallowing safety: A new procedure. *Dysphagia, 2*(4), 216–219.

Leder, S., Ross, D., Brinskin, K., & Sasaki, C. (1997). A prospective, double-blind, randomized study on the use of a topical anesthetic, vasoconstrictor, and placebo during transnasal flexible, fiberoptic endoscopy. *Journal of Speech-Language Hearing Research, 40,* 1352–1357.

Lester, S., Langmore, S., Lintzenich, C., Carter-Wright, S., Grace-Martin, G., Fife, T., & Butler, S. (2013). The effects of topical anesthetic on swallowing during nasoendoscopy. *Laryngoscope, 123*(7), 1704–1708.

Logemann, J. (1983). *Evaluation and treatment of swallowing disorders.* Austin, TX: PRO-ED.

Logemann, J. (1998). *Evaluation and treatment of swallowing disorders* (2nd ed.). Austin, TX: PRO-ED.

Logemann, J. (2013). *The ultimate videofluoroscopic swallow study symposium—from RADS to riches: An SLP perspective.* Dysphagia Research Society 21st Annual Meeting, Seattle, WA.

Logemann, J., Kahrilas, M., & Vakil, N. (1989). The benefit of head rotation on pharyngoesophageal dysphagia. *Archives of Physical Medicine and Rehabilitation, 70,* 767–771.

Logemann, J., Pauloski, B., Rademaker, A., & Colangelo, L. (1997). Super-supraglottic swallow in irradiated head and neck cancer patients. *Head and Neck, 19,* 535–540.

Mann, G. (2000, July 19). *The Florida Dysphagia Institute* [course]. Orlando, FL.

Martin-Harris, B., Brodsky, M., Michel, Y., Castell, D., Schleicher, M., Sandidge, J., . . . Blair, J. (2008). MBS measurement tool for swallow impairment—MBSImP: Establishing a standard. *Dysphagia, 23*(4), 392–405.

McCullough, G., Leder, S., & Coyle, J. (2015). *Point counterpoint: The clinical swallow examination—is it necessary and is it useful?* American Speech-Language-Hearing Association Convention, Denver, CO.

Murry, T., & Carrau, R. (2001). *Clinical manual of swallowing disorders.* San Diego, CA: Singular.

New Oxford Dictionary of English (2nd ed.). (2010). London, England: Oxford University Press.

Raber-Durlacher, J., Brennan, M., Verdonck-de Leeuw, I., Gibson, R., Eilers, J., Waltimo, T., . . . Spijkervet, F. (2012). Swallowing dysfunction in cancer patients. *Supportive Care in Cancer, 20,* 433–443.

Robbins, J., Kays, S., Gangnon, R., Hind, J., Hewitt, A., Gentry, L., & Taylor, A. (2007). The effects of lingual exercise in stroke patients with dysphagia. *Archives of Physical Medicine and Rehabilitation, 88,* 150–158.

Robey, R. (2004). Levels of evidence. *The ASHA Leader, 9,* 5–7.

Rosenbek, J., Robbins, J., Roecker, E., Coyle, J., & Wood, J. (1996). A penetration-aspiration scale. *Dysphagia, 11,* 93–98.

Sapienza, C., & Troche, M. (2011). *Respiratory muscle strength training: Theory and practice.* San Diego, CA: Plural.

Shaker, R., Kern, M., Bardan, E., Taylor, A., Stewart, E., Hoffmann, R., . . . Bonnevier, J. (1997). Augmentation of deglutitive upper esophageal sphincter opening in the elderly by exercise. *American Journal of Physiology, 272,* 1518–1522.

Swallow Solutions. (2014). Dysphagia treatment. Retrieved from http://www.swallowsolutions.com/dysphagia-treatment

ADDITIONAL RESOURCES
BOOKS

Corbin-Lewis, Kim, and Julie M. Liss. *Clinical Anatomy and Physiology of the Swallow Mechanism* (2nd ed.). Stamford, CT: Cengage Learning, 2015.

Leonard, Rebecca, and Katherine Kendall. *Dysphagia Assessment and Treatment Planning. A Team Approach* (3rd ed.). San Diego, CA: Plural, 2014.

Murray, Joseph. *Manual of Dysphagia Assessment in Adults.* San Diego, CA: Singular, 1998.

Shaker, Reza, Caryn Easterling, Peter C. Belafsky, and Gregory N. Postma. *Manual of Diagnostic and Therapeutic Techniques for Disorders of Deglutition.* New York, NY: Springer, 2013.

Sonies, Barbara C., Ed. *Dysphagia: A Continuum of Care.* Gaithersburg, MD: Aspen, 1997.

Swigert, Nancy B. *The Source for Dysphagia* (3rd ed.). East Moline, IL: LinguiSystems, 2007.

VanDahm, Kelly, and Sally Sparks-Walsh. *Tracheostomy Tubes and Ventilator Dependence in Adults and Children: A Handbook for the Speech-Language Pathologist.* Austin, TX: PRO-ED, 2002.

Yorkston, Kathryn M., Robert M. Miller, Edythe A. Strand, and Deanna Britton. *Management of Speech and Swallowing in Degenerative Diseases* (3rd ed.). Austin, TX: PRO-ED, 2013.

WEBSITES

American Board of Swallowing and Swallowing Disorders. www.swallowingdisorders.org/?page=mission

American Speech-Language-Hearing Association. www.asha.org

American Speech-Language-Hearing Association. Special Interest Group 13, Swallowing and Swallowing Disorders (Dysphagia). www.asha.org/sig/13/

Dysphagia Research Society. www.dysphagiaresearch.org

DysphagiaVideo.com. Educational Video for Individuals with Dysphagia. www.dysphagiavideo.com

GI Motility Online. www.nature.com/gimo/index.html

MedlinePlus. Swallowing Disorders. www.nlm.nih.gov/medlineplus/dysphagia.html

National Foundation of Swallowing Disorders. www.swallowingdisorderfoundation.com

Nestlé Health Science. Dysphagia. www.nestlehealthscience.com/health-management/gastro-intestinal/dysphagia/dysphagia-hcp

Swallow Solutions. Dysphagia Treatment. www.swallowsolutions.com/dysphagia-treatment

DYSPHAGIA SCREENING AND ASSESSMENT MEASURES

Bedside Evaluation of Dysphagia (BED): Hardy, E. (1999). *Bedside evaluation of dysphagia* (Rev. ed.). Bisbee, AZ: Imaginart.

Clinical Observational Dysphagia Assessment (CODA): Campbell-Taylor, I. (2005). *C.O.D.A.: Clinical observational dysphagia assessment.* Stow, OH: Interactive Therapeutics.

Dysphagia Evaluation Protocol: Avery-Smith, W., Dellarosa, D. M., & Rosen, A. B. (1997). *Dysphagia evaluation protocol.* San Antonio, TX: Therapy Skill Builders.

Eating Assessment Tool (EAT-10): Belafsky, P. C., Mouadeb, D. A., Rees, C. J., Pryor, J. C., Postma, G. N., Allen, J., & Leonard, R. J. (2008). Validity and reliability of the Eating Assessment Tool (EAT-10). *Annals of Otology, Rhinology & Laryngology, 117*, 919–924.

Mann Assessment of Swallowing Ability (MASA): Mann, G. (2002). *MASA: The Mann assessment of swallowing ability.* Clifton Park, NY: Delmar Cengage Learning.

National Outcomes Measurement System (NOMS): http://www.asha.org/NOMS/

Quick Assessment for Dysphagia: Tanner, D., & Culbertson, W. (n.d.). *Quick assessment for dysphagia: Complete kit.* Oceanside, CA: Academic Communication Associates. http://www.acadcom.com/scripts/prodList.asp?idcategory=34&sortField=price

Swallowing Ability and Function Evaluation (SAFE): Kipping, P., Ross-Swain, D., & Yee, P. A. (2003). *SAFE: Swallowing ability and function evaluation.* Austin, TX: PRO-ED. http://www.proedinc.com/customer/productView.aspx?ID=2162

Toronto Bedside Swallowing Screening Test (TOR-BSST): Martino, R., Silver, F., Teasell, R., Bayley, M., Nicholson, G., Streiner, D. L., & Diamant, N. E. (2009). The Toronto bedside swallowing screening test (TOR-BSST): Development and validation of a dysphagia screening tool for patients with stroke. *Stroke, 40,* 555–561. https://swallowinglab.com/tor-bsst/

Yale Swallow Protocol: Suiter, D. M., Sloggy, J., & Leder, S. B. (2014). Validation of the Yale Swallow Protocol: A prospective double-blind videofluoroscopic study. *Dysphagia, 29*(2), 199–203.

DYSPHAGIA SCALES AND OUTCOME TRACKING TOOLS

Eating Assessment Tool (EAT-10): Belafsky, P. C., Mouadeb, D. A., Rees, C. J., Pryor, J. C., Postma, G. N., Allen, J., & Leonard, R. J. (2008). Validity and reliability of the Eating Assessment Tool (EAT-10). *Annals of Otology, Rhinology & Laryngology, 117,* 919–924.

Functional Oral Intake Scale (FOIS): Crary, M., Carnaby-Mann, G., & Groher, M. (2005). Initial psychometric assessment of a functional oral intake scale for dysphagia in stroke patients. *Archives of Physical Medicine & Rehabilitation, 86,* 1516–1520.

Penetration–Aspiration Scale: Rosenbek, J., Robbins, J., Roecker, E., Coyle, J., & Wood, J. (1996). A penetration-aspiration scale. *Dysphagia, 11,* 93–98.

SWAL-QOL and SWAL-CARE: McHorney, C. A., Martin-Harris, B., Robbins, J., & Rosenbek, J. (2006). Clinical validity of the SWAL-QOL and SWAL-CARE outcome tools with respect to bolus flow measures. *Dysphagia, 21*(3) 141–148.

APPENDIX

TABLE 6-1 Selected Interventions for Patients with Dysphagia

Name	Type of Intervention	Appropriate For	Physiology	Drawbacks	Therapeutic benefit
Chin tuck or chin down	Posture	Premature loss or swallow delay; caps the airway	Brings tongue base closer to posterior pharyngeal wall and widens vallecular space	Reduces constriction forces of the pharynx; can result in increased residue	Does not change muscle function
Head turn (to weak side)	Posture	Unilateral pharyngeal weakness with aspiration and/or residue	Closes off weakened hemipharynx and directs bolus to stronger hemipharynx	Not appropriate for bilateral residue; need to assess in AP view	Does not change muscle function
Chin up, head back	Posture	Status post glossectomy or severe AP transit issues	Uses gravity to assist in posterior bolus movement	Must be cognitively intact; pair with a breath hold because head back position opens the airway	Does not change muscle function
Mendelsohn	Maneuver	Severe residue in the pharyngeal recesses due to poor cricopharyngeus opening, hyolaryngeal elevation	Prolongs hyolaryngeal elevation, thereby increasing extent and duration of the opening of the cricopharyngeus	Can be difficult to teach and learn; biofeedback helps	Can be used in treatment to increase muscle function

TABLE 6-1 Selected Interventions for Patients with Dysphagia *(continued)*

Name	Type of Intervention	Appropriate For	Physiology	Drawbacks	Therapeutic benefit
Effortful swallow	Maneuver	Enhances pharyngeal constriction forces to assist in clearance of residue	Increases extent and constriction of tongue base to posterior pharyngeal wall		Can be used in treatment to increase muscle function
Supraglottic and supersupraglottic swallow	Maneuver	Closes the airway prior to the swallow for patients who have preswallow or periswallow penetration or aspiration	Supraglottic closes the glottis at the vocal folds; supersupraglottic closes glottis at the level of the vocal folds and tilts arytenoids to petiole of epiglottis (tighter breath hold)	Can be difficult to teach and learn; biofeedback and FEES can assist	Can be used in treatment to increase muscle function
Head raise or Shaker exercise	Exercise	Increases strength and contraction of the suprahyoid muscles that pull the larynx anteriorly to open the cricopharyngeus; residue in the pyriform sinuses—superior to the cricopharyngeus	Lay flat on back and bring chin to chest; hold for 30 seconds and 30 individual repetitions; repeat three times	Not for patients with cervical disease; can enhance reflux if performed after tube feeds or oral feeds	Used to increase muscle function

TABLE 6-1 Selected Interventions for Patients with Dysphagia (*continued*)

Name	Type of Intervention	Appropriate For	Physiology	Drawbacks	Therapeutic benefit
Expiratory Muscle Strength Training (EMST)	Exercise (device)	Improves exhalatory muscle strength for improved cough	EMST device with progressive resistance knob	Must be able to obtain lip seal; must purchase individual device	Used to increase expiratory muscle strength
Iowa Oral Performance Instrument (IOPI)	Exercise (device)	Deficits in tongue strength for swallowing	Press regions of tongue on intraoral bulb	Purchase device and use disposable bulbs	Used to increase lingual strength and function
Madison Oral Strengthening Therapeutic Device (MOST)	Exercise (device)	Deficits in oral tongue and tongue base	Press regions of tongue on molded mouthpiece	Each patient must purchase own device	Used to increase lingual strength and function

CHAPTER 7

Adult Neurogenic Communication Disorders

Julia Yudes-Kuznetsov

Key Terms

Aphasia
Apraxia
Dementia
Dynamic assessment
Dysarthria
Goal development
International Classification of
   Functioning, Disability, and
   Health (ICF) Framework

Neurogenic communication
   disorders
Reimbursement
Right-hemisphere
   dysfunction
Traumatic brain
   injury (TBI)

Introduction

The term **neurogenic communication disorders** describes a group of disorders in which a disturbance in any aspect of communication (cognition, language, or speech) is caused by damage to the nervous system. Communication is a complex behavior based on the interaction of multiple components, such as cognition, language, speech, social–emotional factors, hearing, and vision. The damage to the nervous system could be sudden (as in a cerebrovascular accident [CVA] or **traumatic brain injury [TBI]**), gradual, or progressive (as in dementia, Parkinson disease, multiple sclerosis, etc.). The classification of neurogenic communication disorders is often limited to aphasia, apraxia, dysarthria, right hemisphere dysfunction, TBI, and dementia. Any of the components of communication could be affected at the same time, but there could be varying degrees of involvement. For example, a patient might have **dysarthria** and impaired cognitive skills, which would alter the therapy goals and approaches used to achieve these goals.

Clinicians face challenges in providing assessments and interventions to this population. Some challenges come from organizing, sorting, and interpreting information that is limited or confusing. Other challenges stem from the social, emotional, and cognitive consequences that patients experience as a result of the brain damage and their reaction to the stress. This varies from individual to individual (Brookshire, 2003). In addition, the new forms of service **reimbursement** and regulations influence assessment and therapy considerations.

The T3D approach framework used for children's assessment and therapy decisions (see the *Historical Perspective of Goal Writing and Contemporary Practice* chapter) cannot be applied to adults due to the new changes in the healthcare system today.

The traditional medical framework, in which the goal of assessment is to identify impairment and disability then develop therapy goals based on the patient's diagnosis, is no longer beneficial. The diagnosis itself cannot predict an individual's functioning in daily living activities. The third-party requirements for developing a functional therapy plan, including goals, leads clinicians to consider a different framework. The word *functional* is very broad when considering a therapy plan and goals, and it is viewed differently by providers (in this case, speech-language pathologists) and third-party payers (Brookshire, 2015). To use the same approach and speak a common language, providers and payers should adopt the same framework.

The World Health Organization (2002) developed the **International Classification of Functioning, Disability, and Health (ICF) framework**, which is intended to provide a conceptual framework for health, disability, and functional changes for any health-related domain. It integrates biological, psychological, and social aspects of any disability. According to the ICF model, there are three interacting domains: health condition, activities and participation, and contextual factors. Health condition refers to diseases and disorders and their structural and physiological or functional properties. It includes anatomical issues (structural) and the physiological changes that result from those structural abnormalities. Activities and participation refer to the impact of the disability on a patient's functioning. Contextual factors could be personal and could be environmental. Personal factors include age, gender, education, employment, hobbies, interests, language/culture, future plans, and interrupted plans (such as employment). Environmental factors address family support, type of residence, ease of getting around, safety, driving ability, etc. For example, someone with the diagnosis of **aphasia** (disorder) as a result of a left-hemisphere frontal lobe stroke (structural change) has difficulties communicating with his or her spouse and avoids going to public places (activity and participation). This type of patient is viewed within the physical and social environment. It is now important to consider the patient's personal factors and environment for assessment purposes and **goal development**. Another example is a patient with **right-hemisphere dysfunction** resulting in cognitive–communicative difficulties, impaired awareness, unsteady gait, and weakness in upper and lower extremities who insists on going for outpatient services instead of receiving home care. If the patient has to manage three flights of stairs because there is no access to an elevator, safety becomes the first priority, especially when accounting for his or her impaired awareness of the deficits. Proper documentation of awareness issues becomes a key component in third-party approval for home care services.

ICF is a conceptual tool for decision making in planning and policy development. ASHA has adopted the ICF framework and provides guidance in assessments and goal development based on the framework (American Speech-Language-Hearing Association [ASHA], 2017a).

If a clinician understands the concept behind the ICF framework, he or she can perform assessments and interventions, including developing therapy goals, without difficulty. Kagan and colleagues (2008) developed an assessment and therapy guide for individuals with aphasia based on the ICF framework. It is known as Living with Aphasia: Framework for Outcome Measurement (A-FROM). A-FROM is available in both a descriptive form and a Venn diagram (Kagan, 2011; Kagan et al., 2008). For individuals with aphasia, the diagram is easier to use than the description, which allows them to be involved in therapy planning (a Medicare requirement). Even though it was developed for individuals with aphasia, the diagram and description apply to any individual with neurogenic communication disorders.

Comprehensive Assessment

A comprehensive assessment for neurogenic communication disorders presents numerous challenges. First, the currently available standardized batteries provide limited information. The data can barely grasp the complexity of speech and cognitive–communicative abilities. The captured behaviors can lead to preliminary general diagnoses and may identify only some of the patient's strengths and weaknesses. The tests are not designed to identify needs of a patient outside the testing area, nor can they predict a patient's performance in real-life situations (Turkstra, Coelho, & Ylvisaker, 2005). This is the part of the ICF model that refers to activity and participation.

The second issue in assessing these clients is that the clinician's choice of assessment tools should be based on the outcome goals that are specific to the patient, a so-called backward approach (Kagan & Simmons-Mackie, 2007). The desired outcome goals are not constant and will continually change, depending on the various stages along the continuum of medical and rehabilitation care, context, family and patient perception, and adjustment. For example, the needs of patients and families in the emergency department are different than their needs in inpatient rehabilitation. In an emergency department, the medical diagnosis is still in the working stage because the patient's condition is unstable. The condition could rapidly improve, as in transient ischemic attacks, or it could deteriorate, as in hemorrhagic CVAs. Another possibility is the patient may require an additional intervention, such as brain surgery, which could change the situation completely. Any results of the speech and cognitive–communicative assessment may not be valid the next day, or even the next hour, due to the patient's instability and the limited diagnostic information available or obtained. The patient and family could be overwhelmed by the number of tests and the medical terminology that is explained to them. The medical terms sound like a foreign language to them. In inpatient rehabilitation patients have usually been admitted after their medical work-up indicates they are medically stable. These patients may tolerate test batteries easier, which allows for a more thorough assessment.

The variability in assessment goals is a third challenge. A speech-language pathologist could be involved in the assessment to determine the patient's eligibility for certain programs or benefits. Often a speech-language pathologist does the assessment to determine needs for therapy and to develop a treatment plan. The clinician must strategically choose the appropriate assessment tools based on the goal of the assessment and the patient's ability to participate in the specific assessment tools or measures. The tools could be excerpts from standardized, norm-referenced assessments, questionnaires, or rating scales and should always be supplemented by an informal assessment. The Academy of Neurologic Communication Disorders and Sciences (ANCDS) provides guidelines for the assessment of individuals, who are American English speakers, with various neurogenic speech and cognitive–communicative disorders (refer to the "Additional Resources" section of this chapter).

The fourth issue to consider is that for an increasing number of individuals who speak a language other than English or who are part of another culture, a one-size-fits-all approach is not valid. The Bilingual Aphasia Test (BAT) is a reliable and valid tool for use in the assessment of communication skills of patients who speak multiple languages (Paradis & Libben, 2014). The BAT was initially developed between 1976 and 1982 (Paradis, 2004, 2011) and is currently available in more than 70 languages, with new languages continually being added. Any of the available language versions are easily accessible for free on the McGill University website (McGill University, 2017). According to Paradis (2004), the BAT is not a translational test; the stimuli are culturally and linguistically adapted into another language version. Because a clinician who is fluent in the patient's language is not always available, the test can be administered and scored by a layperson. However, the results should be interpreted by a professional, and they can be analyzed in view of any theory. Note that the BAT samples only linguistic behavior. Social, environmental, cognitive, and cultural areas affecting the individual's communication, as described in the ICF framework, must be explored separately, and usually informally, in addition to the BAT findings.

The fifth challenge is that a patient may not be medically stable or may not have adequate attention skills to participate in standardized testing. A clinician may encounter this type of patient in many different settings, not only on medical units of a hospital. For example, suppose that a 34-year-old home care patient had head trauma 1 year ago due to a fall from a ladder. He had severe pain caused by spasticity and was taking strong medications to alleviate the pain. The patient could not fully participate in therapy sessions, either because of the pain or because he would become drowsy from taking pain medications. The assessment techniques must consider his limited attention skills.

A patient could have multiple comorbidities. An another example, suppose a patient is diagnosed with a right CVA resulting in a severe dysarthria, so her cognitive–communicative abilities cannot be evaluated properly because of the poor speech intelligibility. The cognitive tests must be modified or used later in the rehabilitation process. Because the standardized test is not administered according to the directions—it is being modified—the scoring is no longer valid.

Currently available tests do not reflect recent changes in the rehabilitation model (use of ICF framework), leading to the sixth challenge. According to the ICF model, a patient's background, personality, environment, and caregivers (family, friends, coworkers, etc.) are important components of any speech-language assessment and therapy session. This information is often obtained through questionnaires or rating scales. These tools are emerging in the field of neurogenic communication disorders, and their development presents specific challenges. Because typical questionnaires and rating scales are in a verbal format, developers have to consider the patient's communication difficulties so they can capture valid and reliable information. For example, the Assessment for Living with Aphasia test (available at Aphasia Institute) is a picture-based self-reporting questionnaire that measures the quality of life in a person with aphasia. It is based on the A-FROM framework (Kagan, 2011; Kagan et al., 2008). As described by Irwin (2012), other scales and questionnaires are also available for patients with CVAs. These questionnaires and rating scales require additional time to administer and analyze. To explore additional factors that contribute to the successes and challenges of people with language impairment, and to develop a therapy plan, the clinician needs to use a creative approach that is rooted in strong theoretical knowledge and practices related to speech and cognitive–communicative disorders.

The seventh issue is restrictions dictated by payers. Reimbursement rules are tied to the type of rehabilitation facility where a patient is seen and to the specific insurance policy. Third-party payers that follow Medicare guidelines may not reimburse evaluations separately, but they will cover evaluations as part of a treatment session, such as in a skilled nursing facility or in home care. In some cases, such as in home care, a clinician may receive insurance authorization for only one session, then the clinician must submit a report to either request further therapy or discharge. Any of the reports must include justification for such decisions. The request should specify the number of sessions and the time period that is targeted for goal attainment. After the clinician submits the required paperwork, there is no guarantee that the request will be approved; even if it is approved, the insurance company may limit how many sessions are allowed in a year. It could be that the patient still needs therapy, but the insurance company will not pay for more sessions until the next year, so the patient would have to pay for sessions out of pocket. A patient may reject this arrangement, so the clinician should be prepared to develop a backup plan. The clinician must be flexible and resourceful in prioritizing the patient's assessment needs and developing a tentative therapy plan. This is when the education and training of caregivers becomes extremely valuable.

The eighth challenge is that third-party payers often have to review the speech-language pathologist's documentation. The insurance reviewer is usually a nurse, and the nurse may not know the terminology, abbreviations, or therapy approaches used in speech-language pathology. Therefore, the clinician should use a writing style that reflects the needs of the reviewer, who has never met the patient, to convey the intended message, including the justification for therapy, choice of specific goals, and methodology. Clinicians need to write reports that are short but comprehensive and clear, with details that are relevant to the situation and are important for the recommendations and care plan. It is essential then, for novice clinicians to receive training and guidance on the documentation requirements of the facility and as recommended in ASHA guidelines (ASHA, 2017b).

In view of all of these challenges, a **dynamic assessment** approach is most beneficial for patients with neurogenic communication disorders. A dynamic assessment allows flexibility in therapy by constantly reassessing and modifying the patient's response to treatment (Ylvisaker, 1998). The approach considers changing medical conditions, psychosocial interactions, communication style, cognitive abilities, personality, environment and contexts, various cues, and strategies. A dynamic approach to assessment and therapy allows justification for modifying goals and the therapy design. From a documentation standpoint, any changes in therapy are appropriate as long as the clinician provides proper written documentation.

For example, suppose a patient has limited verbal or gestural communication as a result of severe mixed aphasia with suspected cognitive impairment. The patient attends 45-minute outpatient speech-language therapy sessions. He is medically stable and usually participates in the entire session. One day, however, the patient appears to be in distress, which he indicates by body rocking, unintelligible verbalizations, and the inability to sustain his attention on familiar tasks. The clinician attempts to determine a possible cause of the distress by using yes or no questions and prompting the patient to point to the source of distress. She notices that the patient is not able to communicate, even though this goal (basic yes or no head gestures and basic pointing) was addressed in previous therapy sessions (structured tasks). The patient's caregivers are called from the waiting area to help. The situation is eventually resolved, but it takes about half the session time, so the therapy goals for the day are either modified or not addressed at all. The clinician needs to reflect what happened in the session documentation: "The session was limited and interrupted several times because the patient indicated discomfort (facial and body expression and an inability to attend to tasks). He was unable to point to the location of his discomfort (given maximum cues and prompts) or respond with yes or no head gestures or with words. The caregiver intervened and assisted the patient with bathroom needs." In addition, the clinician needs to report on the goals that were intended for this session, and the upcoming goals need to be reevaluated and modified. They include continuing to address yes and no responses and pointing and providing less structured situations so the patient can practice, which requires the involvement and training of caregivers. These activities are reflected as future goals, and the clinician's documentation should reflect the plan for upcoming sessions.

Data Analysis

It is easier to analyze assessment data if the clinician wisely chooses tools and techniques that consider the patient's outcome needs. The clinician can rely on the framework by Helm-Estabrooks and Albert, in which rehabilitation is "the process by which we attempt to close the gap between an individual's impairments and that individual's functional communication needs and desires" (2004, p.166). The data analysis used in therapy plan development should answer the questions of "what a person cannot do/can do/does do" and "what a person needs to do/wants to do" (Helm-Estabrooks & Albert, 2004, p.166). In comparing this framework to the ICF model, the term *impairment* indicates what the patient cannot do, and *functional communication* includes what the patient can do, does do, needs to do, and wants to do.

The Helm-Estabrooks and Albert model was originally developed for assessment and therapy planning for individuals with aphasia; however, it applies to any individual with neurogenic communication disorders. It allows the clinician to go beyond what is available in standardized and formal assessment tools and to view communication as an integrative multicomponent process, which is part of the ICF model.

Knowledge of a patient's communication deficits is not sufficient to develop a functional therapy plan. The clinician should further observe and probe a patient's verbal and nonverbal communication skills (e.g., body language, gestures, vocalizations, etc.), use of cues, and use of strategies, including whether or not those strategies are successful. Observation is a valuable component of comprehensive assessment (Holland, 1982). It is important to observe how patients manage difficult situations and if they are aware of their difficulties and inabilities. If patients are not aware of their challenges (e.g., patients with TBI, right hemisphere dysfunction, or fluent aphasia), it can be addressed in therapy. Awareness is an important element in training, in the use of strategies and cues, and in motivation during therapy. If patients are aware of their communication difficulties, how do they react? Do patients stop and become frustrated, or do they attempt to use self-generated strategies? Are these strategies successful? Which of the available cues for the particular issue are stimulable? What additional cues are required? These are just some examples of observation goals.

For instance, a patient with severe expressive aphasia and possible **apraxia** may perform better during automatic speech tasks, like reciting digits, than during sound and syllable repetition tasks, but only if the clinician initiates the task and the patient completes it. It could be that the patient can perform this task only in unison with the clinician and with a visual model (the clinician's articulation). This observation may lead to developing functional and measurable goals. It also may lead to developing a hierarchy of goals and tasks. The same patient may be able to successfully identify pictures of common objects in a field of six images (can do and does do), which could be used to develop a basic augmentative and alternative communication (AAC) system so the patient could communicate basic information, and other activities could target verbal communication.

The needs and wants that patients and caregivers expressed during the initial evaluation should also be considered while developing the plan of care. As therapy progresses, adjustments and modifications might need to be made due to new concerns that may arise. For example, the patient's performance may change due to progress that is being made, spontaneous recovery, or new medical or psychosocial issues. The clinician should be aware that the patients' and caregivers' perspectives on disabilities and handicaps will undergo modifications during the rehabilitation process.

Often at the beginning of the rehabilitation continuum, long-term goals expressed by patients and family members may sound unrealistic. The clinician, however, should take them into consideration for several reasons. First, it is possible that during the rehabilitation process, the goals could become realistic (refer to "Case Scenario 1" and "Case Scenario 2" at the end of this chapter). Second, the patient's and family's need for counseling and education about communication abilities and the overall plan could be the most important factor at the present moment. Third, patient's and family's expectations and perception of the disability will influence the rehabilitation therapy (which is part of ICF model) and could either support the therapy plan and methodology or work against it.

Avent and colleagues (2005) analyzed what information the families of individuals with aphasia needed, depending on the time after the onset of aphasia. At the initial stage (onset of the communication disorder), families reported a need for obtaining generic information about aphasia and strokes, "realistic and positive prognostic information" (2005, p. 372), coexisting behaviors, medical changes resulting from a stroke, and available resources to cope with aphasia. At the acute rehabilitation stage, families requested specific information regarding treatment options and guidance about how to maximize interactions with individuals who have aphasia, coexisting behavioral and medical complications (especially depression), and resources (including connection to other families with similar problems). At the chronic stage, individuals with aphasia and their families required more community-based information. Regardless of the stage of aphasia, families reported a need for psychological support, counseling, and hopefulness. The needed information should be incorporated into the therapy session (Holland, 2012).

The counseling part of therapy is very important in the treatment of any neurogenic communication disorder. The clinician has to involve the patient and the caregivers in therapy to learn about their perspectives of the current issues that are caused by the disease and their goals for therapy. The clinician should be aware of the variability in patients' and caregivers' needs, depending on the time since onset, individual personalities, family or caregiver dynamics, culture, and so forth.

For example, consider a patient with the following new therapy goal: "The patient will use yes and no head gestures in response to simple questions in a nonstructured context 70 percent of the time, with prompting and modeling." Due to the type of therapy setting (in this example, an outpatient clinic), the opportunity to create sufficient nonstructured situations for the patient to practice is limited. This is when caregivers become essential to the rehabilitation process. Even though the caregivers observed a video of every therapy session, they were surprised when the clinician explained the need to practice the strategies outside the clinic in the real world. When the caregivers realized that the therapy goal targeted a mutual agenda (i.e., functional communication), they were happy to assist in any way they could.

Educating and counseling the patient's family leads to their support of the therapy agenda and increases practice opportunities for the patient. It also provides training for the caregivers to become communication partners. Various therapy approaches include caregivers as an important component of rehabilitation (Holland, 2012; Kagan & Gailey, 1993; Lyon, 2009; Simmons-Mackie, 2009), which ultimately leads to improving the patient's quality of life. The patient's and caregiver's input (goals) should be documented in the initial assessment and, if they have been modified, in the therapy session. The documentation functions as an explanation and justification to others (such as insurance companies, doctors, and other professionals) for why certain goals, tasks, and methodologies were chosen for therapy.

During the analysis of assessment data, the clinician should be aware of various communication and cognitive skills that underlie specific tasks. For example, the task of naming pictures of common objects relies on sufficient vocabulary, experience with the item, word retrieval, visual acuity, and visual–perceptual abilities. A so-called fluency naming task, or providing members in a category, taps into both word-finding skills and cognitive skills such as divergent thinking, organizational abilities, and the capacity to develop strategies. The clinician should critically analyze data from the assessment tasks and question any discrepancies in the patient's performance on tasks that target similar abilities. As an example, consider a patient who can accurately respond to simple personal WH questions (when, who, why, where, etc.), but he has significant difficulties in naming pictures of common objects (such as apple, bed, pencil, etc.). How is it that a patient can perform so differently on seemingly similar tasks? Both tasks target one-word responses and word-finding abilities, but one relies on an auditory presentation and the other uses a visual presentation.

Collaboration

It is imperative to collaborate with other rehabilitation specialists (neuropsychologists, occupational therapists, physical therapists, etc.) for several reasons. Tests and assessment tools often overlap in assessing similar areas, so collaboration could save time and incorporate findings from other professionals, or the test and assessment results could aid in decision making. For example, a patient might present with difficulties in reading, but not in writing (alexia without agraphia), as a result of a CVA. Because reading involves visual skills in addition to language and memory, an occupational therapist's and a neuropsychologist's assessments of visual–perceptual, constructional, and organizational skills might help the speech-language pathologist with better analysis and decision making.

Approaches to the Plan of Care

After the speech-language pathologist finishes analyzing the assessment data and determines the need for therapy, the next step is to develop and write a therapy plan. This is often the most difficult task for beginning clinicians. Burns and Halper, in their analysis of the most popular therapy approaches, concluded that clinicians should combine three approaches that are *not mutually exclusive*:

1. "to *stimulate* whatever viable language residuals exist during early stages post onset"
2. "to *facilitate* maximal language and speech processing through (the) use of deblocking techniques, cueing, prompting, etc., and to work to ensure that the patient learns to use useful facilitory techniques to restore maximal language potential"
3. "to help the patient to *compensate* for nonremediable deficits in the later stages of treatment by incorporating alternative communication and/or symbolic systems" (Burns & Halper, 1988, p. 10)

Two more approaches should be added to this list. First, recent therapy developments advocate including caregivers and other people who are in the patient's life. This will both aid the patient's rehabilitation and help the people in the patient's life to adjust to the new communication dynamics (Grawburg, Howe, Worrall, & Scarinci, 2013), including helping caregivers learn about what communication techniques to use with the patient. This then is a fourth approach (i.e., to include and assist caregivers in the communication techniques with the patient).

Second, Ylvisaker (1988) stressed the need to consider injury prevention and the prevention of psychosocial and behavioral failures. Therefore, the fourth approach is to prevent injuries and failures in communication, psychosocial, and behavioral aspects. Prevention of injuries highlights the topic of safety. Clinicians should consider if a patient's safety is at risk due to cognitive–communicative or speech issues. For example, if a patient with impaired communication is unable to walk or has an unsteady gait and needs assistance with ambulation, how can he or she get the caregiver's attention when needed? Or how can a patient who is cognitively intact but has severely impaired speech intelligibility make a phone call to get help from the caregiver or emergency personnel?

Because the preceding five approaches are not mutually exclusive, the clinician may combine them at any stage of the rehabilitation process. It is possible to have language stimulation goals and a basic communication board in the acute phase of treatment and, at the same time, address how to prevent communication failures by counseling and educating caregivers and people involved in daily care.

Goals and Documentation

Once the clinician and the patient/caregiver have determined the need for therapy, together they develop the plan of care (POC). The POC includes long-term and short-term goals. Long-term goals (LTGs) can be either final-destination goals or goals for a specific time period. Because most of the rehabilitation therapy is regulated by third-party payer rules, a patient's length of treatment in a particular program is limited. Even if final-destination goals are discussed, some of them may not be realistic at that time. Therefore, long-term goals can include both goals for the current rehabilitation stay and goals for the final destination. For example, preventing communication failures that can lead to social isolation could be the final-destination goal, and communicating basic needs and wants to caregivers and medical personnel could be the current long-term goal. Short-term goals (STGs) could be steps in the hierarchy to achieve the long-term goal, or they could be the various techniques that will aid in the achievement of the long-term goal.

In addition to long-term and short-term goals, the care plan should include recommendations for the type of therapy (individual therapy, group therapy, teletherapy, etc.) and the frequency and duration of the sessions. For example, "individual therapy is recommended two times per week in 45-minute sessions for 6 weeks, with the focus on . . ."

Unfortunately, therapy recommendations, whether for the type of therapy, the frequency, or the duration, are subject to third-party reimbursement regulations that often follow Medicare's lead. Even if a patient is paying out of pocket, the financial aspect of treatment could determine the choice of therapy. Additionally, the requirements for report writing and goals are influenced by reimbursement rules that are subject to change, as well as the care setting (medical unit, inpatient rehabilitation facility, or outpatient).

Cognitive domain is partially under a speech-language pathologist's scope of practice (ASHA, 2016). It may or may not be covered by third-party payers. The Michigan Speech Language Hearing Association, following years of extensive discussions with Medicaid and commercial insurance companies, was able to achieve some progress in this area. Blue Cross Blue Shield (BCBS) expanded its coverage of speech-language pathology services, including cognitive therapy for individuals with CVA or TBI (Ledwon-Robinson, 2016). Any goals that address cognition from a communication point of view, however, are considered part of communication and are written as cognitive–communicative goals. For example, suppose a patient is confused, produces disorganized verbal output, and has impaired short-term memory and problem-solving skills as a result of hemorrhagic CVA. His goals target the use of a memory book to locate and input a basic daily log. The use of a memory book relies on daily routines, as well as organizational structure to input into the daily log and to later recall it in the same manner, thus targeting verbal output.

When writing specific goals, the clinician should reflect a logical culmination of information in the evaluation or progress report and provide justification for the chosen therapy. Details that determine the choice of specific goals, therefore, are important to include. As an example, refer to "Case Scenario 2" at the end of this chapter, in which patient KT2 has mild to moderate expressive aphasia and was planning to go back to work. The plan, therefore, was to prepare the patient to return to work. This information is not sufficient to develop therapy goals and techniques because different jobs require different sets of physical, cognitive, and communication skills. The details, such as "KT2 worked as a field manager at the cable company," are important because a managerial position requires a high level of executive function skills, multitasking abilities, and the capacity to handle a large volume of written communications via emails and the company website. Because "KT2 has to spend most of the time away from his office, most communication is done via smartphone and requires a fast response." These details lead to a list of abilities that KT2 should have mastered in his long-term goals: managing a calendar for inputting and locating meetings (both on paper and in electronic format), comprehending written information in business emails, extracting key information from emails and plotting them into the calendar, composing and typing responses to the emails, verbalizing narrative explanations that are clear enough for his employees and superiors to understand and follow, and using a smartphone and the necessary apps.

The purpose of daily notes is to provide written records of a therapy session. Later, they are used to generate a progress summary or a discharge note. They should be short, clear, and reflect the goals stated in the plan of care or goals that have been modified because of new patient-related additional information or issues. They must be functional, measurable, and justify the need for skilled services (ASHA, 2007). *Functional* reflects the ICF model, and *measurable* is represented in accuracy, consistency, number of times an opportunity is given, amount and type of external help (cues or strategies), time constraints, presence or absence of distractions, and so forth. Skilled services include feedback (cues, strategies, etc.) and analysis provided by the clinician. For example, "The patient read short, simulated business-related emails and accurately responded to written WH questions about details with 75 percent accuracy, improved to 90 percent accuracy with the clinician's minimal cues to rely on written information. The errors were mostly with digits." Another example is, "The patient responded with yes and no head gestures to simple personal questions 50 percent of the time, improved to 80 percent of the time with the clinician's moderate prompts and models." The last goal did not target the accuracy of responses; rather, it targeted the initiation in the use of nonverbal responses because the patient's responses were reliable but rare. As mentioned earlier, details that support a change in the goals should be documented. For example, "the patient continues to be motivated and completes his homework assignments" is as important as "the spouse reported that the patient did not sleep well last night," or "therapy was limited to 25 minutes because the patient indicated a headache and was unable to focus; nurse (name) was informed."

Summary

Goal development and writing should reflect logical culmination of the assessment analysis. Information should be short, concise, and at the same time, include important details. Various factors can impact rehabilitation process in positive and negative ways. These details are important to include to aid the reader with understanding the choice of therapy goals approaches. In addition, reports and goals must adhere to the payor's current regulations and standards for reimbursement purposes. The regulations change periodically; therefore a clinician must pay attention to all the changes. A novice clinician often requires guidance from an experienced clinician.

Case Scenarios

The following case scenarios are based on a real patient during different points of his recovery. All of the patient's identifiable information has been changed to protect his privacy. There were two initial evaluation reports, in two different settings, in the course of the patient's rehabilitation. The format of the descriptions is typical of evaluation reports in a medical setting. These reports may not be written in grammatically complete sentences. In an electronic medical record (EMR), these reports may be even further condensed into checklists with summaries.

Case Scenarios *(continued)*

Case Scenario 1

Patient (pt) is a 54-year-old monolingual English-speaking male, KT. Pt had CVA 1 month ago and is seen for initial evaluation. Pt presents with right upper/lower extremities hemiparesis. KT has received speech therapy (ST), occupational therapy (OT), and physical therapy (PT) in an inpatient rehabilitation facility and is currently discharged to home-care. Pt resides at home with spouse and their two children (25-year-old daughter, N, and 15-year-old son, K). KT had worked as a manager at the cable company and is currently on disability due to physical and communication limitations. KT reports "difficulties with talking," the spouse—difficulties understanding KT. Pt reported that his current goal is to get functional communication to manage daily needs with a possibility to return back to work in the future.

Auditory comprehension: Comprehension of simple yes/no questions was good. Difficulties were noted with syntactically complex questions and structured conversation. Use of repetition, rephrasing, and/or visual cues was helpful.

Reading comprehension: Pt reported that he avoids reading as he feels overwhelmed. Reading to be assessed.

Verbal expression: KT's verbal output is limited to appropriate 1–2 word utterances, produced with hesitations and pauses. Pt indicates that he forgets words. Once cued, pt attempts to describe intended word but he is unsuccessful. He occasionally adds gestures or calls his wife to provide necessary information. Pt is able to accurately name 5 out of 15 pictures of common objects. Pt benefits from phonemic cues (not verbal cues). Pt is aware of his difficulties.

Written expression: Pt is right-hand dominant, unable to write with his right hand because of hemiparesis. Pt uses his left hand to print his name. The writing is slow, legibility is good.

Cognitive abilities: Basic cognitive skills are assessed via simple yes/no questions and visual cues (calendar). KT appears to be oriented x3, some difficulties are noted with identifying accurate information on the calendar as KT was confusing digits.

Oral motor examination: Facial symmetry is present at rest. Labial and lingual strength and range of motion (ROM) and diadochokinetic rates are adequate.

Speech/voice: Articulatory precision and vocal quality are good. Speech intelligibility is good.

Swallowing: Pt has no complaints of swallowing difficulties. Pt is on regular consistency diet with thin liquids. Assessment of swallowing reveals functional swallowing for current diet.

📋 Case Scenarios *(continued)*

Case Scenario Summary

KT presents with moderate mixed aphasia, characterized by good comprehension for simple questions and limited verbal output of 1–2 word utterances. KT has moderate word finding difficulties resulting in hesitations, frustrations, unsuccessful attempts to describe the intended word. Pt states that his current needs are to be able to communicate with family/doctors. Pt is very motivated, with a supportive family.

Recommendations

Individual speech therapy 2×/week for 6–8 weeks with focus on improving receptive and expressive abilities to communicate with family and medical staff.

Exercise 1

Using the framework outlined by Helm-Estabrooks and Albert (2004) and information from the evaluation, define the following:

What KT cannot do:

A. _____

B. _____

C. _____

D. _____

E. _____

What KT can do:

A. _____

B. _____

C. _____

D. _____

E. _____

What KT does do:

A. _____

B. _____

C. _____

D. _____

E. _____

📋 **Case Scenarios** *(continued)*

What KT wants to do (consider his current and future agenda):

A. _____

B. _____

C. _____

D. _____

E. _____

What KT needs to do (what skills he should have to communicate successfully with his family or medical personnel):

A. _____

B. _____

C. _____

D. _____

E. _____

Exercise 2

What therapy approaches will be beneficial for this patient? Refer to the list of five approaches that are not mutually exclusive.

A. _____

B. _____

C. _____

D. _____

E. _____

Exercise 3

Write several goals to address in therapy. Think about various ways to measure the target behavior; for example, you can measure them by accuracy, consistency, type and amount of cues, presence or absence of distractions, task complexity, and so forth. Use the following example as a model:

Pt will _____(describe the goal/task) with ___% accuracy without cues; with _____% accuracy with _____ cues (specify type [verbal, visual, phonemic, written, placement] and amount [min, mod, max]).

Caregiver will _____ (describe the goal/task) _____% of the time without cues, _____% of the time with model (or cues, specify) _____.

A. _____

_____

_____.

📋 Case Scenarios *(continued)*

B. _____

_____

_____.

C. _____

_____

_____.

D. _____

_____

_____.

E. _____

_____

_____.

Exercise 4

Should reading and writing be considered a part of therapy for this patient? What factors and constraints should be considered? What additional information would be needed to make the decision? (Hint: Consider the patient's background, current and future goals, family support, availability of assessment information, physical limitations, etc.)

_____

_____

_____

_____

_____

Case Scenario 2

(This scenario is for the same patient, KT, but it occurs 6 months later. He has had speech therapy in the home and is now being treated as an outpatient in the clinic. To distinguish these two cases, the initials for this case are KT2).

📋 Case Scenarios (continued)

Pt is a 54-year-old monolingual English-speaking male, KT2, with CVA 6 months ago and is being seen for the initial evaluation. Pt has received ST in home care setting and brings his notebook with exercises with him. Pt comes with his spouse who assists with some background information. KT2 reports "difficulties with getting the words out," the spouse—that his messages are sometimes confusing. As per KT2 and his spouse, pt has made good progress in the previous therapy and currently plans to continue ST with the goal to return back to work.

KT2 has worked as a field manager at the cable company and is currently receiving disability benefits. KT2 reports that he had to spend most of the time away from his office and that most of the communication was done via smartphone and required fast responses to the messages.

Auditory comprehension: Comprehension of simple and complex yes/no questions and simple conversations is good. Mild difficulties are noted with syntactically complex sentences/questions. Pt benefits from repetitions.

Reading comprehension: Pt reads common words and identifies matching pictures with 80% accuracy. Spelling cues and refocusing improves his accuracy. Pt occasionally confuses words with close spelling graphemes. Reading comprehension of simple questions is good. Difficulties are noted with syntactically complex questions and short paragraphs.

Verbal expression: KT2 names pictures of common objects with 90% accuracy when given additional time. He provides four items in the common category. KT2 attempts to generate simple descriptive narratives. The narratives are adequate in the organization but are often confusing as KT2 has semantic and phonemic paraphasias, incomplete sentences (lacking grammar words and verbs), moderate hesitations, pauses, and part/whole word repetitions.

Written expression: Pt is right-hand dominant. He reports that he had been unable to use his right hand because of the CVA; however, he notices significant progress in this area. During the assessment pt uses his right hand to write his name and one sentence about himself. Legibility is good. Sentence structure is adequate, grammatical markers are absent. Interesting to note, when pt reads his sentences aloud he produces all the necessary grammatical markers.

Cognitive abilities: KT2 is oriented x3. Some difficulties are noted with specific dates and appeared to relate to word finding difficulties as pt has no difficulty identifying the similar information on the calendar. Pt has good awareness of his difficulties. He has good nonverbal reasoning and problem-solving skills based on observation during the assessment.

Case Scenarios *(continued)*

Oral motor examination: Facial symmetry is present at rest. Labial and lingual strength and ROM are within normal limits (WNL).

Speech/voice: Articulatory precision and vocal quality are good. Speech intelligibility is good.

Swallowing: Pt has no complaints of swallowing difficulties. Pt is on a regular consistency diet with thin liquids.

Case Scenario Summary

KT2 presents with mild to moderate expressive aphasia. KT2's major difficulties are in the areas of verbal and written expression such as generation of complete sentences, organized and cohesive narratives, word-finding difficulties, and impaired reading comprehension for complex material. Pt is very motivated with a supportive family. He is eager to return to work.

Recommendations

1. Therapy is recommended 2 times a week for 6 weeks. However, pt reports inability to attend 2 times per week as he depends on his spouse driving so he asks therapy to be 1 time per week.
2. Long-term goal is to improve KT2's receptive and expressive communication skills to return to work.
3. Findings and recommendations were discussed with KT2 and his spouse and they agreed.

Exercise 1

The following goals have been developed over several therapy sessions. Provide the rationale for each goal.
1. Pt will use strategies to compensate for word finding difficulties (e.g., circumlocution, use of synonyms) with 90% accuracy with cues, 50% without cues.

   Rationale
   _____

2. Pt will verbally generate complete simple sentences with minimal clinician support (e.g., choice of two, interpersonal feedback) with 90% accuracy with cues.

   Rationale
   _____

3. Pt will organize and verbally generate short narratives with 80% accuracy with moderate clinician support/cues.

   Rationale
   _____

4. Pt will write simple complete sentences with 90% accuracy with cues.

   Rationale
   _____

Case Scenarios *(continued)*

5. Pt will identify erroneous spelling (nonsense words) in written sentences with 50% accuracy without cues, and correct the words independently with 50% accuracy and 95% accuracy with clinician cueing.

Rationale

6. Pt will identify erroneous semantic words in written sentences with 60% accuracy without cues. Pt will correct the words with 50% independently, 80% with cues.

Rationale

7. Pt will improve comprehension of 3–7 sentence length business letters as assessed via his responses to WH questions with 90% accuracy without cues.

Rationale

8. Pt will improve comprehension of short passages (e.g., news) and will respond to written closed-ended WH questions with 80% accuracy without cues.

Rationale

Exercise 2

Not all of KT2's goals are listed in Exercise 1. What goals would you add, and why do you think KT2 would benefit from them? Write the goals and provide rationales.

REVIEW QUESTIONS

1. Which of the following is not part of the World Health Organization's ICF framework?
   a. How the disability impacts a patient's functioning
   b. Personal factors
   c. Financial factors
   d. Contextual factors
   e. Environmental factors

2. Which of the following assessment types is most suitable to catch the complexity of speech and cognitive–communicative impairments in individuals with neurogenic communication disorders?
   a. Standardized assessment
   b. Informal assessment
   c. Dynamic assessment
   d. Interview
   e. Questionnaire

3. Why are goals that target the prevention of communicative failures important to include in the rehabilitation process?
   a. They address patient safety.
   b. They prevent social isolation.
   c. They prevent behavioral failures.
   d. They improve the patient's and the caregiver's quality of life.
   e. All of the above are true.

4. In assessment tools, a backward approach takes into consideration the
   a. patient's specific outcome goals.
   b. patient's medical and speech cognitive–communicative diagnosis.
   c. patient's personality and education level.
   d. availability of caregivers.
   e. patient's physical abilities.

5. Written goals should be functional, measurable, and justify the need for skilled services. Which of the following goals includes all three requirements?
   a. The patient will articulate one-word responses with fair intelligibility most of the time.
   b. The patient will point to pictures of common objects in a field of three images with 90 percent accuracy.
   c. The patient will locate required information in the calendar with 90 percent accuracy given moderate verbal cues.
   d. The patient will read titles of newspaper articles with minimal cues.
   e. The clinician will observe how the patient uses a basic communication board.

REFERENCES

American Speech-Language-Hearing Association. (2007). Overview of documentation for Medicare outpatient therapy services. Retrieved from http://www.asha.org/practice/reimbursement/medicare/medicare_documentation/

American Speech-Language-Hearing Association. (2016). Scope of practice in speech-language pathology. Retrieved from http://www.asha.org/policy/SP2016-00343/

American Speech-Language-Hearing Association. (2017a). International classification of functioning, disability, and health (ICF). Retrieved from http://www.asha.org/slp/icf/

American Speech-Language-Hearing Association. (2017b). Medicare coverage of speech-language pathologists and audiologists. Retrieved from https://www.asha.org/practice /reimbursement/medicare/

Assessment with Living with Aphasia (ALA) Shop. (n.d.). Retrieved September 10, 2017, from http://www.aphasia.ca/shop/assessment-for-living-with-aphasia-toolkit/

Avent, J., Glista, A., Wallace, S., Jackson, J., Hishioka, J., & Yip, W. (2005). Family information needs about aphasia. *Aphasiology, 19*, 365–375.

Brookshire, R. (2003). *Introduction to neurogenic communication disorders* (6th ed.). St. Louis, MO: Elsevier Mosby.

Brookshire, R. (2015). *Introduction to neurogenic communication disorders* (8th ed.). St. Louis, MO: Elsevier Mosby.

Burns, M. S., & Halper, A. S. (1988). *Speech-language treatment of the aphasias: An integrated clinical approach.* Rockville, MD: Aspen.

Grawburg, M., Howe, T., Worrall, L., & Scarinci, N. (2013). A qualitative investigation into third-party functioning and third-party disability in aphasia: Positive and negative experiences of family members of people with aphasia. *Aphasiology, 27*(7), 828–848.

Helm-Estabrooks, N., & Albert, M. L. (2004). *Manual of aphasia and aphasia therapy* (2nd ed.). Austin, TX: PRO-ED.

Holland, A. (1982, June). Remarks on observing aphasic people. *Proceedings of the Clinical Aphasiology Conference*, Oshkosh, WI. Retrieved from http://aphasiology.pitt.edu/archive/00000749/

Holland, A. (2012). Counseling around the edges of traditional treatment. In R. Goldfarb (Ed.), *Translational speech-language pathology and audiology* (pp. 343–352). San Diego, CA: Plural.

Irwin, B. (2012). Patient-reported outcome measures in aphasia. *SIG 2 Perspectives on Neurophysiology and Neurogenic Speech and Language Disorders, 22*(4), 160–166.

Kagan, A. (2011). A-FROM in action at the Aphasia Institute. *Seminars in Speech and Language, 32*, 216–228.

Kagan, A., & Gailey, G. F. (1993). Functional is not enough: training conversation partners for aphasic adults. In A. L. Holland & M. M. Forbes (Eds.), *Aphasia treatment: World perspectives* (pp. 199–225). San Diego, CA: Singular Publishing Group, Inc.

Kagan, A., & Simmons-Mackie, N. (2007). Beginning with the end: The outcome-driven assessment and intervention with life participation in mind. *Topics in Language Disorders, 27*(4), 309–317.

Kagan, A., Simmons-Mackie, N., Rowland, A., Huijbregts, M., Shumway, E., McEwen, S., . . . Sharp, S. (2008). Counting what counts: A framework for capturing real-life outcomes of aphasia intervention. *Aphasiology, 22*(3), 258–280.

Ledwon-Robinson, E. (2016). The quest for cognitive treatment coverage. *The ASHA Leader, 21*, 20–21.

Lyon, J. G. (2009). Resuming daily life with expressive forms of severe aphasia: Observations of adults who have successfully made life transitions and clinical implications. *SIG 2 Perspectives on Neurophysiology and Neurogenic Speech and Language Disorders, 19*(1), 23–29.

McGill University. (2017). Bilingual aphasia test (BAT). Retrieved from http://www.mcgill.ca /linguistics/research/bat/

Paradis, M. (2004). *A neurolinguistic theory of bilingualism.* Philadelphia, PA: John Benjamins.

Paradis, M. (2011). Principles underlying the bilingual aphasia test (BAT) and its uses. *Clinical Linguistics & Phonetics, 25*(6–7), 427–443.

Paradis, M., & Libben, G. (2014). *The assessment of bilingual aphasia.* New York, NY: Psychology Press.

Simmons-Mackie, N. (2009). Thinking beyond language: Intervention for severe aphasia. *SIG 2 Perspectives on Neurophysiology and Neurogenic Speech and Language Disorders, 19*(1), 15–22.

Turkstra, L., Coelho, C., & Ylvisaker, M. (2005). The use of standardized tests for individuals with cognitive–communication disorders. *Seminars in Speech and Language, 26*(4), 215–222.

World Health Organization. (2002). *Towards a common language for functioning, disability and health: ICF the International Classification of Functioning, Disability and Health.* Retrieved from http://www.who.int/classifications/icf/icfbeginnersguide.pdf

Ylvisaker, M. E. (1998). *Traumatic brain injury rehabilitation: Children and adolescents.* Oxford: Butterworth-Heinemann.

ADDITIONAL RESOURCES

Academy of Neurologic Communication Disorders and Sciences. www.ancds.org
American Speech-Language-Hearing Association. www.asha.org

CHAPTER 8

Augmentative and Alternative Communication

Cindy G. Arroyo

Key Terms

Aided language stimulation
Augmentative and alternative
  communication (AAC)
Communicative competence
Feature matching
High-technology strategies
Low-technology strategies
No-technology strategies

Participation model
Picture Exchange Communication
  System (PECS)
Rate enhancement
Speech-generating devices
System for Augmented Language
Zero-exclusion policy

Introduction

Augmentative and alternative communication (AAC) is an area of clinical practice that implements procedures and processes to compensate for temporary or permanent impairments, activity limitations, and participation restrictions of individuals with severe impairments of speech or language production or comprehension, including spoken and written communication (American Speech-Language-Hearing Association [ASHA], 2005). The concept of AAC has been part of the speech-language pathology field since its inception. As speech-language pathologists, we have always searched for techniques and strategies to improve the expressive abilities of individuals with complex communication needs.

AAC is a system that employs symbols, aids, strategies, and techniques (Beukelman & Mirenda, 2013). Symbols are either unaided or aided. Unaided symbols are characterized by an individual using his or her body to convey the message through the use of gestures, facial expressions, or sign language. Aided symbols require external tools or devices, which may include communication boards or books, memory wallets, or **speech-generating devices**. An AAC strategy contributes to the efficiency and effectiveness of a message, such as **rate enhancement** using word prediction (ASHA, 2004, 2005; Beukelman & Mirenda, 2013). Techniques are methods for transmitting messages (e.g., using direct selection by pointing, typing on a keyboard, or using an eye gaze).

Further classifications of aided AAC modes typically refer to **no-technology strategies**, **low-technology strategies**, and **high-technology strategies**. No-technology strategies involve symbol representations on a board or in a book or wallet. These methods have no voice output, so they depend on the communication partners (e.g., family members, peers, and friends) to be in close proximity to the AAC user so they can interpret the messages. Over the past few decades, increased options in technology have resulted in a wide range of systems that provide voice output, and this has resulted in more efficient communication in a variety of environments and less reliance on communication partners (Light & McNaughton, 2013). Low-technology strategies use devices that provide voice output that is digitized (recorded) rather than computer generated, and there are limitations in the message-generating and storage capabilities. These devices may be an appropriate option for beginning communicators, such as young children or individuals with cognitive limitations. They may also be used as part of a diagnostic evaluation or as a temporary or transitional tool for an individual in a specialized setting, such as an intensive care unit or a rehabilitation facility. High-technology strategies are computer based, with synthesized voice options and limitless messaging and storage capabilities. These devices typically include other options, such as rate enhancement features (e.g., word and phrase prediction) and the ability to operate phones, computer programs, environmental controls, and so forth. The introduction of mobile devices, including iPhones and iPads with AAC apps, have also expanded options for individuals with complex communication needs and have brought AAC into the mainstream, enhancing public awareness and acceptance (Light & McNaughton, 2013). However, these advances in technology have also presented challenges for the evaluation and decision-making process in matching an AAC system to an individual's strengths and needs. As a result, AAC recommendations are sometimes made without careful consideration of the individual's skills, needs, and preferences (Light & McNaughton, 2013).

It has been estimated that more than 3.5 million Americans have such complex communication needs that they cannot communicate effectively using natural speech alone (Beukelman & Mirenda, 2013). Individuals of all ages, who have diverse languages, cultures, and ethnicities, are considered for AAC assessment and intervention (Light & McNaughton, 2014; Soto & Yu, 2014). Both young children and adults with delays or deficits in speech or language development may be considered for AAC, including those with developmental disabilities (e.g., autism spectrum disorders, cerebral palsy, Down syndrome, and other intellectual disabilities) and those who communicate with natural speech but require augmentative strategies to increase their intelligibility and communicative effectiveness (Light & McNaughton, 2013, 2014). Individuals who are striving to recover their speech or language skills due to an acquired disorder (e.g., resulting from traumatic brain injury, stroke, and spinal cord injuries) may also benefit from AAC strategies. Individuals who have been diagnosed with a degenerative neurological condition, such as primary progressive aphasia, amyotrophic lateral sclerosis (ALS), or dementia, experience a loss of speech or language skills; in such cases, AAC may be permanently implemented. In other cases, such as Guillan-Barré syndrome, childhood apraxia of speech, and with intubation, the need for AAC may be temporary (Light & McNaughton, 2013, 2014).

The field of AAC has spread worldwide, as indicated by the designation of the International Society for Augmentative and Alternative Communication as a nongovernmental organization in a consultative status with the United Nations Economic and Social Council (Light & McNaughton, 2014). An emphasis has been placed on the development of communication in the context of social interaction, and the individualized needs and preferences of the AAC user should be paramount. Additionally, the increasing diversity of individuals who may require AAC assessment and interventions must be considered by professionals. This includes age, diagnosis, culture, and ethnicity (Light & McNaughton, 2014; Oommen & McCarthy, 2015; Soto & Yu, 2014).

Comprehensive Assessment

An ASHA position statement (2005) emphasizes the importance of team collaboration in the process of assessing and developing functional goals, with the individual who has complex communication needs being an integral part of the team. Additionally, the individual's family or caregivers and other significant communication partners should be involved in the assessment and intervention process (ASHA, 2004). A primary team member is the AAC specialist, a professional who consistently provides direct AAC intervention services, instructs others about AAC, and formulates and implements specific AAC interventions (Beukelman & Mirenda, 2013). Other team members may include professionals and individuals who can facilitate and support AAC in a variety of environments. For example, a child's classroom teacher may provide important information regarding his or her educational, cognitive, and social skills and needs. Physical therapists or occupational therapists may be important resources with regard to supportive seating and upper extremity function, both of which are essential to maximize effective visual and motoric access to utilize AAC systems. The importance of team collaboration and integration in assessment, service delivery, and goal development has been increasingly recognized, particularly in inclusive settings (Calculator, 2009).

The implementation of AAC should be considered for all individuals with significant communication impairments. In the 1970s and 1980s, an AAC assessment was often based on an individual's eligibility or candidacy. Individuals were often deemed not eligible based on their chronological age (too young or too old), diagnosis (e.g., childhood apraxia of speech, due to concerns that AAC systems might inhibit the development of natural speech), or cognitive level (prerequisite skills, such as object permanence, were expected). Funding restrictions and limiting policies have also impacted individuals' access to AAC assessments and services (Beukelman & Mirenda, 2013). AAC assessment and intervention now stresses a **zero-exclusion policy** in which all individuals are entitled to assessment and consideration for AAC strategies, techniques, and devices, regardless of age, ethnicity, or diagnosis (ASHA, 2005; Lloyd, Fuller, & Arvidson, 1997).

In 1988, Beukelman and Mirenda introduced the **participation model** as a framework for implementing AAC assessments and interventions, eliminating the candidacy model. The participation model was updated in 2013 and is widely used as a guide for AAC assessment. In the participation model, the initial phase identifies the individual's current communication needs and abilities. ASHA also supports a comprehensive needs assessment to identify features that inhibit an individual's ability to communicate effectively, participate in daily activities, and maintain quality of life (ASHA, 2005).

A comprehensive AAC assessment should include background information, including medical and developmental history, cultural considerations, and previous interventions. Visual and audiological assessments should be obtained, and gross and fine motor physical skills should be assessed. A thorough assessment of receptive language skills should include comprehension of messages communicated by natural speech, manual signs, graphic symbols, and other symbolic forms of communication. Expressive communication should be evaluated for adequacy of natural speech and the potential to use or increase natural speech. Semantics, syntax, morphology, and pragmatics should also be assessed. Cognitive functioning may be assessed in young children, through play skills and understanding of cause and effect. Literacy skills, such as spelling, reading, and writing, and the ability to use rate enhancement features like word prediction should be assessed with increased age. Information may be gathered from both formal, standardized assessments and informal, observational assessments. An accurate profile of the AAC user's skills may be challenging due to a lack of appropriate standardized instruments for use with individuals who have significant communication or physical impairments (Beukelman & Mirenda, 2013; Lloyd et al., 1997).

Ideally, assessments should be conducted in natural contexts, including communication environments that the individual will likely encounter and the communication partners who may be involved. This may be accomplished through ongoing or dynamic assessments, rather than a single assessment in one particular setting. Additionally, barriers to implementing effective communication strategies should be identified. These may include policies, practices, attitudes, knowledge, and skills (ASHA, 2005; Beukelman & Mirenda, 2013).

The next phase in the participation model is to conduct a detailed assessment of the individual's future needs to accommodate potential changes in capabilities, lifestyle, and environment (Beukelman & Mirenda, 2013). For example, a young child requires AAC interventions that will support his or her educational needs and the development of language, syntax, and literacy. An individual with a degenerative disease such as ALS may require AAC interventions to accommodate the loss of motoric abilities and changing environments. Beukelman and Mirenda (2013) also suggest conducting a participation inventory, which identifies consistent activities and settings the individual participates in, as well as potential communication partners.

If standardized tests are used, modifications may need to be implemented, such as adaptations for individuals with upper extremity limitations to use eye gaze as a response method. Standardized test scores should never be used to compare individuals with complex communication needs to peers of the same chronological age without disabilities, nor should scores be used to identify an individual as "eligible" for AAC services (Beukelman & Mirenda, 2013).

Feature Matching for Assistive Technologies

The assessment and subsequent intervention should be driven by a systematic process in which the individual's strengths and needs, both current and future, are matched to appropriate tools and strategies (Gosnell, Costello & Shane, 2011). This process is referred to as **feature matching** (Costello & Shane, 1994) and is widely used by AAC specialists (Beukelman & Mirenda, 2013). However, AAC technologies, such as high-technology speech-generating devices and iPad apps, are often selected based on popularity or the clinician's familiarity with them. In this case, the individual may need to adapt to the demands of the technology; however, it is possible that the most appropriate technology was not recommended for that individual (Light & McNaughton, 2013).

Based on the assessment results, the team should be able to identify several AAC devices or techniques that match the individual's needs and abilities, and the devices or technologies should be trialed to determine the optimal recommendation. This process of feature matching requires the AAC specialist or team to know about a variety of AAC options or appropriate resources (Beukelman & Mirenda, 2013). If the clinician does not possess this knowledge and does not have the skills needed to perform an AAC assessment, he or she has a professional responsibility to recognize the need for a consultation or referral to professionals who can provide quality services to individuals with AAC needs (ASHA, 2005).

The frequency and duration of therapy should be determined on an individual basis. Generally, individual treatments sessions are initiated after the AAC strategy or device has been recommended so the treatment team can identify individualized goals. A group intervention may be useful in some environments, such as schools and day treatment centers where individuals may benefit from social interaction and peer modeling.

Policy barriers to AAC implementation have been significantly reduced through advocacy efforts that changed restrictive practices in the United States. For example, the Individuals with Disabilities Education Act of 2004 mandated the provision of AAC devices and services for individuals with complex communication needs. The Assistive Technology Act Amendment of 2004 (PL 108–364) and the Americans with Disabilities Act of 1990 (PL 101–336) secured the right for individuals to have access to assistive technology, which includes speech-generating devices (Beukelman & Mirenda, 2013).

Funding sources for speech-generating devices are available across the life-span (e.g., early intervention programs, school districts, Medicaid, Medicare, and private insurance) and should be explored on an individual basis to ensure access to the recommended device (ASHA, 2005; Beukelman & Mirenda, 2013). As such, recommendations should not be determined based on the cost of a device. It is important to identify and remediate possible barriers to AAC assessment and intervention. Knowledge barriers, characterized by limitations in information, training, and skills, may preclude facilitators, evaluators, and other communication partners from implementing and supporting appropriate communication strategies and decisions. Finally, there may be barriers to AAC implementation based on the attitudes of others (Beukelman & Mirenda, 2013). Unfortunately, there continue to be misconceptions and assumptions regarding individuals with complex communication needs.

Forming Specific Goals

The development of appropriate goals requires a client-centered, individualized approach to ensure positive outcomes and a person–technology fit (Light & McNaughton, 2014; Oommen & McCarthy, 2015).

Individuals who use AAC represent a diverse population in terms of ages, diagnoses, and cultural and linguistic backgrounds. The goals should address the communication needs of the individual with respect to these factors, as well as their communication environments and communication partners. A young child or an individual with developmental disabilities or cognitive impairments may be considered a beginning or emergent communicator. For these individuals, goals often focus on early communicative behaviors using AAC strategies such as using eye gaze or pointing to an object or symbol to reject, request, or respond. An individual with more advanced receptive and expressive language abilities, potentially school-aged individuals, would benefit from goals that focus on expanding semantic, syntactic, and pragmatic skills. An adult recovering from a traumatic brain injury may be in a transitional stage of recovery, and the goals may focus on skills such as the ability to sequence information in a logical manner or to ask and answer a variety of question forms. An adult with an acquired progressive neurological disease like ALS, in which cognitive and receptive language abilities are generally intact, would be considered an independent communicator with AAC needs. This person's goals would be focused on operational competencies, such as using word prediction features or page-linking capabilities on a high-tech AAC device, to maximize their communication efficiency.

AAC may include many different strategies and devices. Oftentimes AAC goals and interventions focus too much on the technology or device and not enough on the individual's needs and skills (Light & McNaughton, 2013). If AAC technologies or devices are used, they should be viewed merely as tools to help develop **communicative competence** (Binger, 2008).

Successful communication requires interaction; therefore, AAC goals and interventions must include the patient's family and other significant communication partners. This includes teaching them the necessary strategies and skills to support interactions and communicative competency (Blackstone, Williams, & Wilkins, 2007; Light & McNaughton, 2013).

The performance levels of goals should be obtained from various sources (e.g., parents, teachers, peers, other communication partners) in multiple environments. This process is called *social validation* (Schlosser, 2003).

Intervention Approaches

Similar to goal development, the implementation of AAC interventions must be individualized. In a broad sense, interventions should consider information and relevant messages for communication, reasons and motivation to communicate, ways in which to communicate, and communication partners and environments (Beukelman & Mirenda, 2013; Lloyd et al., 1997).

Interventions for young children and beginning communicators should follow a developmental model, supporting all aspects of language and communication development. This includes adding vocabulary on a regular basis and facilitating increasingly complex syntactic and linguistic messages (Light & Drager, 2007). AAC interventions have been noted to focus too heavily on the communicative functions of labeling and requesting, and the vocabulary or symbols often reflect a preponderance of nouns. In longitudinal and retrospective studies, AAC users were reported to have pragmatic deficits, limitations in morphology and syntax, reduced length of utterance, and phonological and literacy deficits (Light, 2003).

Parents may be reluctant to implement AAC strategies for their young children because they think it could impede the development of natural speech (Cress & Marvin, 2003; Romski & Sevcik, 2005). However, extensive evidence disputes this assumption; in fact, it shows that, where possible, AAC intervention may facilitate gains in speech production (Millar, Light & Schlosser, 2006; Romski et al., 2010). AAC interventions should always be multimodal, and they should simultaneously target both aided AAC strategies and unaided strategies, such as gestures and natural speech (Oommen & McCarthy, 2015).

Several AAC intervention strategies have focused on encouraging clinicians and communication partners to model the use of a child's aided language system. These include **aided language stimulation** (Goossens, 1989; Harris & Reichle, 2004) and the **System for Augmented Language** (Romski & Sevcik, 1996). Aided modeling provides verbal modeling and modeling the use of the child's communication device (Kent-Walsh, Binger, & Buchanan, 2015). Improvements in the production of multisymbol messages have been seen in investigations using aided modeling as an intervention strategy (Binger & Light, 2007; Kent-Walsh, Binger, & Malani, 2010).

The **Picture Exchange Communication System (PECS)** is a widely used training tool that was originally developed for children with autism spectrum disorders to facilitate self-initiated functional communication (Bondy & Frost, 2001). It utilizes principles of applied behavior analysis, with prompts, reinforcement, and error correction strategies specified at each training phase. Children are trained to request desired items from a variety of communication partners by exchanging a picture or symbol with the partner. The system progresses to building sentences and developing the ability to comment (Bondy & Frost, 2001). Although more research is needed, some empirical evidence supports PECS as an effective intervention for individuals across the life-span who are considered beginning communicators (Beukelman & Mirenda, 2013; Preston & Carter, 2009).

Traditionally, AAC interventions have focused on providing strategies to express wants and needs. The field has grown to recognize that effective communication must foster the development of social relationships with a variety of partners, utilizing a variety of communicative functions. Communication partners should be included in the intervention process so they can learn ways to successfully support communicative interactions (Kent-Walsh & McNaughton, 2005; Light & McNaughton, 2014).

The importance of including literacy in AAC interventions has been increasingly recognized to provide the AAC user with skills for educational and vocational purposes, along with the ability to participate in mainstream social media (Light & McNaughton, 2014; Ruppar, Dymond, & Gaffney, 2011).

The integration and use of AAC in the classroom setting can be facilitated by developing goals that specify interactions or activities that the child typically encounters in that environment. Classroom personnel should be trained to ensure their support of AAC use in the classroom (Calculator, 2009; Schlosser, 2003).

Interventions for the adult and geriatric populations should focus on meaningful life outcomes and address the demands of daily living and functional tasks (ASHA, 2004; Fried-Oken, Beukelman, & Hux, 2011). Across the life-span, changes in quality of life as a result of AAC interventions should be recognized by the AAC user and his or her family and other relevant communication partners (ASHA, 2004). Additionally, increased globalization has expanded the need for some individuals to develop AAC skills and communicative competencies in more than one language and across different environments, with different communication partners (Light & McNaughton, 2014).

The National Joint Committee for the Communicative Needs of Persons with Severe Disabilities stated that

> all persons, regardless of the extent or severity of their disabilities, have a basic right to affect, through communication, the conditions of their own existence. Beyond this general right, a number of specific communication rights should be ensured in all daily interactions and interventions involving persons who have severe disabilities. These basic communication rights are as follows . . . the right to have access at all times to any needed augmentative and alternative communication devices and other assistive devices, and to have those devices in good working order.
>
> (1992, pp. 42–43)

An ASHA position statement says that communication is the essence of human life and that all people have the right to communicate (ASHA, 2005). However, the definition of communication has evolved, particularly in the area of AAC. Light proposed that communicative competence requires the integration of knowledge, judgment, and skills in the linguistic, operational, social, and strategic domains (Light, 1989). Linguistic competence involves the development of skills in the native language that is spoken in the individual's family and social community. The ability to produce unaided symbols like gestures, to open a communication book, to turn pages, or to access symbols on a speech-generating device contributes to operational competence. Social competence is evaluated by an individual's ability to participate in interactions, be responsive to his or her partners, and produce a full range of communicative functions.

The purpose of AAC is to facilitate efficient and effective communicative interactions in a variety of environments to communicate wants and needs, transfer information, achieve social closeness and social etiquette, and conduct an internal dialogue (Beukelman & Mirenda, 2013; Light, 1988).

Summary

AAC encompasses a variety of strategies, processes, and techniques designed to supplement or replace natural speech. Individuals with a wide range of disabilities across the life-span can benefit from using AAC. Speech-language pathologists are primarily responsible for conducting AAC assessments and developing intervention plans and goals; however, team and family collaboration is essential. The implementation of AAC should facilitate and support language and literacy development, communicative competence, and the overall quality of life.

 ## Case Scenarios

Case Scenario 1

Jessica is a 5-year-old child with a diagnosis of autism spectrum disorder and childhood apraxia of speech. She uses gestures, signs, and a limited number of word approximations to communicate. She has also been using a high-tech, speech-generating AAC device to augment her use of sign and natural speech; the limited intelligibility of these methods is impacting her academic performance and personal–social relationships. Jessica is ambulatory and was assessed by an occupational therapist to have age-appropriate fine-motor skills for pointing and keyboarding. Her receptive language and cognitive skills are within age expectations, as indicated by a standard score of 100 (mean) on the auditory comprehension section of the Preschool Language Scale, Fifth Edition (PLS-5). Jessica's expressive language, using her AAC device and other modalities, is significantly delayed and is characterized by one- or two-word messages, limited vocabulary, and syntactic delays. Standardized testing (PLS-5) revealed a score more than 2 standard deviations below

📋 **Case Scenarios** *(continued)*

the mean on the expressive communication section. Additionally, Jessica is a passive communicator; she rarely initiates communication with her peers, and she relies on limited gestures and signs with her family at home, where the primary language is Spanish. Jessica's teacher has expressed concern with her limited participation during morning circle. Her teacher has identified music as a motivating activity for Jessica. Jessica's family has expressed frustration because they did not receive training on the AAC device, and all the messages are in English.

Jessica's use of her high-tech AAC device in the classroom must be facilitated through consultation with the teacher and in consideration of the academic curriculum.

Long-Term Goal 1

Jessica will increase her participation in the classroom and her interaction with peers using her high-tech communication device.

Short-Term Goals 1

1. During morning circle, Jessica will gesture or vocalize her desire to take a turn and will use her AAC device to indicate the day of the week or the weather three times per class period.
2. During morning circle, Jessica will spontaneously use her AAC device to greet a peer using a two-word message (e.g., Hi Amy) two times per class period.
3. Jessica will sequence three symbols, given aided language modeling, to indicate a preference during music (e.g., I want piano) two times per class period.

Jessica's family must also be involved in the training and use of the high-tech AAC system so it can be integrated into the home. A no-technology communication book, with frequently used Spanish words and phrases accompanying the symbols and pictures, will be developed for use at home to support Jessica's cultural diversity.

Long-Term Goal 2

Jessica will communicate requests and comments using her no-technology communication board at home.

Short-Term Goals 2

1. Jessica will indicate a choice by pointing to a symbol on her no-technology communication board three times during mealtimes.
2. Jessica will respond to questions posed by her mother or father by pointing to a symbol on her no-technology communication board three times per day.

Case Scenarios *(continued)*

Case Scenario 2

John is 65 years old and has recently been diagnosed with ALS, which is a progressive, degenerative disease that affects the motor neurons of the brain and spinal cord (Mitchell & Borasio, 2007). John is experiencing dysarthria (a motor speech disorder), which is associated with ALS. John's wife and family estimate that they can understand his speech 50 percent of the time in known contexts and less than 25 percent of the time in unknown contexts. His ability to communicate effectively is rapidly declining, and he is increasingly frustrated and experiencing communication breakdowns. John's primary physician has referred him for an AAC evaluation due to the progressive nature of his disease.

The clinician used the framework of Beukelman and Mirenda's participation model (2013) to gather background and medical information from John's family during the initial assessment. The results of a recent audiological evaluation revealed normal hearing; additionally, John wears glasses due to restrictions in visual acuity. His receptive language, cognitive, and literacy skills were judged to be within normal limits, based on informal and standardized measures. His motoric abilities were assessed by using a team approach that included a physical therapist and an occupational therapist. John is nonambulatory and uses a motorized wheelchair, which he operates with a joystick. His fine-motor abilities are progressively declining, but he is presently utilizing direct selection by typing on a keyboard, although his accuracy is variable.

John is a retired history professor, but he continues to publish articles, and he uses email and social media to maintain contact with former colleagues and students. He lives at home with his wife, and his daughter lives a few hours away. John enjoys trips to the university to visit with his colleagues and going to restaurants with his family.

Following the participation model (Beukelman & Mirenda, 2013), John's present and future communication needs are assessed and considered as part of the AAC recommendations. Following a comprehensive assessment and trials with several high-tech AAC devices, a funding report was submitted by the speech-language pathologist who conducted the evaluation. John received the prescribed AAC device, which accommodates his present access method (direct selection via keyboard) and will accommodate his future needs (direct selection via eye gaze) as his motoric abilities decline.

The intervention goals focused on John's communication environments, partners, and operational competence using eye gaze as a selection modality.

Case Scenarios *(continued)*

Long-Term Goal

John will use his high-tech AAC device to communicate effectively with a variety of communication partners in a variety of communication environments.

Short-Term Goals

1. John will access preprogrammed messages on his high-tech AAC device, using eye gaze, to engage in conversations with his colleagues at the university in 9 out of 10 conversational turns.
2. John will utilize the rate enhancement feature of word prediction on his high-tech AAC device, using eye gaze, with 90 percent accuracy, in formulating messages in a conversation with his wife.
3. John will initiate a conversation with the server in a restaurant and indicate his choices from the menu on his high-tech AAC device, using eye gaze, with 90 percent accuracy.
4. John will access email and social media on his high-tech AAC device, using eye gaze, and will formulate messages to his daughter with 90 percent accuracy.

REVIEW QUESTIONS

1. Which AAC strategy is *not* an example of aided communication?
   a. Communication board
   b. Speech-generating device
   c. PECS
   d. Sign language
   e. Memory wallet

2. Communicative competence includes which of the following domains?
   a. Linguistic
   b. Social
   c. Strategic
   d. Operational
   e. All of the above

3. A systematic process that assesses an individual's strengths and needs and matches them to the appropriate tools and strategies is known as which of the following?
   a. Aided language stimulation
   b. Feature matching
   c. Assistive technology
   d. PECS
   e. Communicative competence

4. A comprehensive AAC assessment should include which of the following?
   a. The individual's current and future communication needs and abilities
   b. Visual, auditory, gross, and fine-motor skills

c. Receptive and expressive language skills

d. Cognitive skills, including literacy

e. All of the above

5. Goals for the implementation of AAC strategies should consider which of the following?

a. The individual, including communication partners and environments

b. Only basic wants and needs

c. Cultural and linguistic considerations

d. A and C

e. A and B

REFERENCES

American Speech-Language-Hearing Association. (2004). *Roles and responsibilities of speech-language pathologists with respect to augmentative and alternative communication: Technical report.* Retrieved from http://www.asha.org/policy/TR2004-00262/

American Speech-Language-Hearing Association. (2005). *Roles and responsibilities of speech-language pathologists with respect to augmentative and alternative communication: Position statement.* Retrieved from http://www.asha.org/policy/PS2005-00113.htm

Beukelman, D., & Mirenda, P. (2013). *Augmentative and alternative communication* (4th ed.). Baltimore, MD: Paul H. Brookes.

Binger, C. (2008). Classroom-based language goals and interventions for children who use AAC: Back to basics. *SIG 12 Perspectives on Augmentative and Alternative Communication, 17,* 20–26.

Binger, C., & Light, J. (2007). The effect of aided AAC modeling on the expression of multi-symbol messages by preschoolers who use AAC. *Augmentative and Alternative Communication, 23,* 30–43.

Blackstone, S., Williams, M., & Wilkins, D. (2007). Key principles underlying research and practice in AAC. *Augmentative and Alternative Communication, 23,* 191–203.

Bondy, A., & Frost, L. (2001). The picture exchange communication system. *Behavior Modification, 25*(5), 725–744.

Calculator, S. N. (2009). Augmentative and alternative communication (AAC) and inclusive education for students with the most severe disabilities. *International Journal of Inclusive Education, 13*(1), 93–113.

Costello, J., & Shane, H. (1994, November). *Augmentative communication assessment and the feature matching process.* Miniseminar presented at the annual convention of the American Speech-Language-Hearing Association, New Orleans, LA.

Cress, C., & Marvin, C. (2003). Common questions about AAC services in early intervention. *Augmentative and Alternative Communication, 19*(4), 254–272.

Fried-Oken, M., Beukelman, D., & Hux, K. (2011). Current and future AAC research considerations for adults with acquired cognitive and communication impairments. *Assistive Technology, 24*(1), 56–66.

Goossens, C. (1989). Aided communication interventions before assessment: A case study of a child with cerebral palsy. *Augmentative and Alternative Communication, 5,* 14–26.

Gosnell, J., Costello, J., & Shane, H. (2011). Using a clinical approach to answer "what communication apps should we use?" *SIG 12, Perspectives on Augmentative and Alternative Communication, 20,* 87–96.

Harris, M., & Reichle, J. (2004). The impact of aided language stimulation on symbol comprehension and production in children with moderate cognitive disabilities. *American Journal of Speech-Language Pathology, 13,* 155–167.

Kent-Walsh, J., Binger, C., & Buchanan, C. (2015). Teaching children who use augmentative and alternative communication to ask inverted yes/no questions using aided modeling. *American Journal of Speech-Language Pathology, 24,* 222–236.

Kent-Walsh, J., Binger, C., & Malani, M. (2010). Teaching partners to support the communication skills of young children who use AAC: Lessons from the IMPAACT program. *Early Childhood Services, 4,* 210–226.

Kent-Walsh, J., & McNaughton, D. (2005). Communication partner instruction in AAC: Present practices and future directions. *Augmentative and Alternative Communication, 21,* 195–204.

Light, J. (1988). Interaction involving individuals using augmentative and alternative communication systems: State of the art and future directions. *Augmentative and Alternative Communication, 4,* 66–82.

Light, J. (1989). Toward a definition of communicative competence for individuals using augmentative and alternative communication systems. *Augmentative and Alternative Communication, 5,* 137–144.

Light, J. (2003). Shattering the silence: Development of communicative competence by individuals who use AAC. In J. Light, D. Beukelman & J. Reichle (Eds.), *Communicative competence for individuals who use AAC* (pp. 3–38). Baltimore, MD: Paul H. Brookes.

Light, J., & Drager, K. (2007). AAC technologies for young children with complex communication needs: State of the science and future research directions. *Augmentative and Alternative Communication, 23,* 204–216.

Light, J., & McNaughton, D. (2013). Putting people first: Re-thinking the role of technology in augmentative and alternative communication intervention. *Augmentative and Alternative Communication, 29*(4), 299–309.

Light, J., & McNaughton, D. (2014). Communicative competence for individuals who require augmentative and alternative communication: A new definition for a new era of communication? *Augmentative and Alternative Communication, 30,* 1–18.

Lloyd, L. L., Fuller, D. R., & Arvidson, H. H. (1997). *Augmentative and alternative communication: A handbook of principles and practices.* Needham Heights, MA: Allyn and Bacon.

Millar, D. C., Light, J. C., & Schlosser, R. W. (2006). The impact of augmentative and alternative communication intervention on the speech production of individuals with developmental disabilities: A research review. *Journal of Speech, Language, and Hearing Research, 49,* 248–264.

Mitchell, J. D., & Borasio, G. D. (2007). Amyotrophic lateral sclerosis. *The Lancet, 369,* 2031–2041.

National Joint Committee for the Communicative Needs of Persons with Severe Disabilities. (1992). Guidelines for meeting the communication needs of persons with severe disabilities. *National Student Speech Language Hearing Association Journal, 19,* 41–48. Retrieved from http://www.asha.org/uploadedFiles/asha/publications/cicsd/1992GuidelinesforMeeting.pdf

Oommen, E. R., & McCarthy, E. W. (2015). Simultaneous natural speech and AAC interventions for children with childhood apraxia of speech: Lessons from a speech-pathology focus group. *Augmentative and Alternative Communication, 31*(1), 63–76.

Preston, D., & Carter, M. (2009). A review of the efficacy of the picture exchange communication system intervention. *Journal of Autism and Developmental Disorders, 39,* 1471–1486.

Romski, M., & Sevcik, R. (1996). *Breaking the speech barrier: Language development through augmented means.* Baltimore, MD: Paul H. Brookes.

Romski, M., & Sevcik, R. (2005). Augmentative communication and early intervention: Myths and realities. *Infants and Young Children, 18*(3), 174–185.

Romski, M., Sevcik, R., Adamson, L., Cheslock, M., Smith, A., Barker, R., & Bakeman, R. (2010). Randomized comparison of augmented and nonaugmented language interventions for toddlers with developmental delays and their parents. *Journal of Speech, Language, and Hearing Research, 53,* 350–364.

Ruppar, A., Dymond, S., & Gaffney, J. (2011). Teachers' perspectives on literacy instruction for students who use augmentative and alterative communication. *Research and Practice for Persons with Severe Disabilities, 36*(3–4), 100–111.

Schlosser, R. W. (2003). *The efficacy of augmentative and alternative communication: Toward evidence-based practice.* San Diego, CA: Academic Press.

Soto, G., & Yu, B. (2014). Considerations for the provision of services to bilingual children who use AAC. *Augmentative and Alternative Communication, 30,* 83–92.

CHAPTER 9

Aural Rehabilitation and Habilitation

Susan Antonellis

Key Terms

Auditory training
Aural rehabilitation and
   habilitation
Categorical phrases
Competing messages
Everyday sentences

Hearing handicap surveys
Listening and Communication
   Enhancement (LACE) program
Minimal pairs
Speechreading

Introduction

Aural rehabilitation and habilitation refers to services and procedures for facilitating adequate receptive and expressive communication in individuals with hearing impairment or deafness. These services and procedures are intended for persons who demonstrate a loss of hearing sensitivity or function in communication situations. The services and procedures include, but are not limited to, monitoring hearing aid performance and the use of hearing aids or cochlear implants, **speechreading**, **auditory training**, and counseling hearing-impaired individuals and their families. An ideal aural rehabilitation or habilitation session should include auditory and speechreading activities.

According to Hipskind, speechreading is "when a listener uses visual cues by observing the speaker's mouth, facial expressions and hand movements to help perceive what is being said" (2017, p. 140). Laypersons use the term *lipreading*, but that means only the lips of the speaker provide visual cues; professionals use the term *speechreading*.

Unfortunately, aural rehabilitation and habilitation is not utilized enough. It should be used as a supplement for any hearing aid or cochlear implant user. Speech-language pathologists and audiologists can provide aural rehabilitation and habilitation services together or independently because they are within the scope of practice for both disciplines. When possible, individuals participating in aural rehabilitation should be exposed to both individual and group sessions.

Research has supported the need for aural rehabilitation and habilitation. Most recently, Kirkwood (2005) reported that today's instruments provide more patient satisfaction compared to those from 10 years earlier and that hearing aids do not play the primary role. In fact, only 6 percent of the 674 dispensing professionals in Kirkwood's survey (2005) reported hearing aids as the most important component of a successful fitting; 39 percent of the respondents reported that the counseling skills of the dispenser were most important; 26 percent identified the dispenser's fitting and programming skills as the most important; 17 percent believed the patient's personality was the number one factor in achieving satisfaction; and 12 percent identified the type and degree of the hearing loss as the most important factor of a successful fitting. Kirkwood further stated that the industry has regarded patient satisfaction a high priority; it is not really the product, but the people involved in the hearing aid fitting that are the main determinants of success (2005).

In addition, Kelly and colleagues (2013) reported that older people want more information than they receive both before and after a hearing aid fitting. Information about and attention to psychosocial aspects of care are key factors that enable people to adjust to and optimize the benefits of hearing aids. This supports the benefit of aural rehabilitation for any client with a hearing aid.

Clients who wear hearing aids would benefit from any form of aural rehabilitation and habilitation, including activities like speechreading, auditory training, using the instrument, and counseling with or without family members. The sessions should be tailored to the client's individual needs. Kobosko, Jedrzejczak, Pilka, Pankowska, and Skarzynski (2015) examined the relationship between cochlear implant satisfaction and the level of psychological distress, stress coping strategies, and self-esteem in adults who are postlingually deaf. The participants were asked to complete a mailed personal inquiry form seeking socio-demographic data, one question related to cochlear implant satisfaction, and the following questionnaires: General Health Questionnaire-28, Brief Coping Orientation to Problems Experienced, and Rosenberg Self-Esteem Scale. The study included 98 patients with postlingual deafness between the ages of 19 and 85 years who had unilateral cochlear implants. The results revealed that psychological factors—self-esteem, distress, and coping strategies—are important for cochlear implant satisfaction in postlingually deaf cochlear implant users and that there are advantages to widening the availability of various tailored forms of psychological intervention for patients with postlingual deafness after receiving a cochlear implant. These results indicate the need for additional strategies in communication to increase self-confidence in communication tasks. Skills in speechreading and the improvement of considering contextual cues would assist cochlear implant users, the same as hearing aid users.

Because understanding speech is a cognitive process—it happens in the brain—untreated hearing loss is associated with accelerated cognitive decline and a higher risk of dementia. The greater the untreated hearing loss, the greater the risk of dementia (Oticon, 2016). Clearly there is a need for services beyond choosing a hearing aid, programming the hearing aid, using the hearing aid, and maintaining the hearing aid.

Comprehensive Assessment

Before clients begin an aural rehabilitation or habilitation program, the clinician needs to assess their needs. Several diagnostic instruments are available to achieve this goal. First and foremost, every client must be seen by an audiologist to evaluate the degree and type of hearing loss. A clinical treatment plan should then be put in place before aural rehabilitation or habilitation can begin. Audiological evaluations should be guided by the following procedures that are recommended by ASHA:

- Pure-tone and speech audiometry is conducted to determine the existence, type, and degree of hearing loss on the basis of behavioral responses to acoustic stimuli.
- Acoustic immittance procedures are conducted to assess middle ear function.
- Results from the audiologic assessment will be interpreted and may result in no recommendations or further audiologic assessment/evaluation; audiologic (re)habilitative evaluation; speech-language evaluation; or medical, psychological, and/or educational referral.

Basic audiologic assessment is prompted by self-referral, family/ caregiver referral, failure of audiologic screening, or referral from other professionals.

Assessment includes the following:

- a case history
- external ear examination
- otoscopic examination
- acoustic immittance procedures (tympanometry, static immittance, and acoustic reflex measures)
- air-conduction and bone-conduction pure-tone threshold measures with appropriate masking
- speech reception thresholds or speech detection/awareness thresholds with appropriate masking
- word recognition measures with appropriate masking
- speech-language screening

Other procedures may be completed to supplement the basic audiologic assessment:

- otoacoustic emissions screening
- communication inventories and needs assessment inventories
- screening for central auditory processing disorders or other auditory disorders

Interpretation of the assessment may indicate one or more of the following:

- hearing within normal limits
- identification and degree of hearing loss
- hearing loss identified but further testing required
- patient could not be tested using standard procedures

Evaluation may result in one of the following:

- discharge and/or recommendations for routine follow-up
- referral for audiologic rehabilitation evaluation
- referral for further audiologic evaluation and/or other services (American Speech-Language-Hearing Association, 2006, pp. 14–15)

Even though speechreading tests are old, they are still beneficial. The two most common speechreading tests are the Barley Speechreading Test (1971) and the Utley Lipreading Test (1989). The Barley Speechreading Test consists of 22 unclued sentences, drawn from the CID Everyday Sentence test (Davis & Silverman, 1970), that clients are not familiar with. A score of less than 20 percent indicates little use of visual cues, and a score of greater than 60 percent indicates a good use of visual cues; there are no data for scores between 20 and 60 percent.

The Utley Lipreading Test is also a sentence test, with 32 sentences the client is not familiar with. A score is obtained after each test is performed. Generally, each sentence is presented two times with visual cues only—no voice cues. It is preferable for the client to respond in writing. The client receives a point for every word he or she speechreads. A total score is obtained and divided by the number of words in the test so a percentage can be calculated.

In addition to evaluating a client's speechreading skills, clinicians should assess the client's psychosocial skills that will play an important role during the intervention and management process. Several instruments are available for this purpose, including **hearing handicap surveys** and longer, more traditional questionnaires. Their features include relevance, diagnostic utility, compatibility with normal interviewing techniques, and good test–retest reliability, which makes them suitable for routine clinical use.

For example, the Hearing Handicap Inventory (HHI) was developed in 1990 by Newman and colleagues. The client answers questions related to hearing and responds with one of three choices: yes, no, or sometimes. A pass or fail is determined by the client's score. The HHI can be adapted for both adult and pediatric populations, but it is used mostly for adults (Newman, Weinstein, Jacobson, & Huq, 1990). After the HHI has been administered, the clinician can begin to prepare an aural rehabilitation plan for the client. The first step is to determine the need for aural rehabilitation therapy. There are several determining factors: fail score on the HHI; if the psychosocial environment is affected daily; and a score of 20 to 55 percent on either speechreading test.

Another scale is the Client Oriented Scale of Improvement (COSI), which was developed in 1997 (Dillon, James, & Ginis, 1997).

> In this method, the client effectively writes the self-report questionnaire by nominating up to five listening situations in which help with hearing is required. At the conclusion of rehabilitation, reduction in disability and the resulting ability to communicate in these specific situations is quantified. Based on correlation analysis, the COSI method is as statistically valid as the much longer, more traditional questionnaires. Other features, such as relevance, diagnostic utility, compatibility with normal interviewing techniques, and good test–retest reliability, make it particularly suitable for routine clinical use.
>
> (Dillon et al., 1997, p. 27)

Because these guidelines determine need, it is of utmost importance that each client is considered on an individual basis. Another important consideration is if the services are eligible for reimbursement. Reimbursement should always be a consideration when treating clients.

Sweetow developed the **Listening and Communication Enhancement (LACE) program** with the belief that hearing is only one element of communication ability (Neurotone, n.d.). Sweetow says that hearing is a passive function, and listening is an active process requiring intention and attention (Sweetow, 2013). Therefore, the use of proper communication strategies can shape both hearing and listening. Weinstein (2014) says that communication breakdowns associated with hearing impairment hinder a person's ability to remain socially engaged. Given the importance of social network size and the quality of social interactions, removing the barriers posed by hearing impairment has the potential to promote healthy aging.

Therapy Plan

Using the assessment scales as a guide, the clinician first needs to decide which mode of therapy—individual, group, or both—is appropriate for the client. Then the clinician must determine whether treatment will include auditory and visual training or just one of these modalities. Ideally, a speech-language pathologist and an audiologist will collaborate to develop a therapy plan. The speech-language pathologist can help plan modifications for a child in a school setting or make a plan that fits into an adult's everyday activities, and the audiologist can address auditory skills and modifications that are necessary for better hearing. Examples of such modifications are as follows:

- Adults: Assistive devices can be used, such as those for watching television, or a telephone with captions and an amplifier to help clients keep in touch with their families and friends. Preferential seating at meetings and gatherings will also help clients interact socially.
- School-aged child: Environmental modifications, such as preferential seating, a separate location for testing, and additional time for testing, can help children in school. In addition, FM transmitters and teachers for the deaf can accommodate children.

In both examples, the expertise of both speech-language pathologists and audiologists can be leveraged to make a better plan for hearing-impaired individuals.

- Aural rehabilitation can be performed on an individual basis or in a group.
- Some group sessions are conducted with spouses or children of the hearing-impaired person.
- Individual sessions can include a combination of speechreading and auditory training skills.
- Everyone has some form of speechreading skills.
- Each client brings individual needs to the sessions.
- The clinician will determine the client's needs from the speechreading tests and a thorough case history and evaluation.

Forming Specific Goals

This section contains example goals for individual and group aural rehabilitation sessions. In actual sessions, the goals would be flexible depending on the client's needs and abilities. Goals that are typical for most hearing-impaired clients are noted.

Individual Aural Rehabilitation Session

Long-Term Goal

- The client will improve communication skills utilizing both visual and auditory modalities.

    This goal would be typical in most instances in preparing an individual aural rehabilitation session. The clinician could elaborate based on other information obtained from the client during the history or from assessment scales. In working with the deaf population, this goal may be altered.

Short-Term Goals

- The client's amplification system will be assessed to ensure it is working properly.

    This goal would be addressed during each session, whether the client uses a hearing aid or has a cochlear implant. Amplification systems—both hearing aids and cochlear implants—should be checked to be sure they are in working order. Universal precautions should be used when checking the systems. A listening stethoscope and a battery tester should be available when checking the integrity of the client's instruments.

- The client will auditorily discriminate **minimal pairs** /p/ and /b/ in the initial position to obtain baseline data with 50 percent accuracy.

  This is an auditory discrimination task. A screen is used to cover the clinician's lips so the client has no visual cues. The client has a list of minimal pair words to work with. The client must identify which word he or she hears from the pairs of words presented, as shown in the following example:

Pair	Bear	Pane	Bane
Pete	Beat	Pole	Bowl
Pile	Bile	Putt	Butt
Pail	Bail	Pit	Bit
Pat	Bat	Pill	Bill

- The client will utilize speechreading abilities to identify **categorical phrases** with a specific theme to obtain baseline data with 50 percent accuracy.

  This is a speechreading task. The client will speechread phrases that belong to the assigned theme of the session. The phrases are presented in the following manner: (1) with visual cues only; (2) with auditory cues only (the clinician's lips are covered with a screen); and (3) with visual and auditory cues combined. Note the following example:

> Theme: Spring
> 1. Springtime 2. May flowers 3. Fresh air
> 4. Baseball season 5. Pastel colors 6. Birds chirping
> 7. Flowers blooming 8. April Fools' Day 9. Green grass
> 10. Blue skies 11. Tulip blossoms 12. Rain boots

- The client will utilize speechreading abilities to focus on **everyday sentences** that follow a dialogue based on the theme of the session to obtain baseline data with 50 percent accuracy.

  This is a speechreading task. The client will speechread sentences that follow dialogue. The client is reminded to take advantage of contextual cues and to concentrate on meaning and not worry about speechreading every word. The sentences are presented in the following manner: (1) with visual cues only;

Total Wght:	# Items Shipped:	#Backorder:	Delivery Instructions:
.95 LB	1	0	

JBCOMPS   1/19/18 11:43:59 Job:PRINTERBA2/880418 User:SCHEDULER   31-606597 00023 00000000 Page:00635

Complimentary Copy

PBDPICJO   JRCOMPS   1/19/18 11:43:59 Job:PRINTERBA2/880418 User:SCHEDULER   31-606597 00023 00000000 Page:00635

JONES & BARTLETT LEARNING
5 WALL STREET
BURLINGTON, MA 01803
(800) 832-0034 FAX (978) 443-8000
www.jblearning.com customerservice@jblearning.com

Customer #:	930150
Invoice#:	BO952562
Order Date:	1/18/18
Page #:	1

Ordered By:

P.O. #: 87F137C3-27FF-40DC-AC46-0
Ship Via: FedEx Ground Prepaid

Ship To #: 930150   48670820.00023

Bill To:
CASEY KECK
ARMSTRONG ST UNIVERSITY
REHABILITATION SCIENCES
11935 ABERCORN ST., SUITE 217
SAVANNAH, GA 31419
(912) 3442576

Ship To:
CASEY KECK
ARMSTRONG ST UNIVERSITY
REHABILITATION SCIENCES
11935 ABERCORN ST., SUITE 217
SAVANNAH, GA 31419
(912) 3442576

FedEx Ground Prepaid

QTY ORD	BACK ORDER	QTY SHP	ITEM #	LOCATION	DESCRIPTION	UNIT PRICE	DISC. PRICE	EXT. PRICE
					Dear CASEY KECK			
					Enclosed is your complimentary copy. Thank you very much for your interest. If you have any questions, please feel free to give us a call.			
					Sincerely,			
					LORETTA LORUSSO			
					This backorder was released against invoice # 3772527.			
1		1	EA 10480-6	JB43A.3	GOAL WRITING FOR SPEECH-LANG PATHOLOGIST & SPECIAL EDUCATO CTN @ EA		.00	.00
					9781284104806, GOZDZIEWSKI			
				Loose Pick: 1 Carton Pick:				

(2) with auditory cues only (the clinician's lips covered with a screen); and (3) with visual and auditory cues combined. Note the following example:

1.	**The weather is so beautiful today!**
2.	I know, we can finally sit outside and enjoy the sun.
3.	**After this freezing winter it's good to have some warm weather.**
4.	But all of next week it is supposed to rain!
5.	**That's typical spring weather.**
6.	I love the spring, but I can't deal with all the rain!
7.	**Is spring your favorite season?**
8.	Absolutely!
9.	**What do you love the most?**
10.	I love the beautiful flowers and the smell of fresh air.
11.	**I can't wait for my flowers to start blooming!**
12.	It's wonderful! Do you plant your own flowers?
13.	**Yes, I have a small garden in my yard.**
14.	What do you have in your garden?
15.	**For now, I only have tulips, lavender, and daffodils.**
16.	Tulips are beautiful! They're one of my favorites.
17.	**Yes, they are beautiful! I want to plant more flowers.**
18.	What else do you want to plant?
19.	**I really want to plant vegetables too!**
20.	That would be great! Good luck with your garden!

This dialogue should be presented with two speakers so the client can speechread more than one person. Nonverbal gestures should be used when presenting this dialogue.

- The client will distinguish between two **competing messages** with 100 percent accuracy and answer three out of five questions correctly.

This is an auditory task that is typical for most hearing-impaired clients. The client will listen to two different passages that are presented simultaneously. The client is instructed to concentrate on one of the two passages. The client will be given both visual and auditory cues. The client is told to concentrate on the main ideas and not to concentrate on hearing every word. After the passages are presented, the clinician asks the client some questions from the main passage to see what he or she has retained. The passage should be related to the theme of the session. As the client progresses, the passages should address the same topic to make the task more challenging.

Clinicians should encourage clients to practice these skills in everyday situations so they can carry over what they learn in the therapy session to their everyday interactions. Their families and friends become a canvas for clients to practice their speechreading skills.

Family members often ask what they can do at home to help the client. Many applications are available for hearing-impaired individuals, both children and adults. In addition, computer and web-based programs are available to assist hearing-impaired persons (refer to the "Additional Resources" section of this chapter).

Group Aural Rehabilitation Session

The following goals are for a typical aural rehabilitation session in a group setting. The most important aspect of group sessions is shared empathy among clients. Each client can share experiences that most clinicians cannot share, notably what it is like to be hearing impaired or deaf. These individuals can share their experiences of frustrating moments, impossible communication situations, and difficult listening conditions. Group sessions give clients information, and information is power.

Long-Term Goal

- The clients will improve communication skills utilizing both visual and auditory modalities.

  This goal would be typical in most instances in preparing a group aural rehabilitation session. The clinician could elaborate based on other information obtained from the clients who are participating in the group or from assessment scales.

Short-Term Goals

- The clients' amplification systems will be assessed to ensure they are working properly.

  This goal would be utilized each session, whether the clients use hearing aids or have cochlear implants. Amplification systems— both hearing aids and cochlear implants—should be checked to be sure they are in working order. Universal precautions should be used when checking the systems.
- The clients will establish rapport with one another and share their communication struggles.

  Each group should be formed with careful consideration. There should be no more than eight people in a group due to time constraints. The groups should be arranged by age and severity of hearing loss. Groups are not for everyone; some hearing-impaired or deaf individuals are not comfortable in a group situation. This should be determined during the assessment process. This goal would be utilized during each session because new clients may join at any time.

- The clients will participate in a discussion about a current event that the clinician will introduce from a news report.

  This goal will help strengthen auditory skills and speech and noise skills. It also fosters confidence in communicating within a group situation. An aural rehabilitation group allows opportunities for people to connect and share their feelings about dealing with hearing loss.

The following is another example of a group session format:

- At the first meeting, asking each hearing-impaired person and SO [significant other] to note "the worst thing about having a hearing loss." At this point, these are just noted; possible solutions come later. People are surprised how often their problems are shared by others.
- Types of hearing loss; understanding the audiogram (basically this should be a review of the information covered during the hearing aid selection process).
- Using hearing aids effectively; introduction and explanation of special features.
- Overview of the various hearing assistive technologies other than hearing aids themselves (e.g., for telephones, TV listening, smoke alarms, special purpose devices).
- Introduction to speech reading and auditory relearning. Home training programs. (Ross, 2011, para. 8)

Summary

Aural rehabilitation and habilitation is an integral part of the treatment plan for a hearing-impaired or deaf individual. The preparation and setting of goals are unique to the client's needs and wants. There is no right or wrong plan; what matters is appropriateness for an individual client. Clinicians need to devise and revise the treatment goals based on the client's struggles. Aural rehabilitation and habilitation involves not only fitting hearing aids or cochlear implants, but also providing tools to clients so they can maximize the performance of their amplification system.

Case Scenarios

Case Scenario 1

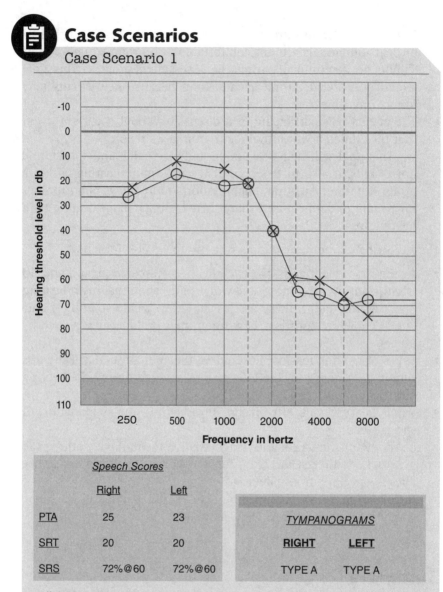

	Speech Scores				
	Right	Left			
PTA	25	23		TYMPANOGRAMS	
SRT	20	20		**RIGHT**	**LEFT**
SRS	72%@60	72%@60		TYPE A	TYPE A

Sally is 58 years old and has a bilateral mild, sloping to severe sensori-neural hearing loss (loss of the inner ear or nerve). Her speech recognition is depressed, and her middle ear function is normal. She currently wears two RIC BTE hearing aids.

Sally is working as a teacher's assistant in a special education pre-school. She has difficulty hearing both the children and, sometimes, instructions given by the teacher. Sally has social limitations. She cannot go to many employee functions because there are too many people and too much background noise. She feels embarrassed when she misunderstands.

Case Scenarios *(continued)*

Rehabilitation Plan

Sally should be enrolled in both individual and group aural rehabilitation sessions. Her goals should be measurable based on speechreading test results and baseline data collected at the initial session.

Sally's goals should include the following:

1. Good use of amplification
2. Evaluate current speechreading skills
3. Improve speechreading skills
4. Improve auditory skills in noisy environments
5. Give carry-over exercises to improve listening skills

Case Scenario 2

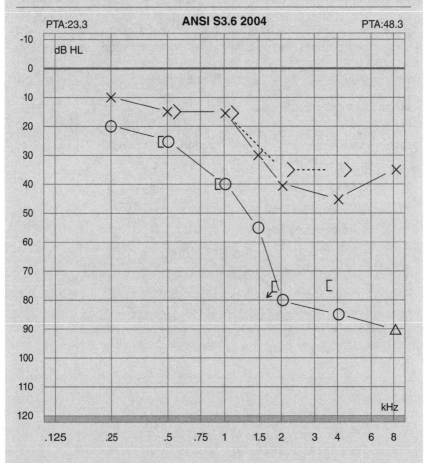

Case Scenarios *(continued)*

Speech Scores		
	Right	Left
PTA	48	23
SRT	50	20
SRS	10%	56%
AIDED SRS-AS	50%	

TYMPANOGRAMS	
RIGHT	**LEFT**
TYPE A	TYPE A

Marlene is 76 years old and has been retired for 10 years. She is depressed because her hearing has declined, and she has little speech recognition in her right ear. Her middle ear function is normal. She currently wears a hearing aid in her left ear, and it performs fairly well. In 2 weeks Marlene has an appointment for a consultation to see if she is a candidate for a cochlear implant. She does not interact socially because she cannot understand average conversational speech in most situations.

Marlene's goals should be measurable based on speechreading test results and baseline data collected at the initial session.

Rehabilitation Plan

Marlene should be enrolled in both individual and group aural rehabilitation sessions. Her goals should include the following:

1. Obtain information regarding cochlear implants
2. Discuss expectations of cochlear implants
3. Evaluate current speechreading skills
4. Improve speechreading skills
5. Improve auditory skills in noisy environments
6. Give carry-over exercises to improve listening skills

As you can see in Case Scenario 1 and Case Scenario 2, the goals are different based on the client's unique needs.

Case Scenarios *(continued)*

Case Scenario 3

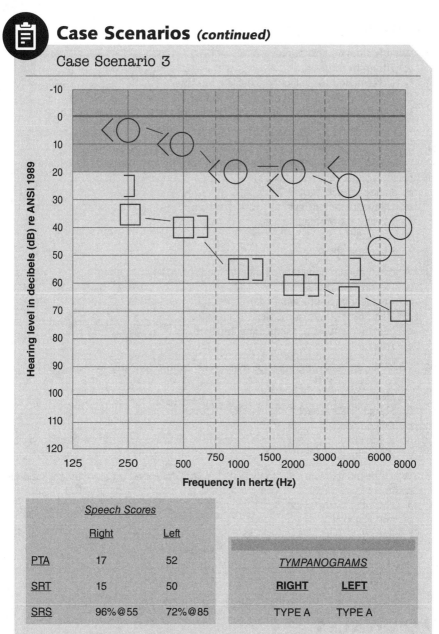

	Speech Scores	
	Right	Left
PTA	17	52
SRT	15	50
SRS	96%@55	72%@85

TYMPANOGRAMS	
RIGHT	**LEFT**
TYPE A	TYPE A

Billy is 10 years old. He experienced a sudden left sensorineural hearing loss and has depressed speech recognition in the left ear. He is having difficulty in school, especially in the presence of background noise and in larger classes. He cannot hear clearly when he sits at the back of the room. He is also losing some hearing in the right ear, and it may be progressive.

Prepare a rehabilitation plan for Billy.

REVIEW QUESTIONS

1. What is aural rehabilitation?
   a. Fitting hearing aids
   b. Determining candidacy for cochlear implants
   c. Providing services and procedures to facilitate adequate receptive and expressive communication in individuals with hearing impairment or deafness
   d. None of the above

2. Which of the following is a speechreading test that can be used to evaluate a person's speechreading ability?
   a. Barley Speechreading Test
   b. Utley Lipreading Test
   c. Mosley Speechreading Test
   d. A and B
   e. All of the above

3. Who can aural rehabilitation be performed for?
   a. Hearing aid users
   b. Cochlear implant users
   c. Significant others of the hearing impaired
   d. Family members of the hearing impaired
   e. All of the above

4. Which of the following are apps that adults can use for carry-over and to improve listening?
   a. Hearwell
   b. Starkey Hear Coach
   c. Oticon Medical
   d. B and C
   e. All of the above

5. Which of the following are tools that clinicians may need for aural rehabilitation sessions?
   a. Listening stethoscope
   b. Loudspeaker
   c. Battery tester
   d. Hearing aid batteries
   e. None of the above
   f. A, C, and D

REFERENCES

American Speech-Language-Hearing Association. (2006). *Preferred practice patterns for the profession of audiology*. Retrieved from http://www.asha.org/uploadedFiles/PP2006-00274.pdf

Dillon, H., James, A., & Ginis, J. (1997). Client oriented scale of improvement (COSI) and its relationship to several other measures of benefit and satisfaction provided by hearing aids. *Journal of the American Academy of Audiology, 8*, 27–43. Retrieved from https://www.audiology.org/sites/default/files/journal/JAAA_08_01_04.pdf

Hipskind, N. M. (2017). Visual stimuli in communication. In R. L. Schow & M. A. Nerbonne, *Introduction to audiologic rehabilitation* (Kindle ed.; pp. 127–166). Boston, MA: Pearson.

Kelly, T. B., Tolson, D., Day, T., McColgan, G., Kroll, T., & Maclaren, W. (2013). Older people's views on what they need to successfully adjust to life with a hearing aid. *Health & Social Care in the Community, 21*(3), 293–302.

Kirkwood, D. (2005). Dispensers surveyed on what leads to patient satisfaction. *The Hearing Journal, 58*(4), 19–22.

Kobosko, J., Jedrzejczak, W. W., Pilka, E., Pankowska, A., & Skarzynski, H. (2015). Satisfaction with cochlear implants in postlingually deaf adults and its nonaudiological predictors: Psychological distress, coping strategies, and self-esteem. *Ear & Hearing, 36*(5), 605–618.

Neurotone. (n.d.). LACE–listening and communication enhancement. Retrieved from https://www.neurotone.com/lace-interactive-listening-program

Newman, C. W., Weinsten, B. E., Jacobsen, G. P., & Huq, G. A. (1990). The hearing handicap inventory. *Ear & Hearing, 11*(6), 430–433.

Oticon. (2016). Oticon Opn: Proven to make it easier on the brain. Retrieved from http://www.oticon.com/solutions/brainhearing-technology

Ross, M. (2011). Are group aural rehabilitation (AR) programs for adults effective? Retrieved from http://www.hearingresearch.org/ross/aural_rehabilitation/are_group_ar_programs_for_adults_effective.php

Sweetow, R. (2013). Aural rehabilitation builds up patients' communication skills. *The Hearing Journal, 68*(4), 8–14.

Weinstein, B. (2014). On hearing loss and healthy aging. *The Hearing Journal, 67*(12), 6.

ADDITIONAL RESOURCES
WEBSITES

Advanced Bionics and Phonak. The Listening Room. www.thelisteningroom.com
Emily Fu Foundation. Angel Sound. http://angelsound.tigerspeech.com
Neurotone. LACE: Listening and Communication Enhancement. www.lacelistening.com

TABLE 9-1 Apps for Hearing-Impaired Adults

Brain Noise; Free	Sound Relief; Free
Brain Noise; $0.99	Starkey Hear Coach; Free
Brainwell; $1.99	Starkey HLS; Free
Caption Call; Free	Starkey Relax; Free
Ibaldi Lite; Free (English and Spanish)	TV Louder; Free
Imagine VS; Free	Whistle Tinnitus; $1.99
Noise Room; $0.99	White Noise Market; $1.99
Oticon Medical; Free	

TABLE 9-2 Apps for Hearing-Impaired Children

Academy Teacher Squadron; Free	PIC Sentence Lite; Free
Bop It; Free	Planet Hearwell; Free
Listen GR 4–8 Lite; Free	Simon Says; Free
More Fun with Directions Lite; Free	Sound Explorer; Free
Oticon Medical; Free	Starkey Hear Coach; Free
Phonak Leo Interactive Stories; Free	STT Lite; Free

Fluency Disorders

Florence L. Myers

Introduction

Insightful clinical questions help us bridge the gap between assessment and treatment goals. To understand what questions to ask and what treatment goals to develop, clinicians need foundational knowledge about the disorder. This chapter addresses the fluency disorders of **stuttering** and **cluttering**. Although there are instances of pure cluttering and, of course, pure stuttering, many individuals both stutter and clutter. It is, therefore, important to understand the nature of both stuttering and cluttering, how they overlap, and how they are different. Most clinicians view the essence of stuttering to comprise physiological tension, in which the speaker has difficulty transitioning from one sound or syllable to the next for a word or phrase he or she intends to express. This difficulty leads to fragmentations in the production of an utterance—such as sound or syllable repetitions and tense pauses—as well as discoordination of the speech production system. Of particular note is the manner of initiation of vocal fold vibration and coordination of phonation with the outgoing airstream.

The classic core features of stuttering include some type of repetition, such as sound or syllable repetitions (the more fragmented, the more stuttering like), prolongations, and tense pauses. Secondary behaviors, such as eye blinks and head movements, can also arise as the speaker exerts greater effort to produce the desired utterance.

Pure cluttering, on the other hand, is marked by a rate that is *perceived* either to be excessively fast—or at least faster than the speaker can manage—leading to misarticulations, disfluencies, and language disorganization. Because pausing is often not at appropriate linguistic junctures, such as at clause or phrase boundaries, the rate can be perceived as irregular as well (St. Louis & Schulte, 2011). An example of an utterance leading to the perception of an irregular or erratic rate is "I pledge (pause) allegiance to the (pause) flag of (pause) the United (pause) States of America." Because the speaker is speaking at a rate that is faster than he or she can handle, other aspects of speech and language are also compromised. Therefore, the evaluation of cluttering needs to encompass an assessment of speech rate, speech intelligibility, organization of language and narratives, disfluencies, and even pragmatics. These dimensions function interactively.

It is sometimes the case that with rate modulation and moderation, the other aspects of communication improve (Myers, 2011). Yet for many people who clutter (PWC), it is difficult to sustain a slower rate. They profess that their natural temperament inclines them to speak excessively fast, even as they are sorting out what they want to encode. A major distinction between the two fluency disorders is that people who stutter (PWS) know what they want to say but have difficulty coordinating the speech production system to encode what they want to say. Importantly, most PWC have multiple competing—often partially formulated—thoughts and words and have difficulty deciding what to say or which word to use, but they keep on speaking anyway. In a sense, cluttering is marked by a degree of disinhibition that precludes optimal organization and monitoring of output (Alm, 2010). To formulate treatment goals, it would be helpful to assess the executive functions (Diamond, 2013) that transcend the thinking and speaking behaviors of a client who clutters.

Comprehensive Assessment and Analysis and Interpretation of Assessment Results

Stuttering

Unlike an assessment for child language disorders, for which there are a number of standardized tests, relatively fewer standardized formal assessment tools exist for stuttering. Notable exemplars of formal stuttering assessments include the following:

- Behavior Assessment Battery CAT–Communication Attitude Test (Brutten & Vanryckeghem, 2006)
- Overall Assessment of the Speaker's Experience of Stuttering (OASES): Documenting Multiple Outcomes in Stuttering Treatment (Yaruss & Quesal, 2010)
- Stuttering Severity Instrument, Fourth Edition (SSI-4) (Riley, 2009)

An assessment of stuttering should be based on multiple fluency samples to arrive at quantitative and qualitative indices of the client's disfluencies. Multiple samples are needed because the degree of fluency varies depending on the psychosocial context and the psycholinguistic demands during the sampling. Stuttering severity is likely to differ, for example, if the client is speaking to a family member compared to delivering an oral presentation in front of class, or reading versus extemporaneous speech. The length and complexity of utterances, semantic and pragmatic loading of utterances (e.g., explaining why one is late for school versus a description of family members), and complexity of narratives impact fluency as well.

A comprehensive assessment of stuttering should also take into account the psychosocial dynamics unique to clients and their family and peers. These dynamics include intrapersonal and interpersonal variables that would impact the therapy goals. Intrapersonal variables include clients' feelings and attitudes about themselves, their stuttering, and their inner perception of how others view their communication. Interpersonal variables include peer and family relationships and how these relationships impact the clients' speech and sense of self-esteem.

A stuttering assessment should also consider any co-occurring speech and language disorders (Wolk & LaSalle, 2015). For example, does the child have a co-occurring speech and language delay or disorder? Children with autism spectrum disorder or some genetically based syndromes, for example, can exhibit stuttering and/or cluttering symptoms (Van Borsel & Tetnowski, 2007). The assessment and treatment of a child who stutters and has co-occurring language problems are markedly different than the language-typical child who stutters. The strategy while formulating goals for such a child is to lower the language demands to facilitate fluency. For the child with misarticulations, the goals to promote fluency should include words containing phonemes that are already in the child's repertoire. Attention should also be given to whether words in the fluency activities require oromotor tension, such as plosives, or words that begin with vowels requiring the initiation of vocal fold vibration with the outgoing airstream.

Fluency analyses must pivot around both quantitative and qualitative measures. Quantitative data include such measures as percentage of disfluent syllables (including both typical and stuttering-like disfluencies), percentage of stuttered syllables, and duration of blocks if remarkable. Although there are published quantitative thresholds that help a clinician determine if a client is someone who stutters, this is only one element of the clinical profile. Clinicians must weigh the interplay between quantitative (such as percentage of stuttered syllables) and qualitative (such as degree of perceived laryngeal tension and degree of anxiety associated with speech) aspects of the disfluencies. In some instances, the qualitative aspects of the client's blocks may carry more perceptual weight with severe supralaryngeal discoordination and laryngeal tension, or the presence of secondary behaviors such as eye blinks and head jerks.

While formulating goals, the clinician must also consider the client's feelings associated with his or her stuttering and his or her degree of control over the various types of blocks. The latter can be classified as those that are shared by typical speakers—hence *typical disfluencies*—such as fillers and revisions. Although these disfluencies disrupt the flow of speech and reduce the aesthetics of speech, they are not pathological. In contrast, stuttering is marked by atypical disfluencies, including tense pauses, sound and syllable repetitions, and prolongations. Typical speakers do not exhibit these types of disfluencies. The clinician should compare the pattern of quantitative and qualitative findings across the multiple fluency samples. This will enable the clinician to obtain a fuller range of data, depending on the discourse context and degree of linguistic loading of the utterances.

Before moving on to planning behavioral objectives, the clinician should also consider the psychosocial dynamics experienced by the client in various speaking situations with various speaking partners. Clinicians should not give the client the impression that near-perfect fluency is expected in all or even most situations because this is not the case even for typical speakers. Particularly with older children and adolescents or adults, it is often best to partner with the client—and especially with parents and teachers for preschoolers or school-age children when feasible—in formulating goals so they make sense from the client's perspective. The client's feelings and attitudes must be taken into account. For example, a school-age child may find it worthwhile to aim for fluency when reading aloud in class or when speaking to the teacher.

Cluttering

Cluttering is often considered a microcosm of many speech and language impairments. The mechanism is speaking at a rate faster than one is able to manage. The resultant disorganization, or cluttering, can occur at the thought, language, or articulatory levels. PWC say that multiple thoughts and fragments of thoughts speed through their minds, and they have a difficult time organizing and sequencing the thoughts. At the language level, they have a difficult time encoding their language output systematically, largely because of the barrage of directly or tangentially related thoughts. Sometimes even the selection of a lexical item is challenging. Linguistic maze behaviors (such as incomplete phrases and revisions) occur. PWC may even exhibit stuttering-like disfluencies, such as part-word repetitions. It is important to ask clients what is motivating these stuttering-like disfluencies. That is, are they exhibiting the disfluencies because they are experiencing difficulty in transitioning from syllable to syllable for a known word they are trying to produce, a scenario typically associated with stuttering? Or are they repeating a syllable even as they are trying to decide between two or more words they are trying to encode? If the latter, cluttering is likely indicated. Pure cluttering is not marked by the struggle behavior experienced in pure stuttering, which is associated with the effortfulness of sequencing motor gestures of a known and intended word; instead, it is marked more by excessive and multiple encodings of thoughts and utterances that are not synergistic and cohesive, due to a speaking rate that is excessively fast or erratic.

It is conjectured that PWC have a temperament that propels them to undertake tasks quickly, including an inclination to exceed their capacity to execute their thought, language, and speech processes in an organized fashion. This conjecture is founded on the introspection of individuals with pure cluttering. An analogy is the fact that some drivers are compelled to exceed the speed limit. Likewise, some PWC claim they are not in their comfort zone unless they multitask several endeavors at a fast rate. It is important to acknowledge that the articulatory rates of some PWC are not necessarily faster than typical speakers (Bakker, Myers, Raphael, & St. Louis, 2011) and that the physical reality of the articulatory rate may or may not be the same as perceptual reality (Myers & St. Louis, 2006). Cluttered speech may be perceived as fast in part because of the over-coarticulations exhibited, so that the message is not entirely intelligible or comprehensible. A classic example of over-coarticulation is "Jeet?" for "Did you eat?"

Additionally, it is often said that PWC are not aware of their excessive rate leading to reduced speech intelligibility and language comprehensibility. However, we need to enlist the insight of PWC to decipher where the breakdown is in monitoring and self-adjusting the communication output (Myers, 2014). This capacity to monitor can range from no awareness at all, to being aware but only after observing the verbal and nonverbal feedback of the listener, to being able to self-adjust one's output when one self-detects communication breakdowns. Whereas PWS would, if they could, speak more fluently to engage in the smooth transition from syllable to syllable of the intended target words, many PWC seem to have a degree of disinhibition that thwarts their attempts to slow down, organize what they intend to say, select the lexical items, and speak more clearly. A prime area to assess, therefore, is the degree to which the PWC can monitor the output first in terms of overall rate and then in terms of the consequence of the fast rate on various speech and language dimensions. A common observation with stuttering, in contrast, is that PWS are often very good at anticipating—or premonitoring—upcoming difficulties in producing a word (Cholin, Heiler, Whillier, & Sommer, 2016).

A comprehensive assessment of cluttering should include the following dimensions: overall speech intelligibility; speech rate; whether the speech rate is perceived to be erratic or spurted, due largely to pauses at unexpected linguistic junctures; articulatory precision; presence of nonstuttering disfluencies, such as fillers and revisions; language organization, especially during extemporaneous narratives; and discourse management, such as excessively dwelling on a conversational point or frequently interrupting the conversational partner's turn (Myers & Bakker, 2011). As with an assessment of stuttering, it is paramount to take multiple speech samples of cluttering.

Cluttering severity varies greatly depending on the nature of the speech task and the degree of informality of the speaking situation. The following speaking tasks generally produce less severe cluttering: shorter utterances, structured speaking tasks, and when the PWC is aware that his or her speech is being judged. The more informal and extemporaneous the speech, the greater the opportunity to observe cluttering. As with stuttering, it is imperative to take multiple fluency samples using different speaking tasks in various pragmatic contexts.

There is no standardized test to assess cluttering. Because cluttering is largely determined behaviorally, many clinicians use the Daly Predictive Cluttering Inventory (Daly & Cantrell, 2006) or perceptual rating scales, such as the Cluttering Severity Instrument (CSI) or the Real-Time Continuous Perceptual Scoring tools (Bakker & Myers, 2014;

Myers & Bakker, 2011). The Daly Predictive Cluttering Inventory item-
izes behaviors in various domains often associated with cluttering.
The clinician, perhaps with insights from the client and client's family
member, notates which behaviors or traits apply to the client. Scores
are suggested, depending on how many behaviors are associated with
the client that would be considered pure cluttering, cluttering and
stuttering, and stuttering. The perceptual scales by Bakker and Myers
(2014), on the other hand, provide opportunities to rate cluttering per-
ceptually based on speech samples. The CSI, for example, allows clinicians to arrive at a score based on the percentage of speaking time
that is considered to contain cluttering, and the severity is judged on
the following dimensions: overall intelligibility, speech rate regularity,
speech rate, articulation precision, presence of typical disfluency, language organization, discourse management, and use of prosody.

Because cluttering can be considered a microcosm of various
speech and language impairments, it is prudent to consider the disorder from a systems approach; that is, the various aspects of the speech
and language system function either in a well-timed (synchronous)
and well-integrated (synergistic) way or not (Myers, 1992; St. Louis,
Myers, Bakker, & Raphael, 2007). As the word *cluttering* implies, the
communication output is cluttered and is compromised in organization, intelligibility, and comprehensibility.

Cluttering and Stuttering

Some clients with disfluencies may exhibit symptoms of both cluttering and stuttering. Until relatively recently in the United States, individuals with disfluencies were often assumed to stutter only because
the field of cluttering had not been well established in this country.
Cluttering as a field was more widely known and received in Europe,
particularly among logopedists in eastern Europe (Myers, 2010). Some
individuals with disfluencies have been misdiagnosed as exhibiting
pure stuttering when, in fact, they exhibited pure cluttering or both
cluttering and stuttering symptoms. When a person is misdiagnosed,
the goals and subsequent treatment goals would not fit the outward
symptoms and inward motivations or causes for these symptoms.

For example, a client may exhibit sporadic stuttering-like symptoms
such as sound repetitions. These fragmentations are often classified
as atypical disfluencies, hence stuttering. However, this classification
needs to be confirmed by asking the client about the epigenesis of
the sound repetitions. If the client indicates that the reason for the
fragmentations is that the mouth is still going, even as he or she is

trying to figure out what word to use or what thought to encode, the symptoms seem more like cluttering than stuttering. Classic stuttering, in contrast, occurs when fragmentations are associated with trying to transition from sound to sound, or syllable to syllable, of a known or intended word.

Although misdiagnoses occur, clinicians should be aware that a **differential diagnosis** of stuttering versus cluttering is sometimes not readily evident or easy to determine. Several reasons may account for this diminished transparency. It is essential that clinicians first have a good understanding of the inherent nature of the two fluency disorders to understand when there may be overlaps or interactions. Cluttering severity, even within the same individual, may be quite variable, depending on the degree of formality versus spontaneity of speaking; the degree to which clients are aware that their speech is in the spotlight, such as when being recorded; and the complexity of the narrative. In some individuals with cluttering, the speech may vary from greatly cluttered to greatly eloquent, depending on the nature of the speaking task and the context.

Clinicians should be mindful that improved speech requires vigilance to maintain because the slower and more articulate speech may go against a person's natural tendency to do everything fast. A critical question to answer is whether disfluencies are present because a person is attempting to transition smoothly from syllable to syllable of a word, or if they reflect ambiguity, indecision, or disorganization about what words or thoughts to encode. The former reflects stuttering, and the latter reflects cluttering. The same client can exhibit both, and it is important for the clinician, in consultation with a client who both clutters and stutters, to decipher the root of given disfluencies. For example, one PWC who exhibited a great number of part-word repetitions produced with great velocity and intensity—normally considered a stuttering-like disfluency due to a high degree of fragmentation—indicated that the underlying cause of the stuttering-like disfluencies was that he was still trying to decide which word to encode even as he iterated syllables.

Forming Specific Goals

The formulation of goals is also based on an analysis of the client's strengths and weaknesses. Because the degree of fluency is the culmination of many variables, it is helpful to organize the strengths and potential weaknesses into three categories: psychosocial, psycholinguistic, and physiological (Wall & Myers, 1995). Psychosocial variables include such variables as degree of self-esteem, degree of support from family and peers, degree of resilience and maturity of the client, as well as the client's attitudes and feelings related to stuttering and talking in general. Psycholinguistic variables relate to degree of phonological and language proficiency, how pragmatic variables affect the client's feelings and, in turn, fluency, and impact of degree of syntactic and semantic loading on the client's fluency. The interaction of fluency and language is pervasive for both children and adults, and this interplay is in continuous flux. In formulating goals, the clinician needs to develop sensitivity to this interaction, especially if the client has delayed speech or language. Clinicians must be mindful that, all things being equal, the fluency with which people speak is determined by the speech, language, and cognitive infrastructure. If the client has word-finding issues, for example, disfluencies are likely to surface. If a client who stutters also has an underlying oromotor issue, this concomitant problem may aggravate the physiological discoordination and tension of the speech production system, compounding stuttering severity.

There are occasions when the client exhibits borderline stuttering. For example, a child may exhibit a higher than usual percentage of disfluent syllables. However, if the disfluencies comprise primarily typical disfluencies, such as fillers and phrase repetitions, the clinician should consider goals that reinforce the child's fluency through activities such as reciting nursery rhymes. The activities have a slower cadence and more exaggerated prosody, and there is not much language loading because the child is reciting nursery rhymes that have preplanned scripts. The therapy goals would be different for a child whose disfluencies are atypical (i.e., stuttering-like) with physiological tension, fragmentation of speech units, awareness and concern, effortfulness, and perhaps even avoidance. Examples of atypical disfluencies include sound and syllable repetitions (s-s-s sunshine), tense pauses in the middle of a word (s—unshine), and a word said with a fixed articulatory posture, such as bilabial pursing on the /m/ when attempting to say "mother." In these instances, therapy should aim to produce speech with a smooth transition between sounds and syllables. It would be prudent for children with severe stuttering to receive individual therapy, preferably three times a week. As necessary, the parents, in consultation with the clinician, may consider group therapy as well to gain peer support and opportunities to generalize one's fluency skills.

Several challenges, therefore, beset the transition from assessment to goal setting for cluttering. Because cluttering is a largely perceptual phenomenon, the severity of which is a confluence of various speech and language dimensions that interact with one another, some dimensions are likely to be more salient to the perceiver than other dimensions (Myers & Bakker, 2014). That is, even though a client may exhibit numerous interjections, the disfluency dimension may not detract from the integrity of overall communication as much as the dimensions of speech intelligibility or erratic rate. A second challenge in goal setting based on assessment is that cluttering severity is not consistent within the same sample, much less across speech samples. In certain speaking contexts, some PWC can exhibit immensely severe cluttering and yet sound quite fluent, intelligible, and comprehensible in other situations. A third related challenge is that some PWC can normalize their speaking, albeit for very short periods of time, in structured tasks if they intuit that clarity of speech matters; this is despite the fact that many, if not most, PWC either resist slowing down or seem not to be aware of the reduced intelligibility and comprehensibility of their communication output. Additionally, although we can count the number of blocks in stuttering, we cannot count the number of clutters because cluttering is not comprised of discrete entities. Yet another challenge for both client and clinician is the need to prioritize which speech and language dimension to work on first.

Meeting these challenges requires partnership with the client to answer the following questions:

- In what speaking situations and speech tasks am I especially vulnerable to cluttering?
- In what speaking situations am I more aware of my cluttering?
- What communication dimension or dimensions most impact my cluttering severity?
- What speaking situations or speaking tasks ameliorate the severity of my cluttering?
- To what extent does my fluency disorder affect my quality of life?

Insight into these questions will help guide goal setting. Establish a hierarchy of goals that start with speaking situations and speech tasks that are least vulnerable to cluttering; namely, start with highly structured speaking situations and speaking material, such as reading phrases while being recorded. The rationale is that highly structured tasks do not tempt the client to encode a multitude of rapid-fire uncensored thoughts into language.

In the foreword to what is now considered a classic volume on cluttering (Myers & St. Louis 1992), Van Riper described cluttering as analogous to watching fish in a feeding frenzy. The overriding impression by a layperson is that cluttering personifies unharnessed energy.

Toward the goal of harnessing and gating this energy, reading provides a means to scaffold thoughts, language, and hopefully speech as the language of a reading passage is preprogrammed so the client can more readily focus on the rate and clarity of his or her speech. Most PWC indicate they have many related and tangential thoughts racing through their mind, yet they do not take the time to select and sequence the thoughts into a coherent and cohesive set of utterances. Ward, Connally, Pliatsikas, Bretherton-Furness, and Watkins (2015), for example, discuss the possibility of cluttering symptoms secondary to disinhibition of the basal ganglia output, possibly influenced by a hyperactive dopaminergic system based on their sparse-sampling functional MRI study of 17 adults with cluttering and 17 controls on a reading task and a spontaneous speech task.

Being recorded while reading structured and scripted material promotes monitoring, which in turn slows down one's rate and reduces cluttering severity. As indicated previously, many PWC have a tendency to make their speech more deliberate if they know their speech is in the spotlight. This occurs even for typical speakers; most people are more conscious of their speech when they know they are being recorded. By the same token, recordings should be made to capture segments with more severe cluttering, such as describing a recent vacation that had a number of complications. Cluttering symptoms for multiple dimensions are likely to surface when encoding a narrative of high interest or excitement with complex story grammar containing numerous episodes and dilemmas requiring resolution.

Types of Intervention Approaches

A useful model to guide goal setting is **Myers's A-frame model for therapy** (**FIGURE 10-1**) (Myers, 2011). The foundation for this A-frame structure is the development of meta-awareness of one's cluttering behaviors. Specifically, what are the distinctive features of the client's cluttering? Due to the multidimensionality of cluttering, PWC have unique profiles. The clinician engages in dialogue with illustrations regarding the dimensions of speech and language impacted by the cluttering. One PWC may have poor speech intelligibility and relatively few disfluencies. Another may have both poor speech intelligibility and narrative skills. Therefore, a major goal that serves as the foundation to the A-frame model for therapy—and all subsequent therapy—is to help the client become aware of and articulate the specific behaviors that result in his or her unique cluttering profile. Additionally, the so-called insulation

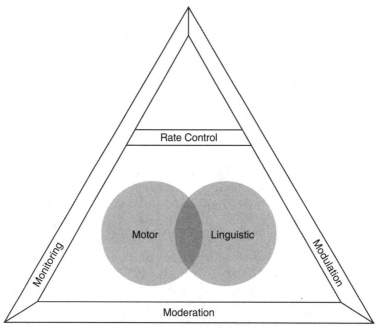

FIGURE 10-1 Myers's A-frame model for therapy.
Cluttering: A Handbook of Research Intervention and Education (2011) Edited by David Ward and Kathleen Scaler Scott, Psychology Press

of the A-frame house is made of goals that enhance the client's ability to *moderate or slow* the rate, to *monitor* the communication output, and to *modulate* or change the behaviors to decrease cluttering severity. As illustrated in Figure 10-1, the center beam of the A-frame is **rate control**. Work toward this one goal, though often easier said than done, will support the rest of therapy. To optimize success, the client needs to be aware that rate control can impact the motoric output (such as articulation), or the linguistic output (such as word retrieval and coherency of narratives), or both. A multitude of goals can emanate from this A-frame model, which is tailored after the individualistic profile of speech-language behaviors assessed based on Bakker and Myers's perceptual rating scales, discussed earlier (Bakker & Myers, 2014; Myers & Bakker, 2011).

Summary

Fluency is a complex and multidimensional phenomenon. In a sense, fluency is suprasegmental and overarches all aspects of speech and language. It is governed by the timing of events—from the thought level, to the semantic and syntactic level, to the articulatory level—and the coordination of these events that occur rather quickly as we utter five to six syllables per second in pragmatically dynamic and changing contexts. This chapter has focused on two of the major disorders of fluency: stuttering and cluttering. Challenges abound in projecting goals for these two disorders. However, a good grounding of the nature of stuttering and cluttering will undoubtedly facilitate thoughtful goals. One needs to be mindful that these disorders occur in the context of the psychosocial, psycholinguistic, and physiological aspects of communication. No singular program or set of goals will address the needs of all fluency clients. Goals should be individualized and prioritized, and they may shift in priority as the client progresses and, indeed, at times regress. Meeting these challenges brings an inordinate degree of fulfillment to the speech-language pathologist and can provide a large measure of gratitude in the clients we serve.

Case Scenarios

Case Scenario 1

Synopsis

John is a 10-year-old child who stutters. From a psychosocial perspective, John has strong self-esteem except when it comes to his stuttering. John comes from a very supportive and loving family; however, because both of his parents work, the household is often frenetic, and his parents are not always able to give him the time he needs to interact with them. The stress of this time pressure, in addition to sibling rivalry for talk time with the parents at the dinner table, worsens his stuttering. Except for a particular classmate who sometimes taunts John for his stuttering, his friends are supportive. The predominantly positive support John receives from his parents and most peers has been an asset. However, John's parents are not aware of variables that impact his disfluencies, such as time pressure at home, having a busy household, and sibling competition for parental attention. John excels academically, but his teacher indicates that he is often reticent to contribute in class discussions because of his stuttering. This reluctance to participate in class discussions or give oral reports in class has academic consequences, even though John has the intellectual competence to meet the curricular demands at school.

    The clinician took three fluency samples to assess John's fluency in various speaking situations. John exhibited the least percentage of stuttered syllables when speaking with his mother and the most percentage of stuttered syllables when doing an oral presentation in front of his class. The qualitative dimensions of his disfluencies range from easy repetitions of words to occasional hard blocks that produce tense pauses and prolongations. He does not evidence any secondaries.

Case Scenarios *(continued)*

John is quite aware that he stutters, but he is not in tune with the specific behaviors that lead to a block or how various pragmatic situations impact the severity of his stuttering. He expresses great frustration that one classmate bullies him in front of his friends, and he becomes quite anxious when he has to respond to the teacher in class or when he has to give oral reports.

Approach

Based on the client profile, therapy should take a three-pronged approach: (1) facilitate greater fluency first in short, structured speech units and then in longer utterances; (2) counsel the parents; and (3) collaborate with John's teacher to improve peer support and reduce bullying and teasing. Because John is generically aware of his stuttering, therapy should focus on helping him adopt an easier manner of producing syllables so that words come out fluently. To fully comprehend the rationale for behavioral change, John must first understand what it is that he does that results in a stutter and how he can change the way he manages his speech helpers so the words come out fluently. Speech is a motor act, and stuttering results when there is a blockage or discoordination of the speech production system. For John, the culprits are extraordinary tension at the level of the vocal folds so that both abductors and adductors contract simultaneously during a tense pause, as in "ba—thtub," and a fixed articulatory posture that results in prolongation of attempted sounds such as sssssssun." The effective treatment of stuttering is intimately tied to illustrating the behaviors that result in blocks that are unique to the client so he or she can gain increased awareness of the sensorimotor feedback associated with the stutters and, subsequently, less severe blocks.

Long-Term Goal 1

John will improve his fluency.

Short-Term Goal 1

John will be able to read a grade-appropriate passage in the speech classroom, as judged by the speech-language pathologist, by the end of the semester.

Daily Goals 1

1. John will be able to describe the behavioral symptoms of his blocks (e.g., his voice box tenses up, his lips get stuck) as he reads a list of phrases with 90 percent accuracy, as judged by the speech-language pathologist.

📋 Case Scenarios *(continued)*

2. John will be able to repeat read phrases on which he exhibited a block with a gentler valving of the articulators or voice onset with 90 percent accuracy, as judged by the speech-language pathologist.
3. John will be able to describe the behavioral symptoms of his blocks as he reads four sentences from a grade-appropriate passage with 90 percent accuracy, as judged by the speech-language pathologist.
4. John will be able to repeat read sentences on which he exhibited a block with gentler valving of the articulators or voice onset with 90 percent accuracy, as judged by the speech-language pathologist.
5. John will be able to read a grade-appropriate passage in the speech classroom with 90 percent accuracy, as judged by the speech-language pathologist, by the end of the semester.

Parent education and counseling is paramount when working with pediatric stuttering. The Stuttering Foundation (http://www.stutteringhelp.org/) provides numerous excellent resources for clients, parents, and teachers. Clinicians should partner with parents, to the extent possible, to provide a fluency-enhancing home environment. Clinicians need to help parents realize that the home environment impacts the child's fluency. Specifically, John's fluency is impacted when he feels rushed or when he feels the need to compete for talk time at the dinner table. Thus, in addition to direct therapy (that is, clinical work with the child), indirect therapy is needed (i.e., partnering with significant others in daily environments).

Long-Term Goal 2

John's parents will provide a fluency-enhancing environment at home.

Short-Term Goal 2

John's parents will provide speaking situations in the home that are fluency enhancing.

Daily Goals 2

1. John's parents will be able to identify three speaking situations that disrupt fluency in the home (e.g., competition for talk time among siblings at the dinner table, when they rush John to speak, and when too many concurrent tasks are taking place at home).
2. John's parents will be able to discuss why these three speaking situations provoke disfluencies (such as being rushed or stressed).
3. John's parents will be able to provide speaking situations in the home that mitigate fluency disruptions.

The third prong of this integrated approach to enhance John's fluency is through collaboration with the classroom teacher, who is instrumental in preparing a speaking environment that reduces stress for John and reducing teasing and bullying by classmates. Negative attitudes toward speaking are well documented in children who stutter (Guttormsen, Kefalianos & Naess, 2015). These

Case Scenarios *(continued)*

two objectives go hand in hand; that is, reducing teasing and bullying by developing classmate sensitivity to the emotional needs of children who stutter cultivates a more nurturing speaking environment in the classroom, both for spontaneous contributions to class discussions and, eventually, more fluency and increased self-esteem during class presentations.

An effective way to promote respect among classmates is through a curriculum developed for teasing and bullying related to stuttering (Langevin, 1998). In addition to the one-on-one fluency-enhancing therapy sessions with John, both John and his teacher may engage in desensitization activities. Desensitization therapy attempts to build up a client's tolerance to stimuli that are anxiety provoking, hence breaking down barriers to fluent speech. In close consultation with the client, the therapy goals should align a hierarchy of three to five situations, ranging from least to most anxiety provoking. For example, the least anxiety-provoking situation might be for John to respond to his teacher's questions using 5- to 10-word answers when speaking with the teacher alone. The most anxiety-provoking situation, based on John's input, is for John to deliver a 5-minute book report in the language arts class. In addition to fluency therapy, John will incorporate relaxation techniques that the clinician models so he can maintain a sense of control and a relatively relaxed state as he progresses through the anxiety-provoking situations. Collaboration between John's teacher and the clinician is paramount. Of note is that the hierarchy of anxiety-provoking situations works on generalization of both fluency behaviors and a sense of well-being in functional speaking situations outside the therapy room.

Long-Term Goal 3

John will maintain fluency when speaking in academic settings.

Short-Term Goal 3

John will be able to speak with 10 or fewer disfluencies when presenting a 5-minute book report in the language arts class.

Daily Goals 3

1. John will be able to speak with two or fewer disfluencies when answering the teacher's short-answer questions using 5 to 10 words, as charted by the student.
2. John will be able to speak with three or fewer disfluencies when answering the teacher's open-ended questions using several sentences, as charted by the student.
3. John will be able to speak with three or fewer disfluencies when initiating his own comments using several sentences during class, as charted by the student.
4. John will be able to speak with five or fewer disfluencies when reading aloud a 250-word passage during class, as charted by the student based on a recording of his speech.
5. John will be able to speak with 10 or fewer disfluencies when presenting a 5-minute book report during class, as charted by the student based on a recording of his speech.

📋 Case Scenarios *(continued)*

This case scenario reflects some basic principles of goal setting for a fluency client: the reduction of severity in the quantitative and qualitative dimensions of stuttering severity; the need to facilitate an awareness and understanding of the nature of one's disfluencies and variables that influence one's vulnerability to disfluencies; the incorporation of a team approach that includes the child's parents and teachers; the realization that a fluency client's psychosocial well-being (both intra- and interpersonal dynamics) plays an important part in treatment; and the need to adopt a holistic approach to fluency that goes beyond the quantification of stuttering symptoms to incorporate the impact of language loading, self-awareness and attitudes, the qualitative aspects of stuttering, and the need to involve peer, parent, and teacher consultations. Goal setting for stuttering therapy is not simply the reduction of a single quantitative index, such as percentage of stuttered syllables.

Case Scenario 2

Synopsis

Peter is 36 years old and has had chronic stuttering since he was 3 years old. Although he was enrolled in therapy at elementary school, he did not think the therapy helped much, largely because he did not see much of a need for going and felt self-conscious about being taken out of the classroom for speech therapy. However, he now realizes that his stuttering is holding him back socially and professionally. He realizes that his stuttering is not likely to be cured because both his father and grandfather were moderately severe stutterers. Peter is now seeking therapy to help him manage his fluency, at least in work situations. He is perceptive of situations that provoke stuttering and their impact on his speech and psychological state. He experiences a great deal of stress when speaking with coworkers and, in fact, avoids speaking whenever possible.

Approach

Three attributes need to be considered, given Peter's case study. Goal setting needs to take into account chronicity, Peter's long-standing and moderately severe stuttering, and the high degree of anxiety associated with his stuttering in work situations. The goals for a moderately severe, chronic stutterer should aim to help the client stutter more easily. It may be unrealistic to aim for complete fluency—as might be the goal for the fluency shaping approach—given the family history and chronicity. Nonetheless, it will be highly beneficial to help Peter to posture and transition movements of the speech production system that have been found to facilitate greater ease and fluency during or in anticipation

Case Scenarios *(continued)*

of blocks. Primarily these include gestures, such as easy onset of vibration of the vocal folds, smooth transition or blending of successive sounds and syllables, and a gentler valving of the supralaryngeal structures to make sounds such as /m/ (bilabial valving) and /t/ (articulating the tongue tip at the alveolar ridge). These goals will help Peter gain better control over the mechanics of fluency.

Long-Term Goal

Peter will speak with greater fluency.

Short-Term Goal

Peter will speak fluently with 95 percent accuracy when using the stuttering modification technique of pullout when he anticipates an upcoming block, as jointly judged by the speech-language pathologist and the client.

Daily Goals

1. Peter will use easy onset and loose contacts when reading a list of multisyllabic words that begin with voiced sounds with 95 percent accuracy, as jointly judged by the speech-language pathologist and the client.
2. Peter will use easy onset and loose contacts when producing self-initiated phrases with 95 percent accuracy, as jointly judged by the speech-language pathologist and the client.
3. Peter will use easy onset and loose contacts when describing common objects with 95 percent accuracy, as jointly judged by the speech-language pathologist and the client.
4. Peter will use easy onset and loose contacts with 95 percent accuracy when he anticipates an upcoming block in conversational speech in the therapy room, as jointly judged by the speech-language pathologist and the client.
5. Peter will use easy onset and loose contacts with 95 percent accuracy when he anticipates an upcoming block during a conversation with a friend at work, as judged by the client.

Simultaneously, therapy should address Peter's speech-related anxieties. These anxieties have accumulated over the decades and are likely to be deeply rooted. It would be prudent for Peter to engage in counseling as well as fluency therapy. The bridge that solidifies gains made in counseling and in fluency is desensitization therapy. The basic rationale of desensitization is to systematically strengthen a client's resistance to negative feelings, such as anxiety, by purposely and purposefully subjecting oneself to feared stimuli, starting with low dosages. The ideal is to couple desensitization therapy with counseling and some form of relaxation therapy. The goal is to build up resistance to feared stimuli while engendering a calmer state of mind. Evidence-based efforts are underway to help PWS reduce social anxiety through counseling approaches, such as

📋 **Case Scenarios** *(continued)*

cognitive-behavioral therapy (CBT). Although CBT has been conducted primarily through face-to-face counseling, the efficacy of a seven-module CBT program delivered through the Internet has been demonstrated through clinical trials to reduce social anxiety and depression in PWS (Menzies, O'Brian, Lowe, Packman, & Onslow, 2016).

Case Scenario 3

Synopsis

Susan is a 16-year-old student who is considered by peers to be quite extroverted and bright, though at times a bit scatterbrained, and very much a divergent thinker. Although she readily engages in social interactions with her peers and teachers, Susan is puzzled that they often ask her to repeat what she just said. Her friends, especially new acquaintances, seem to wear a frown with a tinge of impatience on their face when she tells them a story or tries to explain something. Sometimes they do not understand her, even after she repeats what she just said. It was not until her teacher recommended that she receive speech therapy that Susan realized the primary source of miscommunication might be a lack of clarity and coherence of her speech, particularly when she engages in an exciting narrative. Poor speech intelligibility and language comprehensibility of oral narratives, as two major criteria for service eligibility, can have severe impact on academic and social well-being. For Susan, this impact would continue during adulthood and when she seeks promotions in her profession.

Approach

The speech-language pathologist collected and analyzed three fluency samples from Susan. The samples varied in degree of structure, formality, and extemporaneousness of speaking task. It is commonly noted that cluttering increases with less structured and more informal speaking situations. In fact, to the extent feasible, it is desirable to sample speech when clients are not aware that their speech is being monitored. Susan's three samples revealed that her cluttering varies in severity.

Upon reflection, guided by her clinician, Susan came to the realization that she needs to work on modulating her speech rate first in structured speech tasks, then in speaking tasks that are more extensive, less structured, and informal. Slowing down one's rate is easier said than done for everyone, but exceedingly so for PWC. This is analogous to driving at 55 miles per hour when we habitually drive closer to 65 miles

Case Scenarios *(continued)*

per hour. It is likely to be counterproductive to ask a client to simply slow down because the request may be too abstract and generic. Therapy to slow down speech requires more creative and more concrete activities.

An effective therapy activity is pausing at appropriate linguistic junctures. Several reasons underlie the power of pausing. First, pausing at appropriate linguistic junctures slows down the rate because it makes the speaker more conscious of the speaking process and allows them to plan what to say next. Second, speakers are less likely to speed through a clause or phrase when they know they will pause between clauses. This is analogous to speeding up for a short spurt while driving, then stopping, then resuming a fast speed for another short distance and stopping again. Third, appropriate pausing enhances the effectiveness of speaking. Have the client listen to a famous orator (such as President John F. Kennedy) to help them realize that speech is less effective if rushed, especially if intelligibility and comprehensibility is sacrificed.

Although multiple speech and language dimensions need to be addressed, it is reassuring that the process of slowing speech through activities that promote pausing and rhetoric (such as poetry, nursery rhymes, and skits) will likely also improve the other dimensions. An array of therapy activities and goals are available (Myers, 2011) to address the rate and other dimensions of speech and language.

Long-Term Goal

Susan will use an appropriate rate during conversational speech in an academic setting.

Short-Term Goal

Susan will be able to use an appropriate rate in conversational speech in the speech room through the use of pausing with 90 percent accuracy, as judged by the speech-language pathologist.

Daily Goals

1. Susan will be able to correctly identify the locations of pauses in a reading passage by putting a slash (/) at commas and a double slash (//) at periods to indicate a longer pause with 95 percent accuracy, as judged by the speech-language pathologist.
2. Susan will be able to identify the locations of pauses in a poem by putting a slash (/) at the end of each line with 90 percent accuracy, as judged by the speech-language pathologist.
3. Susan will be able to read a prose passage or poem using the slash marks as indicators for pauses with 95 percent accuracy, as judged by the speech-language pathologist.

📋 **Case Scenarios** *(continued)*

    4. Susan will be able to converse with the speech-language pathologist about a neutral topic (such as describing her routine during a school day) using pauses at the end of clauses or phrases for 3 minutes with 95 percent accuracy, as judged by the speech-language pathologist.

5. Susan will be able to converse with the speech-language pathologist about an exciting or high-interest topic (such as the surprise 16th birthday party that her parents gave her) using pauses at the end of appropriate clauses or phrases for 3 minutes with 90 percent accuracy, as judged by the speech-language pathologist.

REVIEW QUESTIONS

1. Stuttering consists of which of the following?
   a. Effortfulness in the speech production system
   b. Fragmentations of an intended word
   c. Speech that is accompanied by secondary behaviors
   d. All of the above

2. Goals to desensitize anxiety associated with stuttering
   a. should be planned in a hierarchical way, ranging from most to least anxiety provoking.
   b. should be planned in a hierarchical way, ranging from least to most anxiety provoking.
   c. should be used only for adults.
   d. should be used only as a last resort.

3. Cluttering can best be described as a disorder
   a. in which the individual speaks faster than he or she can manage.
   b. that can be characterized by a speaking rate that is faster than the norm.
   c. that is unidimensional.
   d. that is best assessed using acoustical analyses of the fluency samples.

4. Which statement is true of both stuttering and cluttering?
   a. They are two disorders that share commonalities and have distinctive features.
   b. They can coexist.
   c. They can both have other co-occurring disorders, such as autism.
   d. All of the above are true.

5. Which statement is true of goals for the treatment of stuttering and cluttering?
   a. They should be multidimensional to include other considerations, such as the client's language functions.
   b. They should be based on multiple samples in various speaking contexts.
   c. They should be individualized to the client's interpersonal and intrapersonal profile.
   d. All of the above are true.

REFERENCES

Alm, P. A. (2010). The dual premotor model of cluttering and stuttering: A neurological frame-work. In K. Bakker, L. Raphael & F. Myers (Eds.), *Proceedings of the first world conference on cluttering, 2007* (pp. 207–210). Katarino, Bulgaria: International Cluttering Association.

Bakker, K., & Myers, F. L. (2014). *Real-time perceptual tracking of cluttering severity.* Paper presented at the 2nd World Congress of International Cluttering Association, Eindhoven, the Netherlands.

Bakker, K., Myers, F. L., Raphael, L. J., & St. Louis, K. O. (2011). A preliminary comparison of speech rate, self-evaluation, and disfluency of people who speak exceptionally fast, clutter, or speak normally. In D. Ward & K. S. Scott (Eds.), *Cluttering: A handbook of research, intervention and education* (pp. 45–66). New York, NY: Psychology Press.

Brutten, G., & Vanryckeghem, M. (2006). *Behavior assessment battery for school-age children who stutter.* San Diego, CA: Plural.

Cholin, J., Heiler, S., Whillier, A., & Sommer, M. (2016). Premonitory awareness in stuttering scale (PAiS). *Journal of Fluency Disorders, 49,* 40–50.

Daly, D. A., & Cantrell, R. P. (2006). *Cluttering characteristics labeled as diagnostically significant by 60 fluency experts.* Paper presented at the 6th IFA World Congress on Disorders of Fluency, Dublin, Ireland.

Diamond, A. (2013). Executive functions. *Annual Review Psychology, 64,* 135–168.

Guttormsen, L. S., Kefalianos, E., & Naess, K. (2015). Communication attitudes in children who stutter: A meta-analytic review. *Journal of Fluency Disorders, 46,* 1–14.

Langevin, M. (1998). *Teasing and bullying: Unacceptable behavior. Helping children handle teasing and bullying* [Monograph]. Edmonton, Alberta: Institute for Stuttering Treatment and Research (ISTAR) and Communication Improvement Program.

Menzies, R., O'Brian, S., Lowe, R., Packman, A., & Onslow, M. (2016). International phase II clinical trial of CBTPsych: A standalone internet social anxiety treatment for adults who stutter. *Journal of Fluency Disorders, 48,* 35–43.

Myers, F. L. (1992). Cluttering: A synergistic framework. In F. L. Myers & K. O. St. Louis (Eds.), *Cluttering: A clinical perspective* (pp. 71–84). Leicester, UK: FAR Communications.

Myers, F. L. (2010). Conference overview and purpose. In K. Bakker, L. Raphael & F. Myers (Eds.), *Proceedings of the first world conference on cluttering, 2007* (pp. 15–17). Katarino, Bulgaria: International Cluttering Association.

Myers, F. L. (2011). Treatment of cluttering: A cognitive-behavioral approach centered on rate control. In D. Ward & K. S. Scott (Eds.), *Cluttering: A handbook of research, intervention and education* (pp. 152–174). New York, NY: Psychology Press.

Myers, F. L. (2014). *Role of monitoring in the treatment of cluttering.* Keynote address at the 2nd World Congress of International Cluttering Association, Eindhoven, the Netherlands.

Myers, F. L., & Bakker, K. (2011). *The assessment of cluttering severity in research and clinical practice.* Seminar presented at the American Speech-Language-Hearing Association, San Diego, CA.

Myers, F. L., & Bakker, K. (2014). Experts' saliency ratings of speech-language dimensions associated with cluttering. *Journal of Fluency Disorders,42,* 35–42.

Myers, F. L., & St. Louis, K. O. (Eds.). (1992). *Cluttering: A clinical perspective.* Leicester, UK: FAR Communications.

Myers, F. L., & St. Louis, K. O. (2006). Disfluency and speaking rate in cluttering: Perceptual judgments versus counts. *Bulgarian Journal of Communication Disorders, 1,* 28–35.

Riley, G. (2009). *SSI-4: Stuttering severity instrument* (4th ed.). Austin, TX: PRO-ED.

St. Louis, K. O., Myers, F. L., Bakker, K., & Raphael, L. J. (2007). Understanding and treating cluttering. In Conture, E. G. & Curlee, R. F. (Eds.), *Stuttering and related disorders of fluency* (3rd ed., pp. 297–325). New York, NY: Thieme Medical Publishers.

St. Louis, K. O., & Schulte, K. (2011). Defining cluttering: The lowest common denominator. In D. Ward and K. S. Scott (Eds.), *Cluttering: A handbook of research, intervention and education* (pp. 233–253). New York, NY: Psychology Press.

Van Borsel, J., & Tetnowski, J. A. (2007). Stuttering in genetic syndromes. *Journal of Fluency Disorders, 32*, 279–296.

Wall, M. J., & Myers, F. L. (1995). *Clinical management of childhood stuttering.* Austin, TX: PRO-ED.

Ward, D., Connally, E. L., Pliatsikas, C., Bretherton-Furness, J., & Watkins, K. E. (2015). The neurological underpinnings of cluttering: Some initial findings. *Journal of Fluency Disorders, 43*, 1–16.

Wolk, L., & Lasalle, L. R. (2015). Phonological complexity in school-aged children who stutter and exhibit a language disorder. *Journal of Fluency Disorders, 43*, 40–53.

Yaruss, S., & Quesal, R. (2010). *Overall assessment of the speaker's experience of stuttering (OASES).* McKinney, TX: Stuttering Therapy Resources.

CHAPTER 11

Voice Disorders

Ciara Leydon

Key Terms

Acoustic

Aerodynamic

Aphonia

Auditory–perceptual

Dysphonia

Hygienic therapy

Laryngoscopy

Motivational interviewing

Phonation

Phonotrauma

Physiologic approach

Self-perception

Symptomatic therapy

Voice

Voice disorder

Introduction

A **voice disorder** is defined as abnormal or absent pitch, loudness, quality, or flexibility for a person's age or gender (American Speech-Language-Hearing Association [ASHA], 1993), as determined by our sociocultural norms. A disorder can result from dysfunction in the respiratory, phonatory, resonance, or neural systems. Impaired voicing can negatively impact a person's ability to orally communicate effectively and efficiently. Disruption to **voice** is called **dysphonia**, whereas **aphonia** describes the absence of voicing, such as during whispered speech. The prevalence of voice disorders in the United States is estimated at 6.2 to 9 percent of adults (Ramig & Verdolini, 1998; Roy et al., 2004), and 6 to

24 percent of children (Maddern, Campbell, & Stool, 1991). Among professional voice users, such as teachers, lawyers, sales personnel, and performers, the proportion is even higher. For example, close to 60 percent of teachers experience a voice disorder over the course of their career, compared to approximately 30 percent of nonteachers (Roy et al., 2004). Voice disorders represent an important public health problem; they are associated with significant personal psychosocial costs, absenteeism, and short-term disability and work productivity losses (Cohen, Kim, Roy, Asche, & Courey, 2012).

Dysphonia is perceived as negative by a listener. For example, adults with voice disorders may be viewed as less healthy (Maryn & Debo, 2014) or less attractive (Amir & Levine-Yundof, 2013). A child may be judged negatively by peers (Lass, Ruscello, Stout, & Hoffman, 1991) and teachers (Zacharias, Kelchner, & Creaghead, 2013). For a child, a voice disorder can negatively impact educational performance because of its deleterious impact on academics, socialization, and emotional well-being (Ruddy & Sapienza, 2004). Specifically, the child may present with poor **self-perception** (Connor et al., 2008), reduced concentration (Andrews & Summers, 2002), difficulty being heard in a school setting, and he or she may experience reduced opportunities to engage in academic activities, including public speaking, classroom discussions, oral reading (Ruddy & Sapienza, 2004), and social interactions (Connor et al., 2008).

Regardless of the work setting (e.g., health care, school, private practice), a speech-language pathologist may work with individuals with voice or resonance disorders. The clients may be seen in specialized voice clinics or in healthcare, educational, or private practice settings. About one in five school-based speech-language pathologists serve children with voice disorders (McNamara and Perry, 1994). Speech-language pathologists who work with adults report spending 5 percent of their time treating voice or resonance disorders (ASHA, 2011). Given the impact of the voice on all aspects of life—including self-perception, self-actualization, and academic, social, and personal endeavors—a competent evaluation and the development of an appropriate treatment plan for a client with a voice disorder are warranted.

There are many causes of voice disorders. These disorders have been classified as functional or organic. A functional disorder is one for which a physical pathology has not been identified, and the cause is attributed to use patterns. **Phonotrauma** is vocal behaviors that contribute to physiologic or tissue changes in vocal folds (Verdolini, 1999). This term replaces the words *misuse*, *overuse*, and *abuse*, which may be perceived as blaming to the client. Phonotraumatic behaviors have been attributed to stress and psychosocial concerns (Aronson, 1990), in addition to extensively using the voice, straining injured vocal folds, speaking over noise, speaking at an inappropriate pitch, excessively clearing the throat, and coughing (Colton, Casper, & Leonard, 2011). An organic disorder is caused by a disease process or trauma. This classification of disorders as either functional or organic allows for a simple, though imperfect, attribution of a disorder to a proposed etiology.

The ASHA Special Interest Group 3 developed a categorization framework for voice disorders that is based on medical diagnosis and vocal fold function. The framework includes structural, inflammatory, trauma, systemic, aerodigestive, psychiatric or psychological, neurological, and other disorders of voice use (Verdolini, Rosen, & Branski, 2006). The system, purportedly based broadly on the framework of the American Psychiatric Association's *Diagnostic and Statistical Manual of Mental Disorders*, was developed to facilitate consistent communication among practitioners involved in care of the voice and to provide a source of information about the many causes of voice disorders.

Comprehensive Evaluation

A person may be referred for a voice evaluation by a physician (e.g., pediatrician or otolaryngologist), parent, or other source, including oneself, after failing a voice and resonance screening (e.g., in a school setting). Regardless of the referral source, the client will undergo an assessment for a potential voice disorder. The assessment must be multifaceted to reflect the complex interactions among anatomy; physiology; psychology; self-image; and physical, emotional, and communicative environments. This comprehensive approach is consistent with the World Health Organization's International Classification of Functioning, Disability and Health framework, which warrants the assessment of "body structures/functions, activities/participation, and contextual factors" (ASHA, 2004; p. 130).

Regardless of the nature of the voice disorder, "all patients/clients with voice disorders are examined by a physician, preferably in a discipline appropriate to the presenting complaint" (ASHA, 2004; p. 99). Given the focus on laryngeal and vocal tract anatomy and physiology, a laryngeal evaluation by an otolaryngologist is warranted prior to beginning therapy. The physician evaluation can take place before or after the completion of a voice assessment by a speech-language pathologist, but it must occur before treatment. The roles of the otolaryngologist and speech-language pathologist are complementary; the physician establishes a medical diagnosis and formulates a treatment plan that may include behavioral, medical, or surgical treatment, or "watchful waiting" (Schwartz et al., 2009, p. S3). The speech-language pathologist performs a comprehensive assessment of the voice, which can help determine the etiology and pathology of the disorder and characterizes the nature and severity of the functional impact of a vocal pathology on voice production and communication. When behavioral intervention is warranted, the speech-language pathologist develops and implements that plan, determines the prognosis, and makes referrals as appropriate (ASHA, 2004).

Components of a Voice Evaluation

An evaluation characterizes the vocal dysfunction (Baken & Orlikoff, 2000), uncovers a possible etiology, characterizes the effect on the voice, and identifies behaviors that maintain or exacerbate a voice disorder. The speech-language pathologist should gather a thorough case history, including familial, personal, professional, social, educational, pharmaceutical, medical, and surgical histories; voice use in home, work, educational, and social settings; and vocal hygiene (e.g., water intake and exposure to commonly recognized airway irritants, such as smoke and chemicals). An evaluation of the perceived impact of a voice disorder on the client's well-being and quality of life, and the client's motivation for change, is also warranted. An oral–peripheral examination would permit the assessment of anatomical and physiological integrity, including assessment of cranial nerve function. The vocal tract structure, and the rate, range of motion, precision, and coordination of the musculature (function) can also be assessed. Diagnostic data on **aerodynamic**, **acoustic**, and perceptual voice ratings, may be gathered, in addition to laryngeal imaging.

The Individuals with Disabilities Education Act (IDEA) Amendments of 1997 (PL 105-17), and subsequent amendments in 2004 (Individuals with Disabilities Education Improvement Act; IDEA), regulate the provision of services in public schools for children with voice disorders when those disorders incur demonstrable negative impacts on academic and nonacademic educational performance (Ferrand, 2012; Ruddy & Sapienza, 2004). Assessments for voice disorders in children, therefore, should include an evaluation of the voice and voice use in academic and nonacademic school settings. School therapists may perceive barriers in developing and implementing a treatment plan. These perceived barriers include a lack of access to laryngoscopic examinations (Hooper, 2004) and a lack of clarity regarding the type of voice disorders that warrant speech-language pathologist services in the school setting (Ruddy & Sapienza, 2004). Given the negative impact of voice disorders on a child's academic, social, and emotional well-being, these barriers must be overcome by the speech-language pathologist through information gathering, education, and advocacy (Ruddy & Sapienza, 2004). The speech-language pathologist must attain competence in pediatric voice evaluation and treatment, be well informed of service eligibility for voice disorders, and be knowledgeable about community resources available for the child and family. In a study of voice therapy by speech-language pathologists in a school setting, those who reported adequate and effective training in the treatment of voice disorders were more confident in working with voice disorders (McNamara & Perry, 1994). It is therefore important that speech-language pathologists seek education or mentorship in the evaluation and treatment of voice disorders if they lack knowledge, skills, or confidence in this area.

Assessment and Plan of Care

The goal of an assessment is to identify and describe the functional impact and severity of a voice disorder. By assessing the structural and physiologic integrity of the mechanisms underlying voice production, the speech-language pathologist can identify and treat acoustic dysfunction (Baken & Orlikoff, 2000). To do this, the speech-language pathologist must add the communicative context and the client's cognitive, psychological, and motivational attributes and self-image. The evaluation can be completed alone or alongside an otolaryngologist. Upon completion of the assessment, the speech-language pathologist will formulate a plan of care that is consistent with the physician's recommendation and is aligned with the client's perceived needs. Depending on the disorder, voice therapy may be provided alone or in conjunction with medical or surgical treatment.

Compare Formal and Informal Testing and Observations

A comprehensive evaluation can permit a characterization of the nature and severity of a voice disorder based on the integration of data that were gathered through interviewing, educational and medical reports, instrument assessments, and clinical judgment. However, the clinician's role extends beyond identifying and describing a disorder and its underlying physiological impairments. As recommended by ASHA's support for the World Health Organization framework, the role of the speech-language pathologist is to identify and describe a disorder, with a focus on understanding how performance impacts communication and participation. The clinician must probe how a voice disorder impacts an individual's participation in work, academic, social, and personal activities. For children, the clinician must also assess how a voice disorder impacts educational performance.

Formulate a Prognostic Statement and Treatment Plan

Upon completion of an evaluation, a prognostic statement and treatment plan can be formulated. The areas of strengths and weaknesses will be identified. A strength can offer a platform from which to scaffold improvements, providing a starting point for the treatment of impairments. For example, a person with aphonia (a weakness) may show voicing during vegetative tasks (a strength), such as during throat clearing. Voicing during these tasks can be shaped into speech. A person with muscle tension dysphonia who presents with hard glottal attack (weakness) may be able to discriminate between target voice productions (e.g., easy onset) and less desirable productions (e.g., hard glottal attack). The ability to discriminate (strength) is an important skill for developing independence. It allows for future generalization of gains achieved during treatment and continues outside the treatment room. It helps maintain gains after the treatment has ended.

Determine the Context of the Voice and Voice Use

The voice and voice use must be understood in the context of the developing individual, the whole complex person, and the communicative environments. Understanding human development is important for the evaluation and treatment of voice. The voice is a product of anatomy, physiology, and neurology of respiration, **phonation**, and resonance. Life-span changes in these subsystems result in predictable and noticeable changes in the voice. Consequently, vocal function parameters (e.g., pitch, loudness, and vocal stability) must be assessed with respect to age and gender. *Presbyphonia* is a term used to describe age-related changes in the voice. For example, the average fundamental frequency, which is determined by the anatomy of vocal folds (e.g., length and mass), declines from birth through adolescence (most dramatically in males), stabilizes through middle age, and, in males, rises in later years (Baken & Orlikoff, 2000). Dynamic range (Baker, Ramig, Sapir, Luschel, & Smith, 2001) and vocal stability decrease with age (Linville & Fisher, 1985).

Voice disorders are multifactorial. Although the acoustic signal of a voice can be described by the underlying anatomical, physiological, and neurological substrates, it cannot be evaluated or remediated holistically without consideration for hearing status, cognitive-linguistic skills, and psychological well-being. A comprehensive assessment will probe each of these areas. Functional hearing permits the monitoring of vocal output (Lejska, 2003). Hearing impairments are associated with increased pitch and phonatory instability, or jitter and shimmer (Dehqan & Scherer, 2011), and they alter the measures of vocal output. If a hearing loss is suspected, an assessment of hearing by a certified audiologist is recommended. An awareness of cognitive-linguistic impairments will permit the clinician to use appropriate language complexity during instruction and treatment. Psychosocial factors, such as depression, anxiety, conflict, anger, and stress, can alter the measures of vocal output. They can contribute to the development or maintenance of voice disorders (e.g., muscle tension dysphonia), or they can arise in response to voice disorders. Aronson (1990) recommends the inclusion of psychosocial considerations in a thorough evaluation of the voice. A referral for a psychological evaluation may be warranted.

The evaluation data must be gathered and interpreted, with consideration for an individual's social, cultural, and linguistic background. A comprehensive assessment must include the consideration of contexts such as home, school, workplace, and social environments that a person navigates. For example, the Connecticut State Department of Education stipulates that cultural and linguistic influences on a child's voice must be considered during a child's evaluation. Specifically, the speech-language pathologist must consider the "influence of vocal characteristics of native language on voice resonance in English (e.g., tone languages); cultural variations in acceptable voice quality (e.g., pitch, loudness); possible role of insecurity about speaking English on volume of voice in English; possible role of stress from adapting to a new culture on vocal tension affecting voice quality" (Connecticut State Department of Education, 2008, p. 35).

Make a Determination for Services

Upon completion of a comprehensive evaluation, the speech-language pathologist may indicate if the client's voice is typical, different, delayed, or disordered. A typical voice is characterized by pitch, loudness, and quality that are appropriate for the speaker's age and gender, given sociocultural norms. A typical voice is sufficiently flexible to meet all communicative needs, and it presents no handicap to the speaker. A voice may be considered different if the pitch, loudness, or quality do not align with expectations based on age and gender, given the listener's sociocultural norms. For example, the pitch may be perceived to be higher or lower than expected, given age and gender (e.g., glottal fry), but it may be appropriate given the speaker's sociocultural or linguistic norms. A disorder occurs when vocal pitch, loudness, quality, and flexibility are absent or aberrant. The disordered voice may compromise intelligibility, may not meet the communicative needs of the client, and present the client with a handicap. In this case, treatment should be considered.

Apply Clinical Judgment and Professional Experiences

During an evaluation, a speech-language pathologist gathers a case history, including **auditory–perceptual** (e.g., voice quality), acoustic (e.g., pitch and loudness), aerodynamic (e.g., airflow and air pressures), or imaging (e.g., transoral rigid **laryngoscopy**, transnasal flexible fiberoptic laryngoscopy, and videostroboscopy) information. A standard collection of measures and an implementation protocol do not exist currently for performing a comprehensive evidence-based clinical voice assessment (Roy et al., 2013). Consequently, clinical judgment drives the choice of subjective and objective measurement tools to be used, as well as the interpretation of findings and the development of recommendations. Auditory–perceptual measures are one of the most common measures gathered during an evaluation (Behrman, 2005). They are popular, in part, because a voice is an acoustic signal (Oates, 2009) that is judged by a listener to be typical or disordered, based on expectations for pitch, loudness, quality, and flexibility for the speaker's age, gender, culture, and communicative context. These measures require judgment about pitch, loudness, and voice quality (e.g., breathy or hoarse) and can be gathered with or without the use of a scale, such as Consensus Auditory–Perceptual Evaluation of Voice (CAPE-V) (Kempster, Gerratt, Abbott, Barkmeier-Kraemer, & Hillman, 2009) or grade, roughness, breathiness, asthenia, strain (GRBAS) (Hirano, 1981). The judgment of auditory–perceptual measures is influenced by the clinician's experience with rating voice parameters and training. For example, exposure to examples of normal and mild, moderate, and severely disordered voices (i.e., auditory anchors) improves intrarater reliability in the judgment of voice parameters for overall severity and voice effort (Eadie & Kapsner-Smith, 2011).

Develop Recommendations

Following a comprehensive evaluation, the speech-language pathologist will formulate recommendations, including whether or not to treat
the client. If treatment is recommended, the type, duration, and goals
for treatment must be developed. Direct therapy may include individual
or group sessions. Group therapy facilitates generalization and maintenance of goals, offers support, is less expensive, and creates a challenging
environment for clients to hone their skills (Adler, Hirsch, & Mordaunt,
2012; Searl et al., 2011). Examples of voice disorders that are appropriate for group therapy include vocal hygiene for professional voice users
(Timmermans, De Bodt, Wuyts, & Van de Heyning, 2005), voice therapy
for transgender or transsexual clients (Adler et al., 2012), and treatment
for patients with Parkinson disease (Searl et al., 2011). Although an individualized treatment plan may be used for each participant, group goals
may also be established. Some groups provide support and education,
rather than treatment, to individuals with voice disorders and their families. For example, support groups for patients with Parkinson disease or
laryngectomies can be found in many geographic areas.

The recommended frequency and duration of treatment will vary
depending on factors including the etiology, nature, and severity of the
voice disorder, stimulability, and treatment approach. Voice treatment may
be completed in one or two sessions (Roy & Hendarto, 2005); a prescribed
number of sessions (e.g., 16 sessions for Lee Silverman Voice Treatment,
or LSVT LOUD) (Fox et al., 2006); or delivered intensively over the course
of one or more days, such as in boot camp. Voice therapy boot camp,
which consists of multiple hours of individualized treatment, provides the
client with extensive practice to acquire skills and, purportedly, increases
the transfer of skills and client adherence (Patel, Thibeault, & Bless, 2011).

Depending on the nature of the voice disorder, direct therapy may
occur in a traditional clinic, with access to voice instrument equipment, or in other settings that are relevant to the client's communicative context. For example, treatment may occur in the home, on the
playground, or in the classroom; for athletes or coaches, treatment
may occur in the gym, on a treadmill, or poolside. Data suggest that
telepractice for the treatment of voice disorders may be both feasible
and cost effective (Fu, Theodoros, & Ward, 2015; Tindall, Huebner,
Stemple, & Kleinert, 2009), and it may increase access to care. However, reimbursement rates and licensing regulations for telepractice
vary by insurance policy and state. The delivery of therapy can include
high-tech equipment, such as endoscopy or computer programs for
biofeedback, or relatively inexpensive and portable equipment, such as
a digital tuner, stop watch, sound level pressure meter, or app.

Treatment may be direct or indirect. Direct therapy aims to alter the physiology underlying voice production (e.g., breathing, phonation, and vocal tract posturing) to alleviate symptoms and maximize efficient and effective vocal function. In contrast, indirect therapy may involve client and family education about healthy voice behaviors, such as vocal hygiene, diet, vocal rest, and relaxation (Ferrand, 2012), or amplification and manipulating the communication environment to support efficient and effective oral communication (e.g., reducing background noise to allow a child with an asthenic or breathy voice to be heard without the need for vocal strain).

In some cases, treatment may not be recommended, or it may be declined. In that event, monitoring, or "watchful waiting" (Schwartz et al., 2009, p. S3), may be recommended. However, voice treatment, rather than monitoring, is recommended for pediatric dysphonia for two reasons. First, it cannot be assumed that children will outgrow a voice disorder; childhood voice disorders can persist through adolescence (De Bodt et al., 2007). Second, voice disorders can have a long-lasting and far-reaching negative impact on educational performance. Treatment, in the form of direct therapy, family education and involvement, and environment manipulation, may be recommended (Gardner, 2014).

Given the complex nature of speech disorders, the specialization of professionals, and overlapping and complementary skills, interprofessional collaboration provides an efficient way for practitioners to work with and learn from one another when treating clients with multifactorial disorders. Colleagues who may participate in the management of voice disorders include neurologists, pediatricians, oncologists, plastic surgeons, pulmonologists, allergists, psychologists, educators, audiologists, respiratory therapists, physical therapists, athletic trainers and coaches, and vocal coaches.

ASHA developed an online National Outcomes Measurement System (NOMS) that provides a rating scale for clinicians to indicate perceived severity level of a voice disorder in adults and prekindergarten children before and after treatment (ASHA, 2003). The scores range from 1 to 7, with 1 indicating the least functional voice, and 7 indicating the most functional voice. Speech-language pathologists enter pre- and posttreatment NOMS scores into a national database, which provides aggregated data that allow insight into the length of treatment and extent of improvement for a given disorder.

Consider Other Factors

Voice therapy provided by a speech-language pathologist can be covered under Medicare if ordered by a physician and if medically necessary.

Medicaid may cover voice therapy. However, the qualifying criteria vary among states. Private health insurance might cover voice therapy, depending on the insurance company and policy. The CPT codes used for voice evaluation and treatment include 92524 (behavioral and qualitative analysis of voice and resonance); 92520 (laryngeal function studies); 92507 (voice treatment); and 92597 (evaluation for use and/or fitting of voice prosthetic device to supplement oral speech).

Children with voice disorders that are chronic and impact educational services are eligible for services in schools under IDEA. The eligibility criteria vary among states, counties, and school districts. For example, in Connecticut, students may be eligible for voice therapy services if they present with a chronic problem (at least 6 weeks in duration) in phonation, resonance, or prosody (Connecticut State Department of Education, 2008). Adults with voice disorders may be entitled to workplace accommodations under the Americans with Disabilities Act (ADA) Amendments Act of 2008 (ADAAA) (Isetti & Eadie, 2015).

Forming Specific Goals

Goals must be individualized and attainable given anatomical, physiological, and psychological constraints. The goal of treatment may be to restore voice, eliminate vocal handicap, and prevent recurrence of a disorder. Alternatively, when a typical voice cannot be restored, the goal may be to maximize effective and efficient oral communication and minimize vocal handicap in contexts relevant to the client. When habilitation or rehabilitation of voice is not possible, the goal may be to establish an alternative sound source for speech (e.g., esophageal speech).

Assess the Client's Functional Level

A comprehensive assessment of the voice will inform the determination of etiology and pathology and will characterize the nature and severity of the functional impact that a vocal pathology has on voice production and communication. Baseline voice measures gathered during the evaluation provide insight into vocal strengths and weakness and the impact the voice disorders have on functional communication in contexts that are relevant to the client. The prognosis will be determined by the nature of the disorder, awareness of the disorder, motivation to change behaviors, and participation in treatment (Stemple, Roy & Klaben, 2014).

Develop Specific Expectations

Expectations for Therapy

The speech-language pathologist must provide the client and family with realistic expectations for therapy, based on the nature, progression, and severity of the disorder, and based on the data for treatment outcomes, when available.

Expectations for the Client

The speaker judges his or her voice based on the extent to which it reflects that individual's self-image and communication needs and intents. The client's expectations for the voice must be elicited, and his or her goals must be integrated into recommendations. Merely informing the client of expectations may not be adequate (Behrman, 2006). The client's expectations of therapy must be elicited and evaluated for feasibility in the context of anatomical, physiological, neurological, psychological, and treatment constraints.

Expectations for the Family

Family involvement is important for success in treatment. For example, when a student has a voice disorder, the family can advocate for medical and therapeutic services, and the student may need assistance with homework to promote the generalization of therapeutic gains. The home environment may need to be modified, such as carpeting on the floor or curtains on the windows. The speech-language pathologist can provide support and encouragement through education and counseling (Ruddy & Sapienza, 2004). For this to occur effectively, the family must have an opportunity to express their expectations. The speech-language pathologist should assess the expectations to ensure they are realistic and are aligned with the treatment goals; if they are not, the clinician should provide education and counseling when necessary.

Determine How to Reach the Expectations

Goals will be formulated to restore or maximize vocal function in contexts that are relevant to the client. These goals will be formulated in conjunction with the client and family, with consideration to anatomical, physiological, or behavior factors underlying the disorder; knowledge of best practices; the client's desires and motivation; sociocultural considerations; and communicative contexts.

Consider Strong versus Weak Goals

A well-written goal is specific, measurable, attainable, relevant, and timely (SMART) (Torres, 2013). The goal must be individualized to the client and family, pertinent to their needs and wants, and implemented using techniques that are supported by the strongest clinical evidence, when available. The goal must be feasible given an individual's anatomy and physical capabilities. For example, the restoration of a voice to normal may not be possible when the vocal fold tissue is damaged or if breath support is impaired. However, in such cases, the vocal function can be maximized through treatment. For individuals who have undergone a laryngectomy, an alternative vibratory source for oral communication may be identified.

The goal and treatment techniques must be appropriate given the developmental level of the child (e.g., play therapy and environmental manipulation may be most appropriate for a young child with a voice disorder). Treatment may target changes in behavior that have the biggest impact on ease of communication, intelligibility, or self-esteem, or that is most helpful to access educational or social opportunities or is most amenable to change as determined by stimulability testing.

Intervention Approaches

Voice therapy improves voice outcomes (Speyer, Wieneke, & Dejonckere, 2004). After a disorder has been identified, treatment is implemented to restore the voice or minimize impairment. The goal of treatment is to maximize effective and efficient oral communication in contexts that are relevant to the client. Speech-language intervention may be performed alone or in conjunction with medical or surgical intervention. Many treatment options are available for prevention, habilitation, and rehabilitation of the voice. These approaches include education about the vocal mechanism and sound production, and self-awareness and practice will be targeted (Stemple et al., 2014). The main behavioral treatment approaches are hygienic, symptomatic, physiologic, and eclectic. Other approaches are used to treat specific voice disorders (e.g., spasmodic dysphonia or paradoxical vocal fold movement).

Hygienic therapy is an indirect voice therapy that seeks to identify, substitute, or minimize behaviors that cause, maintain, or exacerbate voice disorders. Following a thorough case history in which undesirable voice behaviors are identified, the client is educated in the deleterious effects of behaviors on voice and is given recommendations.

The client is encouraged to implement an individualized plan that may include the following (Adler et al., 2012; Colton et al., 2011):

- Maintain adequate systemic hydration by drinking water (e.g., 64 ounces)
- Minimize dry air by using a humidifier
- Minimize the inhalation of irritants (e.g., improve ventilation)
- Substitute throat clearing and coughing behaviors, which cause forceful closure for behaviors that limit vocal fold adduction (e.g., swallowing or coughing silently with abducted vocal folds)
- Minimize talking over noise (e.g., reduce environmental noise or use amplification)
- Minimize loud sounds (e.g., use hand signals instead of yelling)
- Substitute atypical sounds during speech, such as screeching (e.g., use lip trills or buzzing sounds that reduce laryngeal tension by encouraging forward focus of the voice where vibrations are felt on the face)
- Institute vocal rest

This approach, when used in conjunction with a direct treatment approach, can improve voice outcomes (Roy et al., 2001).

Symptomatic therapy seeks to identify and remediate symptoms of a voice disorder, such as atypical pitch, loudness, voice onset, and breath support, through facilitative techniques (Boone, McFarlane, Von Berg & Zraick, 2013). For example, if laryngeal tension is present, behaviors that reduce hyperfunction are trialed. If glottal fry is noted, pitch is increased. This may include a yawn followed by an audible sigh (yawn–sigh); insertion of the aspirated *h* before a vowel sound to minimize hard glottal attacks (easy onset); exaggerated chewing gestures (Froeschels chewing); or relaxed tongue protrusion during phonation of labial consonant and vowel combinations. Supportive evidence for this treatment approach is lacking.

In contrast to the symptomatic approach, the **physiologic approach** is holistic. It is based on the assumption that vocal physiology can be altered through exercise. Accent, resonant voice therapy (RVT), vocal function exercises (VFE), and LSVT LOUD are examples of this approach (Stemple et al., 2014). The accent method aims to improve respiratory control for speech and establish relaxed phonation with varied pitch and loudness (Kotby, 1995). RVT encourages efficient vocal fold positioning in which the vocal folds are barely adducted or barely abducted, as well as a resonant voice that is experienced as vibrations felt on the face (mask) during phonation (Verdolini-Marston, Burke, Lessac, Glaze, & Caldwell, 1995). Vocal hygiene treatment is incorporated in RVT. VFE are implemented to improve the strength, endurance, coordination, and balance of the respiratory, phonatory, and resonance systems (Stemple, 2005). A series of exercises are organized in a manner similar to physical therapy; that is, vocal muscles are warmed up, stretched, contracted, and cooled down. The speech-language pathologist uses an eclectic approach when using more than one treatment approach to remediate a voice disorder.

Although the strength of evidence supporting these treatments is varied and often lacking, direct treatments tend to produce better results than indirect treatments (Speyer et al., 2004). An important problem associated with each treatment approach is attrition. Ideally, treatment will continue until a client has met the goals and is satisfied with his or her voice outcomes. But in practice, the attrition rates from traditional voice therapy are high, with up to 65 percent of clients discontinuing treatment (Hapner, Portone-Maira, & Johns, 2009). The causes of attrition include costs (e.g., insurance denials), time commitment (e.g., travel distance), and skepticism about the benefits of treatment (Portone, Johns, & Hapner, 2008). To reduce attrition and maximize functional outcomes, Behrman (2006) proposed incorporating **motivational interviewing** into the management of voice disorders. This therapeutic technique goes beyond explaining the benefits of treatment to a client; clients are also guided through empathetic, open dialogue to identify undesirable behaviors, amplify any discrepancy between undesirable behaviors and the desired voice, encourage client-led identification of solutions, and support a client's belief in his or her ability to modify a behavior. Through this process, the client will develop a sense of readiness for change, which is necessary for implementing changes in vocal behaviors to improve vocal function and reduce attrition.

Summary

Voice disorders occur when there is an abnormality in pitch, loudness, quality, or vocal flexibility. They can occur across the life-span and range in severity from mild to severe. The impact of voice disorders on the individual and on society can be substantial and far ranging; voice disorders can be associated with significant educational, psychological, social, professional, and financial burdens. Speech-language pathologists play important roles in identifying, evaluating, and treating voice disorders, as well as advocating for people with these disorders. The treatment choice, duration, and outcomes depend on many factors, including etiology, contributing factors, client preference, perceived impact on quality of life, and readiness for change.

Case Scenarios

A 20-year-old student teacher, Ms. C, works in a first-grade class-room. Ms. C reported hoarseness and discomfort when speaking, and it worsens as the day progresses. At times, she has to strain to project her voice so students can hear her, particularly over classroom noise and outside noise. She attributed this difficulty to her lack of control over student behavior in the classroom and elsewhere. The client reported heavy voice use outside of work; she takes classes two nights per week that require group discussions and presentations, and she socializes two to three times per week and sometimes con-verses with friends at the gym while she exercises. Ms. C is usually talkative, but she has begun to withdraw from participation in class discussions and social conversations due to vocal fatigue, laryngeal discomfort, and embarrassment about her voice, which she feels no longer represents her. She reported that she is conscientious about drinking water frequently throughout the day. Ms. C's medical his-tory is significant for allergies, and she takes over-the-counter anti-histamines as needed.

An otolaryngology evaluation was completed prior to the voice evaluation. The laryngoscopic evaluation revealed ventricular fold medi-alization; small bilateral, pliable vocal nodules at the midmembranous aspect of the vocal folds; and mild erythema. The otolaryngologist rec-ommended voice therapy followed by a return visit for reexamination in 6 to 8 weeks.

A voice evaluation was completed. The Voice Handicap Index was administered and yielded a high score of 72, which is consistent with severe handicap. The CAPE-V yielded the following scores:

- Overall severity: 60
- Roughness: 60
- Breathiness: 50
- Strain: 55
- Pitch: 40
- Loudness: 0

Throat clearing was noted throughout the assessment. An acous-tic analysis revealed fundamental frequency for sustained vowel at 184 Hz (norm: 190–210 Hz), which is a little below the expected

📋 Case Scenarios *(continued)*

value for the client's age and gender. Her measures of vocal stability jitter (2.1 percent; norm: less than 1.04 percent) and shimmer (9 percent; norm: less than 3.5 percent) were elevated. Her harmonic-to-noise ratio was low (17 dB; norm: greater than 20 dB). These parameters are consistent with perception of hoarseness. The pitch variation during spontaneous speaking was reduced, which is consistent with perceived monotone voice, and the pitch range was reduced (10 semitones, norm: 24–36 semitones). The mean loudness during spontaneous speech was appropriate (68 dB). However, the client's voice quality was perceived to deteriorate at louder volumes. Aerodynamic data revealed elevated subglottal pressure for production of *pi* at a comfortable pitch (7.2 cm H_2O; norm: 3 cm H_2O) and reduced breath support for speech maximum phonation time (MPT; 7 seconds; norm: 15–25 seconds).

It was recommended that Ms. C use a personal amplification device in the classroom and participate in weekly treatment to restore her voice and prevent the reoccurrence of vocal nodules. An eclectic treatment approach was used. An individualized voice hygiene plan was developed, with an emphasis on realistic and positive statements to increase adherence; symptomatic therapy was recommended to minimize the most salient symptoms of the voice disorder (pitch); and vocal function exercises were recommended to restore the balance among the respiratory, phonatory, and resonance mechanisms.

Long-Term Goal

Improve voice quality, comfort, and endurance for satisfying personal and professional needs, including classroom activities for up to 45 minutes without symptoms of discomfort or handicap.

Short-Term Goals

1. Demonstrate knowledge of healthy versus maladaptive or unhealthy laryngeal and vocal behavior, as evidenced by 80 percent accuracy in a question-and-answer activity.
2. Use a silent cough or hard swallow as a substitution for throat clearing, with no more than three missed opportunities during a treatment session.
3. Independently use exaggerated vocal variety during a 2-minute conversation, with at least 70 percent accuracy.
4. Complete an at-home vocal exercise program that includes vocal function exercises twice daily, with two repetitions per exercise as documented by the client in a daily log.

Case Scenarios *(continued)*

Case Scenario 2

Ms. Q is 70 years old and presents as outgoing, friendly, and talkative. She works part-time as an accountant. Her work does not require heavy voice use; she participates in occasional phone calls and small group discussions. However, Ms. Q is very involved with her local theater, where she performs many duties including directing, managing, and acting. She also cares for three young grandchildren 1 day per week, during which time she sings, reads, and talks continuously. She complains of a weak voice, difficulty becoming loud, and reduced stamina, as evidenced by fatigue when speaking at work and at the theater. She noted that she frequently has to take a breath when speaking. She reports that her symptoms began about 1 year prior to her evaluation and have become more bothersome over time.

Ms. Q's otolaryngology consult revealed bilateral vocal fold bowing consistent with presbyphonia. The otolaryngologist recommended trial voice therapy to optimize her voice prior to consideration of medical intervention. The voice evaluation revealed elevated airflow (250 mL/s; norm: 200 mL/s); reduced dynamic range (61–82 dB; norm: 50–110 dB); mild to moderate breathiness (30 mm on CAPE-V; norm: 0); mild roughness (15 mm on CAPE-V); reduced breath support for speech and laryngeal valving, as indicated by maximum phonation time (MPT 9 seconds; norm: 15–25 seconds) and s/z ratio (s: 10 seconds, z: 6 seconds, s/z: 1.67; norm: less than 1.4 seconds); and vocal handicap (40 on VHI; norm: 0), consistent with her medical diagnosis and clinical complaints.

Treatment was recommended to maximize effective and efficient oral communication in contexts relevant to the client (e.g., at home and the theater) and minimize her perceived vocal handicap. Symptomatic treatment focused on increasing breath support and control for speech to permit efficient and safe increase in vocal volume and to restore coordination between respiration and phonation. An increased mouth opening was recommended to increase oral resonance. A physiologic approach, resonant voice exercises, was implemented to facilitate efficient production of strong voice.

Long-Term Goal

Optimize voice quality and function for personal, social, and artistic communication.

📋 Case Scenarios *(continued)*

Short-Term Goals

1. Improve breath support for speech by using deep abdominal replenishing breaths in 8 of 10 trials when orally reading short phrases.
2. Improve breathing and phonation coordination by producing a simultaneous vocal attack at the beginning of utterances during utterances within a 3–5 minute conversation, given no more than three errors.
3. Improve voice projection through the use of exaggerated articulation and frontal focused resonance when speaking self-formulated sentences, with at least 70 percent accuracy.
4. Complete an at-home daily vocal exercise program that includes 15–20 minutes of resonant voice exercises using an audiotaped model, as documented by the client in a daily log.

Case Scenario 3

The client, Ms. L, is a 16-year-old high school student who presents at the clinic, accompanied by her mother, with complaints of episodes of difficulty breathing and wheezing. She reports that, during these episodes, she experiences tightness in her neck and sudden difficulty inhaling, typically triggered by exercise. She describes the episodes to be of short duration, but scary and stressful. These symptoms resolve best when she purses her lips on inhalation and exhalation. You gather a thorough medical and social history. Ms. L excels academically and engages actively in extracurricular activities. She is a good athlete who participates on her school soccer and track teams. Ms. L states that prior to visiting the clinic, she was seen by a pulmonologist, who prescribed inhalers for exercise-induced asthma, but they did not provide relief. Her respiratory function values are unremarkable. She denies a history of allergies and reflux. You assess her voice and note that her acoustic, aerodynamic, and perceptual measures are all within functional limits. Upon visualization of the vocal folds through transnasal flexible fiberoptic laryngoscopy by you and an otolaryngologist, a period of vocal fold adduction on inhalation is triggered by physical exertion (running on a treadmill). Based on her symptoms, history, and the endoscopy, Ms. L is diagnosed with paradoxical vocal fold movement (PVFM).

Treatment is recommended. After consultation with Ms. L and her family, you develop a plan to address education, breathing techniques,

📋 **Case Scenarios** *(continued)*

and relaxation exercises. You will educate Ms. L on normal respiration, vocal fold function, and PVFM. The breathing portion of treatment will focus on two techniques: sniff and inhale with abdominal breathing, and inhaling and exhaling while sustaining /s/. For relaxation, the client will learn the yawn–sigh technique, humming, and chewing to reduce laryngeal and jaw tension, and she will learn isometric exercises to reduce neck and shoulder tension. Based on this information, write one long-term goal and three short-term goals.

REVIEW QUESTIONS

1. Which of the following is true of a voice disorder?
   a. It can result from anatomical, physiological, cognitive, psychological, and hearing factors.
   b. It is defined as abnormal or absent pitch, loudness, quality, or flexibility as determined by our sociocultural norms.
   c. It may be perceived differently across cultures.
   d. It is associated with financial, psychosocial, emotional, and educational costs.
   e. It is treated by a speech-language pathologist and otolaryngologist.
   f. All of the above are true.

2. Why is advocacy and treatment for children with voice disorders in school settings warranted?
   a. Voice disorders negatively impact educational performance.
   b. Children do not grow out of voice disorders.
   c. Children's participation in academic opportunities may be compromised.
   d. Children with dysphonia are perceived negatively by their peers.
   e. All of the above are true.

3. Which of the following is not true regarding treatment?
   a. Vocal function exercises and resonant therapy are examples of a physiologic treatment approach.
   b. Symptomatic treatment identifies and remediates the symptoms of a voice disorder (e.g., hard glottal attack).
   c. Accent therapy is an example of a vocal hygiene approach to treatment.
   d. Well-designed studies are warranted to assess the effectiveness of treatment strategies.

4. Which of the following is not true regarding attrition from voice treatment?
   a. High levels of attrition occur with voice therapy (up to 65 percent of clients may discontinue treatment).
   b. Time and financial burdens associated with treatment, and lack of confidence in treatment, may contribute to high attrition levels.
   c. Incorporating motivational interviewing into voice treatment may reduce attrition rates.
   d. A symptomatic treatment reduces the rate of attrition.

5. A good treatment goal must be which of the following?
   a. Specific, realistic, attainable, relevant, and timely
   b. Developed in conjunction with the client and family
   c. Aimed to restore normal physiology
   d. A and B
   e. A, B, and C

REFERENCES

Adler, R. K., Hirsch, S., & Mordaunt, M. (2012). Voice and communication therapy for the transgender/transsexual client: A comprehensive clinical guide (2nd ed.). San Diego, CA: Plural.

American Speech-Language-Hearing Association. (1993). Definitions of communication disorders and variations. *ASHA, 35*(Suppl. 10), 40–41.

American Speech-Language-Hearing Association. (2003). National outcomes measurement system (NOMS): Adult speech-language pathology user's guide. Rockville, MD: Author.

American Speech-Language-Hearing Association. (2004). *Preferred practice patterns for the profession of speech-language pathology*. Retrieved from http://www.asha.org/uploadedFiles/PP2004-00191.pdf

American Speech-Language-Hearing Association. (2011). SLP health care survey report: Patient caseload characteristics trends 2005–2011. Retrieved from http://www.asha.org/uploadedfiles/hc11-caseload-characteristics-trends.pdf

Amir, O., & Levine-Yundof, R. (2013). Listeners' attitudes toward people with dysphonia. *Journal of Voice, 27*(4), 524.e1–524e.10.

Andrews, M. L., & Summers, A. C. (2002). *Voice treatment for children and adolescents*. San Diego, CA: Singular Thomson Learning.

Aronson, A. E. (1990). Importance of the psychological interview in the diagnosis and treatment of "functional" voice disorders. *Journal of Voice, 4*, 287–289.

Baken, R. J., & Orlikoff, R. F. (2000). *Clinical measurement of speech and voice* (2nd ed.). San Diego, CA: Singular.

Baker, K. K., Ramig, L. O., Sapir S., Luschel, E. S., & Smith, M. E. (2001). Control of vocal loudness in young and old adults. *Journal of Speech and Hearing Research, 44*(2), 297–305.

Behrman, A. (2005). Common practices of voice therapists in the evaluation of patients. *Journal of Voice, 19*, 454–469.

Behrman, A. (2006). Facilitating behavioral change in voice therapy: The relevance of motivating interviewing. *American Journal of Speech-Language Pathology, 15*, 215–225.

Boone, D. R., McFarlane, S. C., Von Berg, S. L., & Zraick, R. I. (2013). *Voice and voice therapy* (9th ed.). Boston, MA: Pearson.

Cohen, S. M., Kim, J., Roy, N., Asche, C., & Courey, M. (2012). The impact of laryngeal disorders on work-related dysfunction. *Laryngoscope, 122*, 1589–1594.

Colton, R. H., Casper, J. K., & Leonard, R. (2011). *Understanding voice problems: A physiological perspective for diagnosis and treatment* (4th ed.). Baltimore, MD: Lippincott Williams & Wilkins.

Connecticut State Department of Education. (2008). Guidelines for speech and language programs: Determining eligibility for special education speech and language services under IDEA. Retrieved from http://www.sde.ct.gov/sde/lib/sde/PDF/DEPS/Special/Speech_Language_2008.pdf

Connor, N. P., Cohen, S. B., Theis, S. M., Thibeault, S. L., Heatley, D. G., & Bless, D. M. (2008). Attitudes of children with dysphonia. *Journal of Voice, 22*(2), 197–209.

De Bodt, M. S., Ketelslagers, K., Peeters, T., Wuyts, F. L., Mertens, F., Pattyn, J., . . . Van de Heyning, P. (2007). Evolution of vocal fold nodules from childhood to adolescence. *Journal of Voice, 21*, 151–156.

Dehqan, A., & Scherer, R. C. (2011). Objective voice analysis of boys with profound hearing loss. *Journal of Voice, 25*, e61–e65.

Eadie, T. L., & Kapsner-Smith, M. (2011). The effect of listener experience and anchors on judgments of dysphonia. *Journal of Speech, Language and Hearing Research, 54,* 430–447.

Ferrand, C. T. (2012). *Voice disorders: Scope of theory and practice.* Boston, MA: Pearson.

Fox, C. M., Ramig, L. O., Ciucci, M. R., Sapir, S., McFarland, D. H., & Farley, B. G. (2006). The science and practice of LSVT/LOUD: Neural plasticity-principled approach to treating individuals with Parkinson disease and other neurological disorders. *Seminars in Speech and Language, 27,* 283–299.

Fu, S., Theodoros, D. G., & Ward, E. C. (2015). Delivery of intensive voice therapy for vocal fold nodules via telepractice: A pilot feasibility and efficacy study. *Journal of Voice, 29,* 696–706.

Gardner, H. (2014). Collaborative working between pediatric speech and language therapy and ENT colleagues: What is good practice? *Current Opinion in Otolaryngology & Head and Neck Surgery, 22*(3), 167–171.

Hapner, E., Portone-Maira, C., & Johns, M. M. (2009). A study of voice therapy dropout. *Journal of Voice, 23*(3), 337–340.

Hirano, M. (1981). *Clinical examination of voice.* New York, NY: Springer.

Hooper, C. R. (2004). Treatment of voice disorders in children. *Language, Speech, and Hearing Services in Schools, 34,* 320–326.

Isetti, D., & Eadie, T. (2015). The Americans with Disabilities Act and voice disorders: Practical guidelines for voice clinicians. *Journal of Voice, 30*(3), 1–8.

Kempster, G. B., Gerratt, B. R., Abbott, K. V., Barkmeier-Kraemer, J., & Hillman, R. E. (2009). Consensus auditory–perceptual evaluation of voice: Development of a standard clinical protocol. *American Journal of Speech-Language Pathology, 18,* 124–132.

Kotby, N. (1995). *The accent method of voice therapy.* San Diego, CA: Singular.

Lass, N. J., Ruscello, D. M., Stout, L. L., & Hoffmann, F. M. (1991). Peer perceptions of normal and voice-disordered children. *Folia Phoniatrica et Logopaedica, 43,* 29–35.

Lejska, M. (2003). Voice field measurements–a new method of examination: The influence of hearing on the human voice. *Journal of Voice, 18,* 209–215.

Linville, S. E., & Fisher, H. B. (1985). Acoustic characteristics of women's voices with advancing age. *Journal of Gerontology, 40,* 324–330.

Maddern, B. R., Campbell, T. F., & Stool, S. (1991). Pediatric voice disorders. *Otolaryngology Clinics of North America, 24,* 1125–1140.

Maryn, Y., & Debo, K. (2014). Is perceived dysphonia related to perceived healthiness? *Logopedics Phoniatrics Vocology, 40,* 12–28.

McNamara, A. P., & Perry, C. K. (1994). Vocal abuse prevention: A national survey of school-based pathologists. *Language, Speech, and Hearing Services in Schools, 25,* 105–111.

Oates, J. (2009). Auditory–perceptual evaluation of disordered voice quality. *Folia Phonatrica et Logopaedica, 61,* 49–56.

Patel, R., Thibeault, S. L., & Bless, D. M. (2011). Boot camp: A novel intense approach to voice therapy. *Journal of Voice, 25*(5), 562–569.

Portone, C., Johns, M. M., & Hapner, E. R. (2008). A review of patient adherence to the recommendation for voice therapy. *Journal of Voice, 22,* 192–196.

Ramig, L. O., & Verdolini, K. (1998). Treatment efficacy: Voice disorders. *Journal of Speech-Language and Hearing Research, 41,* S101–S116.

Roy, N., Barkmeier-Kraemer, J., Eadie, T., Sivasankar, M. P., Mehta, D., Paul, D., & Hillman, R. (2013). Evidence-based clinical voice assessment: A systematic review. *American Journal of Speech-Language Pathology, 22,* 212–226.

Roy, N., Gray, S. D., Simon, M., Dove, H., Corbin-Lewis, H., & Stemple, J. C. (2001). An evaluation of the effects of two treatment approaches for teachers with voice disorders: A prospective randomized clinical trial. *Journal of Speech Language and Hearing Research, 44*, 286–296.

Roy, N., & Hendarto, H. (2005). Revisiting the pitch controversy: Changes in speaking fundamental frequency (SFF) after management of functional dysphonia. *Journal of Voice, 19*, 582–591.

Roy, N., Merrill, R. M., Thibeault, S., Parsa, R. A., Gray, S. D., & Smith, E. M. (2004). Prevalence of voice disorders in teachers and the general population. *Journal of Speech Language Hearing and Research, 47*, 281–293.

Ruddy, B. H., & Sapienza, C. M. (2004). Treating voice disorders in the school-based setting: Working within the framework of IDEA. *Language, Speech, and Hearing Services in Schools, 35*, 327–332.

Schwartz, S. R., Cohen, S. M., Dailey, S. H., Rosenfeld, R. M., Deutsch, E. S., Gillespie, M. B., . . . Patel, M. M. (2009). Clinical practice guidelines: Hoarseness (dysphonia). *Otolaryngology– Head and Neck Surgery, 141*(3), S1–S31.

Searl, J., Wilson, K., Haring, K., Dietsch, A., Lyons, K., & Pahwa, R. (2011). Feasibility of group voice therapy for individuals with Parkinson's disease. *Journal of Communication Disorders, 44*(6), 719–732.

Speyer, R., Wieneke, G. H., & Dejonckere, P. H. (2004). Documentation of progress in voice therapy: Perceptual, acoustic, and laryngostroboscopic finding pretherapy and posttherapy. *Journal of Voice, 18*, 325–340.

Stemple, J. C. (2005). A holistic approach to voice therapy. *Seminars in Speech and Language, 26*, 131–137.

Stemple, J. C., Roy, N., & Klaben, B. (2014). *Clinical voice pathology: Theory and management* (5th ed.). San Diego, CA: Plural.

Timmermans, B., De Bodt, M. S., Wuyts, F. L., & Van de Heyning, P. H. (2005). Analysis and evaluation of a voice-training program in future professional voice users. *Journal of Voice, 19*, 202–210.

Tindall, L. R., Huebner, R. A., Stemple, J. C., & Kleinert, H. L. (2009). Videophone-delivered voice therapy: A comparative analysis of outcomes to traditional delivery for adults with Parkinson's disease. *Telemedicine & E-Health, 14*, 1070–1077.

Torres, I. (2013). Make it work: Write targeted treatment goals. *The ASHA Leader, 18*, 26–27.

Verdolini, K. (1999). Critical analysis of common terminology in voice therapy: A position paper. *Phonoscope, 2*, 1–8.

Verdolini, K., Rosen, C. A., & Branski, R. C. (Eds.). (2006). *Classification manual of voice disorders–I.* Mahwah, NJ: Lawrence Erlbaum.

Verdolini-Marston, K., Burke, M. K., Lessac, A., Glaze, L., & Caldwell, E. (1995). Preliminary study of two methods of treatment for laryngeal nodules. *Journal of Voice, 9*, 74–85.

Zacharias, S. R. C., Kelchner, L. N., & Creaghead, N. (2013). Teachers' perceptions of adolescent females with voice disorders. *Language, Speech and Hearing Services in Schools, 44*, 174–182.

ADDITIONAL RESOURCES

American Academy of Otolaryngology–Head and Neck Surgery: www.entnet.org
American Speech-Language-Hearing Association: www.asha.org
National Center for Voice and Speech: www.ncvs.org
National Institute on Deafness and Other Communication Disorders: www.nidcd.nih.gov
Voice Foundation: www.voicefoundation.org
World Professional Association for Transgender Health: www.wpath.org

Reading Disabilities: Skill Development through Assessment, Goals, and Strategic Instruction

Elizabeth Stein

Key Terms

Comprehension
Decoding
Explicit instruction

Metacognition
Phonemic awareness
Reading fluency

Introduction

Developing literacy skills is a complex process based on a multilayered skill set that must blend together with ease so reading is a pleasurable and meaningful experience. Yet for many learners, gaps in mastering specific skill sets result in years of reading struggles. Today's learners need effective instruction across content areas. They need authentic reading, writing, listening, speaking, and thinking experiences in natural environments so they will have deep, meaningful interactions with text beginning at an early age (Gargiulo & Metcalf, 2017). Thoughtful interactions with words and language on a daily basis increase literary development (Schmoker, 2007).

However, compelling research reveals that students at risk for reading disabilities experience significant difficulties in foundational skills, regardless of exposure to literary experiences. In general, students with a reading disorder demonstrate difficulty in **decoding**, word recognition, fluency, or **comprehension** (Hulme & Snowling, 2013).

Comprehensive Assessment

The ultimate goal of reading is to actively and efficiently construct meaning from text. Beginning readers must acquire two important skill sets: recognizing printed words and applying strong reading comprehension skills. To achieve a high level of reading skills, students need effective instruction and abundant practice (Paratore, Cassano, & Schickedanz, 2011). These two important skill sets can be broken down into subskills to guide beginning readers.

The National Reading Panel, which is a group of literacy and reading scholars appointed by the National Institute of Child Health and Human Development and the U.S. Department of Education, identified five "big ideas" (see **TABLE 12-1**) that represent the subskills needed to

TABLE 12-1 Big Ideas for Reading Success

Big Idea	Explanation
Phonemic awareness: The ability to hear, identify, and manipulate sounds in spoken language.	• Phonemic awareness is essential for children to develop before they can learn to read. • Phonemic awareness is the foundation for reading and is a strong indicator of a child's potential to successfully read. • Phonemic awareness rests on the understanding that spoken words are made up of phonemes, which are individual units of sound that influence the meaning of a word. For example, the word *cat* has three individual phonemes: /k/ /a/ /t/. If you replace one of the phonemes, the meaning of the word changes. For instance, if the initial phoneme /k/ is replaced by /b/, the word changes completely. In addition to the awareness that spoken words are made up of small units, readers also need the ability to break down, manipulate, and blend phonemes as they learn to read.

TABLE 12-1 Big Ideas for Reading Success *(continued)*

Big Idea	Explanation
	• The three main aspects of phonemic awareness include syllables, rhymes, and beginning (initial) sounds. Early readers need to be able to identify and manipulate these elements to begin reading.
Phonics: Connecting the letters of written language with the individual sounds of spoken language. Also connected with the alphabetic principle and decoding, which is linking sounds to letter symbols and patterns. Strong skills in phonics allow readers to apply the relationship between written language and spoken language so they can read printed text and spell words.	• As phonemic awareness develops, readers must be able to transfer knowledge of phonemes used in oral language to written language. • In addition to phoneme awareness and letter knowledge, knowledge of sound–symbol associations is vital for success beginning in first grade and beyond. Accurate and fluent word recognition depends on phonics knowledge. • The ability to read words accounts for a substantial proportion of overall reading success, even in older readers. • When effective readers encounter an unknown word, they decode the word, name it, and attach meaning to it. Typically, the context of the text helps the reader get the meaning of the word after a word has been decoded. By the end of second grade, readers should be able to decode almost any unfamiliar word so they can focus on gaining meaning as they read. • Some students need explicit, systematic instruction to guide their phonological development (see the "Types of Intervention Approaches" section in this chapter). Instruction in word recognition includes sound–letter correspondence, sight words, syllabication (breaking words into syllables), and morphology (breaking words into meaningful parts).

TABLE 12-1 Big Ideas for Reading Success *(continued)*

Big Idea	Explanation
Fluency: The automatic reading of text.	• After students are able to decode with accuracy, they apply their decoding skills to reading a text with fluency and automaticity. • Adequate fluency allows readers to be more successful in comprehending what they are reading. Successful readers can read about 95 percent of the words without struggling with decoding. • Readers who have difficulty constructing meaning from text often read too slowly. In addition, some readers need additional support to strengthen their fluency and automaticity, even though they have experienced instruction with basic phonics.
Vocabulary: Understand the meanings of words.	• As readers decode accurately and fluently, meaning is gained from text, and readers begin to expand their vocabulary. This knowledge of word meaning is a critical component of reading comprehension. • Reading widely promotes acquisition of word knowledge. • Most of the words children learn in school are acquired through hearing them read aloud or by reading them in books.
Comprehension: A complex cognitive process that allows intentional interaction between reader and text that results in the reader constructing meaning.	• Comprehension is the ultimate goal of reading. Comprehension depends greatly on a well-developed vocabulary and background knowledge base. • Students' background knowledge starts to develop before they learn to read as they listen to parents and teachers, and through interactive read-aloud experiences. • Teachers expand students' background knowledge by exposing learners to frequent interactive reading experiences of narrative and expository texts to expand children's knowledge of the world.

TABLE 12-1 Big Ideas for Reading Success *(continued)*

Big Idea	Explanation
	• As early as kindergarten, children begin to learn to become active readers as teachers encourage them to apply **metacognition** by thinking about their thinking through generating and asking questions, making connections between the text and their own lives, and making predictions about what they think will happen next in a story.
	• Metacognitive strategies become more prevalent as students shift from learning to read (grades kindergarten through second grade) to reading to learn (grades three and up). The early years set the foundation for the reading skills and metacognitive strategies that students need to become successful readers for life.

achieve ultimate reading success (National Reading Panel, 2000). These big ideas—these skills—must be assessed and be a part of daily effective instructional practices that are important for all students. They are especially important as part of explicit, strategic instruction for students who are at risk for reading disabilities.

Early intervention and remediation of students who are at risk for reading disabilities is critical for academic success later in life. It is far easier to remediate reading deficits in young at-risk children than to remediate deficits in older children who have an identified learning disability (Schatschneider & Torgesen, 2004). Evidence suggests that phonological awareness plays an essential role in reading development and reading disorders, and it is the core deficit in students with reading disorders (Torgesen, 2002). An assessment of **phonemic awareness** typically includes rhyming, blending, segmenting, and phoneme manipulation (Mather & Wendling, 2012).

Rasinski, Rikli, and Johnston (2009) described **reading fluency** as the ability to decode words and symbols rapidly, effortlessly, and automatically. When students apply a high level of fluency, they are able to comprehend the text and predict unknown words based on the context of what they are reading (Pikulski & Chard, 2005). Reading fluency is an essential aspect of reading and was identified as one of the key areas of reading by the National Reading Panel (2000). Fluency consists of three elements. The first is accuracy. Accuracy is the ability to recognize or decode words. Children who have poor word-reading accuracy typically have difficulty with understanding the author's message, and oftentimes they misunderstand the text. The second element in fluency is reading rate, which consists of the ability to recall words quickly with appropriate speed and flexibility (Hudson, Lane, & Pullen, 2005). Children who are poor readers typically read laboriously, which results in struggling with schoolwork and may, in turn, result in lost interest in school (Moats, 2001). Prosody, the third area of reading fluency, is the rhythmic and tonal features of speech demonstrated through expressive reading (Rasinski et al., 2009). Struggling readers often read in a monotone voice that lacks expression or meaningful phrasing (Hudson et al., 2005). The assessment of reading fluency includes measures of accuracy, rate, and prosody (Mather & Wendling, 2012). One of the most effective methods of measuring reading fluency is through oral reading. To assess reading fluency and to make decisions about children's progress in reading, teachers must provide feedback to students regarding both strong areas and areas that need improvement as they provide encouragement and direction for students to read with expression (Mitchell, Rearden, & Stacy, 2011). The process of assessment refers to formal and informal gathering of data to identify a student's areas of strengths and needs. The collected data are then used to make decisions about the next educational steps toward designing instruction for student achievement.

Comprehensive Reading Assessments

Assessing students' reading skills through informal assessments is a natural part of the educational process for all learners. Yet students who are at risk for a reading disability—or those already identified as having one—must be a part of additional and ongoing assessments to frequently monitor their progress so instructional decisions can be made. The federal Individuals with Disabilities Education Act (IDEA) requires that a team of professionals assess a student's broad range of cognitive, academic, and social achievements. IDEA stipulates that the use of formal and informal assessment tools be administered to provide a comprehensive view of a student's performance. School psychologists, teachers, and other educational diagnosticians are responsible for evaluating the student's strengths and needs. Interindividual and intraindividual differences are assessed through the use of norm-referenced and criterion-referenced assessments (Gargiulo & Metcalf, 2017).

Formal Assessments

Norm-referenced assessments are standardized tests and are connected to interindividual differences. The results of the assessment compare the student's performance with a representative sample so the evaluator can see how the student performed in comparison to his or her same-aged peers. Data gathered from norm-referenced tests reveal a ranked ordering of student achievement within the representative sample population from high to low achievement along the bell curve and, therefore, provide limited information to guide instructional decisions. Criterion-referenced tests, on the other hand, assess mastery learning and reveal correct responses and specific student abilities and areas of need that can serve to guide instructional decisions (Salvia, Ysseldyke, & Witmer, 2012).

Examples of formal assessments include the following:

- Brigance Comprehensive Inventory of Basic Skills II—Revised (Brigance, 2010)
- Dynamic Indicators of Basic Early Literacy Skills (DIBELS) (Good, Gruba, & Kaminski, 2002).
- Gray Oral Reading Test (GORT-5) (Wiederholt & Bryant, 2012).
- Test of Phonological Awareness (TOPA) (Torgesen & Bryant, 2004)
- Test of Word Reading Efficiency (TOWRE) (Torgesen, Wagner, & Rashotte, 1999).
- Woodcock Reading Mastery Tests, Third Edition (Woodcock, 2011)

Informal Assessments

Informal assessments provide authentic, meaningful data about how a student approaches the reading process. In addition, they reveal the strategies that a student applies as any part of the reading process breaks down.

Examples of informal assessments include the following:

- Dolch sight word lists: The assessment evaluates a student's ability to read from a list of 220 frequently used sight words. The ability to read sight words accurately plays a part in guiding a student to read fluently because these words are read in context (Gargiulo & Metcalf, 2017).
- Informal Reading Inventory (IRI): This assessment uses a series of passages that are used to determine a student's reading level, strengths, and needs. An IRI assessment provides general skill levels and an overall sense of comprehension level.

- Retrospective Miscue Analysis (RMA): This approach to reading assessment and instruction has a long history of success and is most commonly used with readers who have difficulty constructing meaning from text. The assessment raises the readers' awareness of their thinking during the process of reading (Wurr, Theurer, & Kim, 2009). Typically, a reader records him- or herself reading an unfamiliar text. As the reader listens to the recording, he or she notices the strategies that worked and areas that need new strategies to address weaknesses. The teacher guides the reader through this reflective process by asking four central questions: (1) Did the miscue make sense? (2) Did the miscue interfere with comprehension? If not, then the miscue does not need to be corrected. (3) Did you self-correct, if needed? (4) Why do you think you made that miscue?

Interpreting Reading Assessments

Reading is the foundation for individuals to exchange information. It is also a necessary skill in any learning process. It is critical that educators understand how to translate student performance on assessments into meaningful instructional decisions.

Oral Reading Assessments

To assess the accuracy and fluency of a reader, an oral assessment must be administered. This is a common assessment in primary grades as students are learning how to read. According to Salvia and colleagues (2012), oral reading assessments measure reading behaviors through the documentation of miscues in oral reading. Miscues occur when a reader's perception and reading of words do not match what is actually on the page (Davenport, 2002; Goodman, Watson, & Burke, 1987). These miscues provide insight into understanding the strengths and needs of the reader and facilitate planning for strategic instructional decisions to support the student's future reading success. Common miscues seen on oral reading tests include (but are not limited to) the following:

- Omissions: The reader may skip a word, phrase, or complete sentences.
- Insertions: The reader may add words or groups of words that do not appear in the text.
- Substitution: The reader replaces a word or group of words from the text with something that he or she inserts based on his or her own thinking.

- Inversion: The reader changes the order of words as they appear in the text.
- Pacing: The reader disregards punctuation, which may adversely affect gaining meaning from text.

A miscue is significant only if it interferes with constructing meaning from text. Many miscues are acceptable and are a natural part of the reading process. Miscues become significant when they interfere with comprehension, when words are mispronounced, when students do not self-correct when needed, and when they occur frequently in a manner that adversely affects the reading process (Reschly, Busch, Betts, Deno, & Long, 2009).

Reading Comprehension Assessments

According to Salvia and colleagues (2012), assessments may reveal information about a reader's abilities by evaluating six reading comprehension skills:

- Literal comprehension: The reader may comprehend information that is directly stated in the text.
- Inferential comprehension: The reader must interpret what is read.
- Listening comprehension: The student listens to a text that is read aloud, then responds to questions to demonstrate understanding about what was read.
- Critical comprehension: The reader makes judgments, and evaluates and analyzes the text, to demonstrate higher-level thinking skills.
- Affective comprehension: After reading a text, the teacher evaluates the student's emotions as a result of reading the text.
- Lexical comprehension: The reader's knowledge of vocabulary is evaluated within the context of reading a text.

The IRI is a quick reading assessment that can provide valuable insights into the types of errors and basic comprehension skills demonstrated by the student. The results of the IRI place the reader at one of three levels:

1. Independent: The student was able to read 98 percent of the words, and answered the comprehension questions that followed, with 90–100 percent accuracy.
2. Instructional: The student recognized 95 percent of the words, and answered the comprehension questions, with 70–85 percent accuracy.
3. Frustration: The student recognized less than 90 percent of the words and responded to the comprehension questions with less than 70 percent accuracy.

Word Reading Skills Assessments

Students who recognize many words are said to have good sight vocabularies, or good word recognition skills. According to Ehri (2014), some students who have difficulty with word recognition may have a range of difficulties, including the following:

- Auditory discrimination: The student may mispronounce words, which interferes with expanding vocabulary and word knowledge.
- Auditory–visual memory: The student has great difficulty with sounding out words—he or she does not connect phonemes with printed letters—and often reads a word inaccurately by guessing based on picture clues or the context of the story. The student may give up or substitute a word with minimal success.
- Receptive or expressive language: The student has difficulties either understanding what is said (receptive) or demonstrating understanding through the spoken or written word (expressive).

Determining Eligibility for Special Education Services

Teachers play a key role in deciding whether students' needs may be addressed through effective classroom instructional decisions or if more support is needed through possible special education services. Friend and Bursuck suggest that teachers analyze any unmet needs presented by the student. They outline five questions that teachers should ask themselves:

1. What are the unmet needs? What behaviors or academic performance issues continue to be present in daily class time?
2. Is there a chronic pattern that is negatively impacting student learning?
3. Are the unmet needs becoming more serious over time?
4. Is the student's learning behavior significantly different from his peers in class?
5. Is there an inconsistent presence of learning behaviors that negatively impact learning—yet you cannot predict when these learning actions will occur? (Friend & Bursuck, 2002, p. 45)

After the teacher has a clear vision of what the student's unmet needs are—and evidence to support those concerns—it is time to communicate with parents, colleagues, and the student, if appropriate. During the collaboration time, the teacher should continue implementing specific interventions to try to meet the needs of the student. It is very important to continue documenting the student's unmet needs, the specific communications that were implemented, and the specific instructional strategies that were used to support the student's learning. If progress is not noted after the pre-referral action steps, it may be time for a referral to special education services.

Response to Intervention

The premise of response to intervention (RTI) is providing high-quality, scientifically validated instruction to guide student achievement. RTI is not a special education initiative. Rather, it is a framework of meaningful instruction that ensures learners are provided with high-quality instruction. The RTI process rules out poor or insufficient instruction as a reason for struggling with learning. RTI provides a framework for evaluation on how students are responding to high-quality instructional decisions and practices. Generally, RTI is defined as a three-tier framework of support (**FIGURE 12-1**):

> Tier 1: The first tier is the general education whole class setting where high quality instruction serves to meet the needs of the learners in the room. Tier 1 is always a part of a student's learning process. Tiers 2 and 3 are additional supports for students who demonstrate difficulties in meeting grade level expectations.
> Tier 2: The intensity of instruction increases through this supplemental small group instruction that meet two to three times a week. This small group instruction is additional re-teaching, pre-teaching, or review for students who struggle within the whole class, tier 1 instruction.
> Tier 3: If students continue to struggle within the whole class (Tier 1) and Tier 2—the intensity of instruction increases through more frequent small group—and sometimes one-to-one instructional time. Through ongoing progress monitoring, Tier 3 support is continued or it may be decided to move forward with a referral for special education services. (Stein, 2013, p. 10)

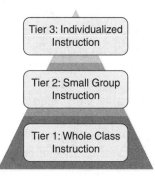

FIGURE 12-1 The three tiers of RTI.

The RTI process can guide the identification of students with disabilities by reducing the number of students that are misidentified. RTI ensures consistent, effective learning experiences for all learners. After weeks or months of providing high-quality instruction and monitoring students' learning—some students continue to struggle—the special education referral process may enter the scene.

Referral Process

In the case of reading difficulties, referrals arise from concern about a child's inability to demonstrate skills that are expected at or near the current grade level. This student has exhibited ongoing learning behaviors that adversely affect his or her ability to successfully participate in grade-level learning. The referral form must express clear, detailed reasons why the request is being made. Teachers must provide documentation in the form of specific classroom examples over time, and they must submit student work samples that provide evidence of the concern. Teachers must be explicit when sharing the instructional practices that were in place to ensure the child was given the very best instruction in efforts to support reading growth. Typically, information is gathered from a multidisciplinary team to paint a full picture of the child's abilities. The team typically consists of the general education teacher, a special education teacher, a speech-language pathologist, a psychologist, a social worker, a school nurse, a principal, and the parent or guardian. If the team decides to proceed, the parent or guardian must sign a written consent for the child to be evaluated through a formal process. After written consent is given, the evaluation process may begin (Gargiulo & Metcalf, 2017).

All speech-language pathologists are trained to diagnose and treat speech- and language-related disorders, which is closely related to a child's ability to achieve mastery in all skills needed for reading. During the evaluation process, the speech-language pathologist will provide a complete language evaluation to assess skills such as receptive and expressive language, phonemic awareness, vocabulary, pragmatic skills, and literal and inferential comprehension skills (Smith & Tyler, 2010). Standardized IQ tests are typically administered by a school psychologist, and an individual achievement test is administered by a special education teacher as part of the decision-making process to see where a child's performance falls in comparison to a standardized, representative sample of same-aged peers. The scores are reviewed, and the child's learning profile is discussed when the multidisciplinary team convenes at a committee on special education meeting to determine eligibility for special education.

Service Delivery Options

It is important to remember that students who are eligible for special education services are general education students first—and always. They require additional supports to help bridge gaps in their personal learning profiles to guide them to meet grade-level expectations to the absolute best of their abilities. The most common placement options for students who struggle with reading are as follows:

- Inclusive, cotaught classroom: The student receives instruction alongside grade-level peers in the general education setting. There are two teachers in the room: one general education teacher and one special education teacher. The two teachers combine their expertise regarding content and strategies to meet the needs of the diverse learners in the room.
- Resource room: The student receives supplemental small-group instruction with a special education teacher and up to four peers. The instruction targets specific, individualized, targeted goals that connect with the general education curriculum.

Forming Specific Goals

Before designing instruction, educators must highlight the learning goal. In addition to grade-level instructional learning goals, students with reading disabilities have specific individualized education program (IEP) goals that serve to drive instruction. IEP goals are generated at the special education committee meeting when the special education teacher shares the areas of need in reading that were identified from the student's performance on academic achievement testing. A strong cycle of learning occurs because the assessment guides the development of goals, which informs instructional decisions, as the instruction and student performance are monitored closely through ongoing informal assessments (**FIGURE 12-2**).

The cycle continues as teachers monitor student progress, and the instructional decisions, to ensure high-quality, meaningful learning to meet the needs of each student.

Present Levels of Performance

The child's strengths are considered along with the baseline data for present levels of academic achievement. The present levels of performance ensure that manageable goals will be created to ensure a student's participation and progress in the general education curriculum.

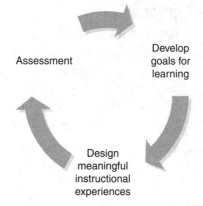

FIGURE 12-2 The cycle of learning.

For example, consider a first-grade student and a sixth-grade student who have specific reading needs to be addressed in the classroom.

- Veronica is in the first grade, and her fluency goal is as follows: In small-group instruction, when prompted to read aloud a grade-level informational text, Veronica will read 100 words with no more than three accuracy or fluency errors in three out of five read-aloud sessions. Veronica's teacher will monitor her fluency progress by keeping anecdotal notes to document her performance over time.
- Billy is in the sixth grade, and his comprehension goal is as follows: After reading a grade-level text, Billy will highlight or underline at least two pieces of text evidence to support the theme or main idea of the text, with 90 percent accuracy over 4 weeks. Billy's teacher will collect a work sample every 4 weeks to monitor his performance.

Veronica's and Billy's IEP goals for reading are monitored by the special education teacher through ongoing monitoring and connecting their goals to high-quality whole class instruction and small-group instruction.

Types of Intervention Approaches

Explicit Instruction

Explicit instruction is systematic, direct, engaging, and one of the most effective research-based instructional approaches for all students (**TABLE 12-2**). It is essential when working with students who have specific needs to guide them through targeted strategies both accurately and successfully. Explicit instruction follows a scaffolding approach—I do, we do, you do—in which teachers gradually release responsibility to students so they can apply strategies independently (Vygotsky, 1978).

TABLE 12-2 Explicit Instruction

	Teacher's Role	Student's Role
I do (direct instruction)	Provides direct instruction by explicitly sharing the goal, modeling a specific strategy, and thinking out loud to express the systematic steps of applying a strategy.	Actively participates by listening, asking questions, and taking notes.
We do (interactive, guided instruction)	Continues to model while including the student to add the student's thinking and ideas. Monitors the student's understanding, and prompts and applies additional modeling as needed.	Works with teacher to apply a specific strategy. Completes the process in collaboration with peers and the teacher.
You do (independent application)	Monitors student's performance, provides support, and clarifies and elaborates as needed.	Takes full responsibility to complete the learning task and asks for clarification as needed.

The teacher begins by modeling the skill or strategy; as the lesson evolves, the teacher interacts with the students; finally, the student applies the strategy independently (Fisher & Frey, 2007).

Direct Instruction

When early reading skills need to be practiced, direct instruction provides opportunities to break down reading tasks into smaller steps that progressively build on prior knowledge and learning. Direct instruction is similar to explicit instruction in that it includes active student participation to practice skills under the teacher's guidance.

The natural flow of a direct instruction lesson is as follows: The teacher reviews a concept that has been taught to make sure the student has sufficient background knowledge to move on to the next phase of learning, which is repeating teaching as necessary. The teacher then presents the new content or skill and guides the student to apply the skill while continuously monitoring his or her performance (**FIGURE 12-3**).

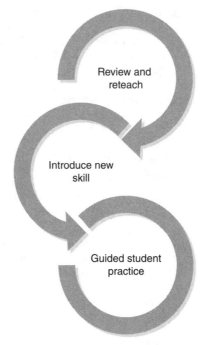

FIGURE 12-3 The natural flow of direct instruction.

In addition to basic reading skills (the big ideas described in Table 12-1), students with reading disabilities need support for reading comprehension. Active reading strategies, such as asking questions, monitoring comprehension, and making predictions and inferences, are a part of evidence-based practices that work effectively through modeling direct, explicit instruction (Fritschmann, Deshler, & Shumaker, 2007).

Collaborative Strategic Reading

Collaborative strategic reading is a cooperative learning approach to increase vocabulary and reading comprehension. It involves four steps that students apply before, during, and after reading (Bremer, Vaughn, Clapper, & Kim, 2002):

1. Preview the text: Students activate their background knowledge by writing down everything they already know about the topic. They skim the text then add their predictions for what they think they will learn.
2. Clicks and clunks: Students read the text and note any places where they read something interesting and where their comprehension made sense (clicks). They also note anywhere they needed clarification or help reading a word or phrase (clunks).

3. Get the gist: Students summarize the important parts of the text and generate a sentence or phrase to share the main idea.
4. Wrap up: Students go back to their thoughts when they previewed the text and add what they learned.

Summary

Reading is a complex process that requires many skills to blend together for a smooth, successful process. All classrooms need high-quality instructional practices in place to build a strong foundational skill set. Some students continue to struggle even if they received years of effective instruction in basic reading skills.

Five big ideas outline critical reading skills that set the foundation for all future reading experiences. Formal and informal assessments inform instructional decisions and manageable goals to meet specific student needs. Explicit, direct instruction is essential for breaking down skills and systematically addressing gaps in a student's ability to meet grade-level expectations.

 ## Case Scenarios

Case Scenario 1

Kyle is a third-grade student who has received special education services since the second grade. He has struggled with gaining basic phonemic awareness and phonics skills since he was in preschool. His parents made sure to immerse him in language and opportunities to connect letters with their related sounds as directed by the preschool and kindergarten teachers. Kyle achieved great gains during first grade, but his efforts to apply basic reading skills resulted in weak comprehension skills. Kyle received additional reading instruction within the RTI process and tier 2 small group instruction with a reading teacher.

The second-grade teacher, Mrs. Kay, was concerned with Kyle's ability to apply basic reading skills with the ease needed to meet grade-level expectations. She also began to think about the increase in curriculum demands for third grade. The focus on reading instruction in third grade has a strong shift from learning to read to reading to learn. Mrs. Kay knew that as Kyle continued to struggle with basic reading skills, his comprehension skills were falling further behind. Mrs. Kay decided to gather documentation and discuss her concerns with Kyle's parents. In addition, she set up a meeting with her school's instructional support team to discuss options for reinforcing Kyle's grade-level performance as he transitions to third grade.

📋 Case Scenarios (continued)

After a few more weeks of meetings and gathering evidence of Kyle's struggles and progress, a referral for special education was in motion. Throughout the weeks, Mrs. Kay continued to collaborate with the reading teacher, who provided direct instruction to guide basic reading skills and comprehension. Mrs. Kay continued to apply explicit instruction. Weeks later, it was confirmed that Kyle was eligible for special education. He was classified as a student with a learning disability who would begin to receive additional support through a resource room. Mrs. Kay would work with a special education teacher to guide Kyle's progress in his overall reading skills.

The goals for Kyle include applying grade-level phonics skills. Specifically, two goals include identifying common prefixes and derivational suffixes and decoding multisyllabic words. In addition, teachers plan to work on Kyle's ability to apply his decoding skills with accuracy and fluency to support comprehension. Kyle's comprehension skills will be assessed through daily reading comprehension tasks to ensure that he is progressing in the area of asking and responding to literal and inferential comprehension questions for literature and informational texts.

Case Scenario 2

Martha is a student with a learning disability that has resulted in difficulties with decoding and reading comprehension when she is required to read independently. Her weakness in reading adversely affects all content area learning. Martha has a long history of family gatherings and conversations that resulted in her rich background knowledge of history. She participated in social studies by connecting concepts and stories her grandfather told her. Martha participated in English class because her mom and dad discussed the books she read in school along with the books they enjoyed reading.

Martha's area of need followed her through the grades as she continued to struggle with decoding. Up until now she always found a way around her disability by connecting her rich background knowledge to discussions. Due to the fast-paced complexity of the middle-school curriculum, the special education teacher needed to find time to provide direct instruction with decoding and word recognition skills to guide Martha to read independently.

It was decided that three times each week Martha would receive direct instruction with specific goals to expand her vocabulary knowledge and fluency to increase word recognition. In addition, decoding skills would be embedded by guiding Martha to approach unfamiliar

📋 **Case Scenarios** *(continued)*

words by breaking the words into syllables to guide word-level reading. Comprehension continued to be an integral focus, so Martha was guided to apply basic reading skills with the ultimate goal of combining her strong background knowledge with text-based evidence. Martha learned to apply this approach in class without the support of the special education teacher. Over time, Martha began to show progress in applying a strategic word attack approach within the context of reading in her content area classes.

REVIEW QUESTIONS

1. The overarching goal of reading is to
   a. expand vocabulary.
   b. master decoding.
   c. construct meaning from text.
   d. respond to questions to demonstrate understanding.

2. Reading success depends on which two main skill sets?
   a. Decoding and comprehension
   b. Fluency and phonemic awareness
   c. Accuracy and decoding
   d. Accuracy and comprehension

3. Goal setting and informed instructional decisions are the result of which of the following?
   a. Ongoing progress monitoring through assessments and daily student performance
   b. Annual scores on formal assessments
   c. Collaboration with colleagues
   d. B and C

4. Why is explicit instruction necessary?
   a. So a student gains knowledge from the content he or she needs to remember
   b. So a student gains the skills he or she needs to apply during the learning process
   c. So a student experiences the process of learning through teacher modeling and strategic application
   d. B and C

5. How do explicit and direct instruction serve to support students' learning goals?
   a. They work on the skills students need to fill in gaps in their learning.
   b. They give students a systematic way to learn so they can memorize and repeat exactly what the teacher modeled.
   c. They provide a step-by-step process to increase students' engagement in the learning process for future applications.
   d. Both A and C are correct.

6. How do the five big ideas work together to set the foundation for all future reading experiences?
7. All effective instruction is driven by assessment. Explain the value of this statement and provide an example.
8. Explicit instruction is good for all learners. Explain why it is necessary for students with disabilities.
9. How does the process of RTI limit unnecessary referrals to special education?
10. Explain one educational approach to teaching students who struggle with reading. How does this approach guide student achievement?

REFERENCES

Bremer, C. D., Vaughn, S., Clapper, A. T., & Kim, A. (2002). Collaborative strategic reading (CSR): Improving secondary students' reading comprehension skills. *Research to Practice Brief, 1*(2), 1–2.

Brigance, A. H. (2010). *Brigance transition skills inventory.* North Billerica, MA: Curriculum Associates.

Davenport, M. R. (2002). *Miscues, not mistakes: Reading assessment in the classroom.* Portsmouth, NH: Heinemann.

Ehri, L. C. (2014). Orthographic mapping in the acquisition of sight word reading, spelling memory, and vocabulary learning. *Scientific Studies of Reading, 18*(1), 5–21.

Fisher, D., & Frey, N. (2007). Implementing a schoolwide literacy framework: Improving achievement in an urban elementary school. *The Reading Teacher, 61*(1), 32–43.

Friend, M., & Bursuck, W. D. (2002). *Including students with special needs: A practical guide for classroom teachers.* Boston, MA: Allyn & Bacon

Fritschmann, N. S., Deshler, D. D., & Schumaker, J. B. (2007). The effects of instruction in an inference strategy on the reading comprehension skills of adolescents with disabilities. *Learning Disability Quarterly, 30*(4), 245–262.

Gargiulo, R. M., & Metcalf, D. (2017). *Teaching in today's inclusive classrooms: A universal design for learning approach.* Boston, MA: Cengage Learning.

Good, R. H., Gruba, J., & Kaminski, R. A. (2002). Best practices in using dynamic indicators of basic early literacy skills (DIBELS) in an outcomes-driven model. In A. Thomas & J. Grimes (Eds.), *Best practice in school psychology* (pp. 699–717). Bethesda, MD: National Association of School Psychologists.

Goodman, Y. M., Watson, D. J., & Burke, C. L. (1987). *Reading miscue inventory: Alternative procedures.* New York, NY: Richard C. Owen.

Hudson, R. F., Lane, H. B., & Pullen, P. C. (2005). Reading fluency assessment and instruction: What, why, and how? *The Reading Teacher, 58*(8), 702–714.

Hulme, C., & Snowling, M. J. (2013). Learning to read: What we know and what we need to understand better. *Child Development Perspectives, 7*(1), 1–5.

Individuals with Disabilities Education Act of 2004 (IDEA), Public Law 108-446, 118 Stat. 2647 (2004).

Mather, N., & Wendling, B. J. (2012). Linking cognitive abilities to academic interventions for students with specific learning disabilities. In D. P. Flanagan & P. L. Harrison (Eds.), *Contemporary intellectual assessment: Theories, tests, and, issues* (3rd ed.; pp. 553–581). New York, NY: Guilford.

Mitchell, E., Rearden, K., & Stacy, D. (2011). Comedy hour: Using audio files of joke recitations to improve elementary students' fluency. *Current Issues in Education, 14*(2).

Moats, L. C. (2001). When older students can't read. *Educational Leadership, 58*(6), 36–40.

National Reading Panel. (2000). *Teaching children to read: An evidence-based assessment of the scientific research literature on reading and its implications for reading instruction.* Bethesda, MD: Author.

Paratore, J. R., Cassano, C. M., & Schickedanz, J. A. (2011). Supporting early (and later) literacy development at home and at school. *Handbook of Reading Research, 4*, 107–135.

Pikulski, J. J., & Chard, D. J. (2005). Fluency: Bridge between decoding and reading comprehension. *The Reading Teacher, 58*(6), 510–519.

Rasinski, T., Rikli, A., & Johnston, S. (2009). Reading fluency: More than automaticity? More than a concern for the primary grades? *Literacy Research and Instruction, 48*(4), 350–361.

Reschly, A. L., Busch, T. W., Betts, J., Deno, S. L., & Long, J. D. (2009). Curriculum-based measurement oral reading as an indicator of reading achievement: A meta-analysis of the correlational evidence. *Journal of School Psychology, 47*(6), 427–469.

Salvia, J., Ysseldyke, J., & Witmer, S. (2012). *Assessment: In special and inclusive education.* Boston, MA: Cengage Learning.

Schatschneider, C., & Torgesen, J. K. (2004). Using our current understanding of dyslexia to support early identification and intervention. *Journal of Child Neurology, 19*(10), 759–765.

Schmoker, M. (2007). Radically redefining literacy instruction: An immense opportunity. *Phi Delta Kappan, 88*(7), 488–493.

Smith, D. D., & Tyler, N. C. (2010). *Introduction to special education: Making a difference.* Boston, MA: Pearson Education.

Stein, E. (2013). *Comprehension lessons for RTI grades 3–5: Assessments, intervention lessons, and management tips to help you reach and teach tier 2 students.* New York, NY: Scholastic.

Torgesen, J. K. (2002). The prevention of reading disabilities. *Journal of School Psychology, 40*(1), 7–26. doi:10.1016/S0022-4405(01)00092-9

Torgesen, J. K., & Bryant, B. R. (2004). *Test of phonological awareness: Examiner's manual.* Austin, TX: PRO-ED.

Torgesen, J. K., Wagner, R. K., & Rashotte, C. A. (1999). *TOWRE: Test of word reading efficiency.* Austin, TX: PRO-ED.

Vygotsky, L. S. (1978). *Mind and society.* Cambridge, MA: Harvard University Press.

Wiederholt, J. L., & Bryant, B. R. (2012). *Gray oral reading tests* (5th ed.). Austin, TX: PRO-ED.

Woodcock, R. W. (2011). *Woodcock reading mastery tests: WRMT-III* (3rd ed.). Bloomington, MN: Pearson.

Wurr, A., Theurer, J. L., & Kim, K. L. (2009). Retrospective miscue analysis with proficient adult ESL readers. *Journal of Adolescent and Adult Literacy, 52*(4), 324–333.

ADDITIONAL RESOURCES

WEBSITES

Eunice Kennedy Shriver National Institute of Child Health and Human Development. What Are Reading Disorders? www.nichd.nih.gov/health/topics/reading/conditioninfo/pages/disorders.aspx

LD OnLine. The Educator's Guide to Learning Disabilities and ADHD. www.ldonline.org

National Center for Learning Disabilities. www.ncld.org

Understood. Learning and Attention Issues. www.understood.org/en/learning-attention-issues

BOOKS

Allington, Richard L., and Patricia Marr Cunningham. *Schools That Work: Where All Children Read and Write* (3rd ed.). Boston, MA: Pearson/Allyn & Bacon, 2007.

Shaywitz, Sally E. *Overcoming Dyslexia: A New and Complete Science-Based Program for Reading Problems at Any Level.* New York, NY: A. A. Knopf, 2012.

CHAPTER 13

Writing Disorders

Margaret M. Laskowski
Terry H. Gozdziewski
J. Reilly Limowski
Anita W. Frey

Key Terms

Alphabet knowledge
Dysgraphia
Dyspraxia
Executive function
Expository writing
Fictional stories
Literacy
Literate language
Macrostructure
Microstructure

Narrative writing
Personal narratives
Persuasive writing
Phonological awareness
Print concepts
Scripts
Self-regulated strategy
   development (SRSD)
Self-regulation
T-unit analysis

Introduction

Writing—it is not a purely motor or primarily visual activity. It is fundamentally Language by Hand, which shares some common processes with other kinds of language (listening, speaking, and reading) but also some distinct processes that are unique to writing. (Berninger et al., 2006, p. 88)

The purpose of this chapter is to provide students, special educators, educational specialists, and speech-language pathologists with basic information that can be used as a starting point to write informed, appropriate goals for clients having challenges with written language. If you ask any student which academic task is most challenging, the response will usually be writing. Because writing is the most complex form of language, this chapter provides sources in the "Additional Resources" section that readers can use as a springboard for increasing their knowledge. Without knowledge of the typical development process, therapists, special educators, educational specialists, and teachers cannot judge what is atypical. Therefore, a basic overview of typical development is provided for writing, the relationship of writing to literacy development, writing processes and products, and assessment methods. This groundwork will aid the analysis required for writing informed, appropriate, and attainable goals. Any information or suggestions from this perspective can easily be modified for use in a variety of settings. Information relevant to the Common Core State Standards (CCSS) and collaboration with other educational professionals is included to facilitate the development of goals for written language to best support student achievement in the classroom and, ultimately, the workplace.

From prehistoric times, people have found ways to record important data and special events. Cave dwellers covered their walls with drawings, perhaps for ceremonial or historical purposes. Hieroglyphics, often referred to as holy writings, were left by Egyptians inside pyramids to chronicle religious events, stories, and myths. Cuneiforms were used by the ancient Greeks to record the history of their times. Today we have more advanced ways to record ideas and chronicle events. Students have a myriad of options—paper, computers, social media platforms, cell phones, tablets, photographs, and other tools—to record data, create stories, and document important events. Regardless of the format, writing remains a primary form of communication and is a critical tool for academic success and vocational opportunities (Fallon & Katz, 2011).

Literacy

Writing is part of the much larger skill known as literacy. **Literacy**, which includes both reading and writing, is one of the cornerstones of education. Most people are unaware that written expression begins as an offshoot of language development. As children develop oral language skills, they start to formulate written expression skills.

The simple act of a child responding to a parent's inquiry of "How was your day?" is a prerequisite for the child's developing narrative skills. "Speaking, reading and writing are interrelated skills because literacy skills are basically language skills. Good oral language skills are a prerequisite for reading and writing. A child or adult with poor oral language skills cannot be a good reader or writer" (Hegde, 2010, p. 457).

Several areas that are critical for literacy development typically emerge in the preschool period and are considered essential foundational skills for the development of reading and writing. **Phonological awareness**, **print concepts**, **alphabet knowledge**, and **literate language** are all considered essential components of emergent literacy experiences that provide children with introductory knowledge of written language (Justice & Ezell, 2004; Justice & Kaderavek, 2004; Pullen & Justice, 2003; Westby, 1991).

Phonological awareness is a metalinguistic skill considered necessary for the development of reading. Phonological awareness is the awareness, knowledge, and ability to manipulate sounds, syllables, and words. It can be viewed as a subdivision of the much broader category of phonological processing (Bauman-Waengler, 2012). The components of phonological awareness are phoneme isolation, sound blending, syllable identification, and sound segmentation (Hegde, 2010). Subcategories of this skill include syllable segmentation, syllable completion, syllable identification, and syllable deletion (Pindzola, Plexico, & Haynes, 2016). The sequence of phonological awareness development is detailed by Shipley and McAfee (2016) and Paul and Norbury (2012).

Children learn about print concepts through exposure to books during shared-reading activities. During these interactions, whether on a one-to-one basis with an adult or within a larger group preschool activity, children learn that words are made up of printed letters and that words convey information. Children learn how to handle books, that there is a left-to-right progression when you read, and that you turn pages to continue reading a story. When children understand letter names and sounds in upper and lower case and that words are made up of groups of letters, they have acquired alphabet knowledge. Children with alphabet knowledge know they can read words by sounding out the individual letters of the word.

During these book-centered interactions, children gain their first exposure to literate language. Literate language describes language that is highly decontextualized (Turnbull & Justice, 2017) in formal written language; it uses abstract vocabulary and complex syntactic and semantic features not found in oral conversational language. Because literate language has no context, the reader must derive meaning from the language itself by making inferences and drawing conclusions from the text to understand the meaning the writer is trying to convey. For example, we encounter slang and jargon in oral conversation, but it is absent in literate language (Nippold, 2007). Oral conversation is usually about the here and now, whereas literate language lacks this supportive context.

Children learn the elements of language, such as phonology, morphology, syntax, semantics, and pragmatics, by learning to talk, or the oral language style. The world of literate language is introduced to preschoolers through shared storybook times when they talk to learn (Westby, 1991).

Writing Process and Product

ASHA acknowledges the central role of language in literacy development (American Speech-Language-Hearing-Association [ASHA], n.d.b) and the roles and responsibilities of speech-language pathologists as they relate to the identification, treatment, and prevention of literacy problems (ASHA, n.d.b, 2001, 2002, 2010).

> **Writing** is the process of communicating using printed symbols in the form of letters or visual characters, which make up words. Words are formulated into sentences; these sentences are organized into larger paragraphs and often into different discourse genres (narrative, expository, persuasive, poetic, etc.).

Writing includes the following:

- **Writing process**—the ability to plan (i.e., "pre-writing"), organize, draft, reflect on, revise, and edit written text; the ability to address specific audience needs and convey the purpose of the text (e.g., persuasion). This process is iterative.
- **Written product**—the end product of the writing process; it can be examined at the **word level** (e.g., word choice and spelling), **sentence level** (e.g., grammar and complexity), and **text level** (e.g., discourse structure, use of cohesive devices and coherence). The written product can also be described in terms of **writing conventions** (e.g., capitalization and punctuation), **communication functions** (e.g., to inform, to persuade), **organizational structure** (e.g., chronological, sequential, compare and contrast), and **effectiveness** in meeting the information needs of the audience. (Nelson, 2014; Puranik, Lombardino, & Altmann, 2007; Scott & Windsor, 2000, as cited in ASHA, n.d.b, Overview section)

Writing is not simple. It is incredibly complex and requires the integration of multiple processes on several levels (Reid & Lienemann, 2006). Students must learn not only the mechanics or conventions of writing (e.g., punctuation, capitalization, spelling, etc.), but also composition (e.g., the process of putting words and sentences together to express thoughts in themes, essays, etc.). The process of writing involves planning, generating content, organizing the composition, and translating content into written language (Bashir & Singer, 2006; Graham & Harris, 2003). Also, students must be able to plan and organize their work. Developing a plan for the completion and revision of a written language assignment requires the use of **executive function** skills and **self-regulation** (Reid & Lienemann, 2006; Scott, 2012).

Executive functions are cognitive processes that allow a student to pay attention, analyze situations, set goals, and organize a plan to complete a task or assignment (Horowitz, 2007; Singer & Bashir, 1999). Self-regulation refers to behaviors that help a person guide and monitor their performance and stay on track to complete a task (Fahy, 2014; Singer & Bashir, 1999). Writing is a skill that can be continually developed and refined over a lifetime through explicit instruction and practice.

Writing as a Fine-Motor Skill

Despite access to computers, handwriting remains an essential tool for school success. Legible handwriting is critical for attaining higher-level academic skills, such as spelling and essay writing (Feder & Majnemer, 2007). Students reportedly spend between 31 and 60 percent of their school day engaging in handwriting or other fine-motor tasks (McHale & Cermak, 1992). Students are required to take notes in class, compose written essays, and complete applications for colleges and jobs.

The ability to physically write develops in parallel with fine-motor skills. Writing begins in infancy as children first reach out for objects to touch and hold. As infants grow and their senses of curiosity and exploration heighten, they start to bring the objects they hold up to their mouths. Babies discover that they can use crayons to scribble and leave marks (Berninger et al., 2006). Toddlers learn to imitate the actions of their parents, caregivers, and teachers using crayons to make isolated horizontal, vertical, and diagonal lines, circles, and simple shapes made from straight lines and circular strokes (Berninger et al., 2006). By creating artwork, children learn about colors and shapes as well as quantitative and spatial concepts (e.g., big, small, more, all, some). Playing with sculptural clay allows children to work in three dimensions.

During their preschool years, children learn to name alphabet letters and develop motor control that is needed to use a pencil by connecting dots in drawings, completing line mazes, and tracing alphabet letterforms. Preschoolers are interested in making alphabet letterforms when their teachers provide a model. In first grade, students learn to copy upper- and lowercase alphabet letterforms accurately and can name all of these forms when presented in random order (Berninger et al., 2006). First graders can accurately write upper- and lowercase letters from memory when dictated by the teacher and can also accurately write the alphabet in the correct order from memory (Berninger et al., 2006). All these skills are prerequisites to putting thoughts on paper. As students move through first and second grade, they can write frequently occurring words more quickly (without thinking). The ability to handwrite quickly without too much conscious thought is necessary for writing basic sentences that will eventually become short stories, then the narrative writing that is expected by third grade.

Learning to Write Specific Genres of Text

Writing is an essential tool for academic success and vocational opportunities (Fallon & Katz, 2011; Price & Jackson, 2015). During the elementary school years, children acquire literate language, or language for learning (Greenhalgh & Strong, 2001; Paul & Norbury, 2012; Westby, 1991). Literate language is the language of lectures, scientific writing, and essays. The CCSS, which are educational standards for students in kindergarten through 12th grade, clearly delineate written language skills in each grade level that students are expected to attain. As of this writing, these standards have been adopted by 43 states and 5 U.S. territories.

There are three written language genres of text that are addressed in the CCSS: **narrative writing**, **expository writing**, and **persuasive writing** (Scott, 2012). Mastery of these written genres typically follows the progress of the school writing curriculum. Students learn to write narratives in early elementary school before moving on to multiple challenges presented by expository and persuasive writing. Each type of writing genre has its own **macrostructure**, or organization, and **microstructure**, or vocabulary and syntactic sentence structure (Nippold, Hesketh, Duthie, & Mansfield, 2005; Scott, 1994; Westby, 2012). When students understand how writing assignments should be organized (the macrostructure) and what vocabulary and syntax (the microstructure) is expected, they are better prepared as writers to successfully complete the assigned task.

Narrative Writing

Narrative writing, or narrative text, tells a story and includes fables, realistic fiction, fantasy, personal memoirs, and folktales. Narrative writing occurs most frequently in the early elementary years because narratives are usually about things that happen to people over time. Because narratives happen over time, temporal and causal events organize the story and provide a framework for the flow of the story. Children usually have firsthand experience with the events or themes of the narratives they write.

Narrative writing is broken down into three subtypes: **personal narratives**, **fictional stories**, and **scripts** (Hughes, McGillivray, Schmidek, 1997; Paul & Norbury, 2017; Scott, 2012).

Personal narratives are children's nonfiction accounts of their own personal experiences. They are centered around a significant personal experience, an activity, or a situation that triggered an emotion.

Fictional stories are centered around a character and problem solving narrative. The main character experiences an exciting situation or has a problem to solve. Everything that happens to the main character is called the plot. The plot follows a predictable sequence: beginning, middle, and end. The main event, which is usually the most exciting part of the story, occurs in the middle of the sequence. The main event is typically the problem to be solved or the significant personal dilemma faced by the main character. The resolution of the problem occurs at the conclusion of the story. The organizational framework, or macrostructure, used for narrative writing is called story grammar.

A script narrative informs the reader about a repeatedly experienced routine. Script narratives are explanations of what happens during day-to-day events.

Expository Writing

Expository writing can be thought of as the language of the school curriculum, and it is the most literate and advanced form of writing. Expository text is nonfiction writing that explains or describes information that is new to the reader. Exposure to reading and writing expository texts increases as students move out of primary grades and into upper elementary grades and high school. Writing expository text assignments is challenging, even for typically developing students, due to the unique macrostructure and microstructure of each type of expository text.

Westby (2012) identifies six expository text types, characteristics, and keywords that the student can look for to determine the type of text and to write an appropriate response:

1. Descriptive: Does the text say what something is? Keywords include **for example**, *such as, to illustrate, characteristics.*
2. Sequence or procedural: Does the text say how to do something or make something? Keywords include *first, next, then, second, third, following this step.*
3. Cause or effect: Does the text provide reasons for why something happens? Keywords include *because, since, then, therefore, for this reason.*
4. Problem or solution: Does the text state a problem and offer a solution to the problem? Keywords include *the problem is, a solution is, so that.*
5. Compare or contrast: Does the text show how two things are the same or different? Keywords include *different, same, alike, similar, although, however.*
6. Enumerative: Does the text list things that are related to the topic? Keywords include *an example is, for instance, another.*

Persuasive Writing

Persuasive, or argumentative, writing attempts to convince the reader that the writer's point of view is correct. This type of writing occurs later in the secondary school level curriculum and is the genre frequently used for many state-level tests and the written section of the SAT. Persuasive writing is considered the most difficult genre for students to master (Nippold et al., 2005).

The basic structure used in schools for persuasive writing is the five-paragraph essay. A topic sentence starts each paragraph by stating the main idea, and a wrap-up sentence ends each paragraph by summing up the paragraph. The thesis is introduced in the first paragraph. The second through fourth paragraphs restate subtopics and provide supportive information using the same structure as the first paragraph. The fifth and final paragraph starts with a topic sentence and ends with a compelling wrap-up sentence that sums up the paragraph.

Typical Sequence of Writing Development

When children enter kindergarten, they embark on their journeys to become writers. They will learn transcription (spelling and writing words) while learning to plan, generate, and revise their written products (Scott,

2012). It is essential that teachers, educational specialists, and therapists know the typical developmental milestones required for motor skills, the writing process, and written products to write intervention goals. **TABLE 13-1** describes the milestones for writing development.

TABLE 13-1 Typical Sequence of Writing Development

Age (Grade Level)	Typical Sequence of Writing Development
3 years	• Scribbles with no discernable letters • Some scribble shows basic knowledge of conventional rules of writing: ♦ May occur in lines, flow from left to right and top to bottom, may show some conventional spacing
4 years	• Writing resembles standard letters and words • Writing must be interpreted for others
5 years (kindergarten)	• Knows basic conventional rules of writing ♦ Scribble may occur in lines, flow from left to right and top to bottom, may show spacing between words • Writes a few meaningful words: common nouns and own name • Most upper- and lowercase letters are written legibly • Use of initial consonants begins • Draws or writes texts for social expression • Writes themes that often are about self, families, or pets

6 years (1st grade)	• Shows knowledge of relationship between letters and sounds
	• Mostly uppercase letters are used
	• Writes strings of letters (not words) with no spacing
	• Only one or some letters in a word are written, usually first consonant, to represent a whole word or syllable
	• Invented spellings are typical; initial and final consonant present but vowels may be omitted
	• Begins sentences with capital letter and ends sentences with period
	• Personal narratives introduced
	  ♦ Subject matter usually expresses feelings, personal ideas, new possessions, holidays, and memories
	• Uses short, simple sentences
	• Grammatical errors are common
	  ♦ Verb tense
	  ♦ Regular, irregular plurals

TABLE 13-1 Typical Sequence of Writing Development *(continued)*

Age (Grade Level)	Typical Sequence of Writing Development
7 years (2nd grade)	• Phonetic spellings decrease as traditional spellings increase; spelling rules applied more frequently • Correctly uses upper- and lowercase letters, space between words, and basic punctuation • Legible writing • Writes simple fiction and nonfiction based on model using a variety of sentence types • Longer, organized stories with a beginning, middle, and end • Familiar words spelled correctly • Morphologic structures in spelling system better internalized
8 years (3rd grade)	• Uses conventional spellings for the most part • Uses dictionary to learn new words or correct spellings • Vowels used correctly most of time • Letters are transposed in less-frequently used words • Writes narratives, letters, and simple expository reports • Stories contain more detail and description • Writing themes may expand to include sports, superheroes, and mythical beasts • Introduction to poetry • Sentence length increases; includes more complex forms
9 years (4th grade)	• Recognizes misspellings; can correctly spell unfamiliar words by using orthographic knowledge • Convention and exception in spelling rules are known • Uses narrative and expository writing • Organizes writing by using a beginning, middle, and end to convey a central idea • Concepts of drafts introduced with emphasis placed on editing character development and plot • Edits work for grammar, punctuation, and spelling
10 years (5th grade)	• Writes for a variety of purposes using a variety of sentence structures • Capable of writing multiepisode narratives • Expansion of writing abilities with more detailed interaction and dialogue among characters • First research paper assigned • Uses vocabulary effectively • Revises and edits own writing
11 years (6th grade)	• Writing becomes more adultlike • Revisions are more challenging

TABLE 13-1 Typical Sequence of Writing Development *(continued)*

Age (Grade Level)	Typical Sequence of Writing Development
12 years (7th grade)	• Writing genres expand to biographies, autobiographies, and world issues (e.g., the environment) • Revising original draft is easier • Cooperative learning for writing process is beneficial
13 years (8th grade)	• Has sense of pride in use of proper grammar and writing mechanics • Able to modify first and second drafts • Improved ability to corroborate facts with supportive details
14–15 years (9th and 10th grades)	• Writing often related to literature • Can write from different points of view
16–17 years (11th and 12th grades)	• Longer, more complex forms of written genres required
18+ years (college)	• Writes persuasive text

Adapted from Berninger et al., 2006; Gentry, 2004; Scott, 2012; and Woods, 1997.

The written language skills of U.S. students have received national attention, and student performance remains a source of concern. The adoption of the CCSS is an attempt to provide uniform standards of skill proficiency to ensure that students are ready for college and career. A report by the National Center for Education Statistics (2012) reported the results of nationwide writing assessments, which showed that the majority of 8th and 12th graders did not write at or above the proficiency level for their grade. According to the report, 74 percent of the 8th graders and 73 percent of the 12th graders did not attain the expected academic performance.

The CCSS for kindergarten through 12th grade details the expectations in English language arts and mathematics for each grade level. Very specific writing guidelines and benchmarks are specified throughout the CCSS, and it is strongly advised that these documents be carefully and thoughtfully reviewed. Clinicians can refer to the Common Core State Standards Initiative (2017), which explains the national standards and provides links to the standards in each state. Speech-language pathologists should use the developmental sequence and the CCSS as a guide for writing goals specifically tailored to a student's needs rather than just writing a laundry list of skills to be taught or selecting generic goals from a commercial goal bank. Depending on the age of the student, thoughtful consideration must be given as to when compensatory strategies may be considered versus following the typical developmental sequence. Guidance in this area is available from ASHA (2004).

Etiologies of Writing Disorders

It is well documented that students with language learning disorders have difficulties with writing, but the causes of writing disorders are not known (ASHA, n.d.b; Berninger, 2000; Paul & Norbury, 2012; Scott, 2012). ASHA (n.d.b) says the etiologies of written language disorders remain unknown at this time. Students who are diagnosed with language learning difficulties typically present with deficits in written language that are evidenced by errors in syntax, semantics, morphology, and spelling. These students also demonstrate difficulty with various aspects of advanced language that are needed for writing narrative, expository, and persuasive texts (Paul & Norbury, 2012; Ward-Lonergan & Duthie, 2016). Writing requires knowledge of higher-level language strategies and executive function skills for editing and revising written work (Bashir & Singer, 2006). In addition to the language processing components, the physical act of writing requires sustained attention and fine-motor control, bilateral and visual-motor integration, and motor planning (Feder & Majnemer, 2007)

ASHA (n.d.b) further says that external and internal factors can negatively impact the development of written language skills. These factors potentially include limited early literacy experience, insufficient or inadequate reading and writing instruction, and insufficient early oral language experience. Internal factors—those that are intrinsic to the child—include genetic and neurological factors. Cognitive, social, emotional, and adaptive development issues, and physical impairments such as blindness and deafness, may also contribute to writing difficulties.

Difficulties with handwriting can also be caused by **dysgraphia**, a learning disability that can have an adverse impact on an individual's ability to write, spell words, use written expression as an effective means of communication, and complete written assignments. Richards defines dysgraphia as "a writing pattern characterized by substantial effort which interferes with a student's ability to convert ideas into a written format" (1999, p. 72). The student has difficulties with automatically remembering and executing the sequence of movements needed in writing. Symptoms of dysgraphia include letter inconsistencies, irregular letter sizes and shapes, problems with spacing, and poor organization on the line and the page. For people with dysgraphia, the physical act of writing is a struggle and is fatiguing. Dysgraphia is diagnosed by professionals, such as developmental pediatricians, neurologists, or licensed psychologists, who are trained in identifying learning disabilities. After diagnosis, a referral is typically made to an occupational therapist for an evaluation to obtain more detailed information regarding fine-motor and visual-motor integration skills and strategies for remediation. **Dyspraxia**, or developmental motor disorder, can affect fine-motor skills, such as handwriting, gross-motor skills, language and perception, and executive functioning (Boon, 2010; Hendrickx, 2010). Again, the child should be referred to a qualified professional for an assessment and diagnosis.

Assessment of Writing Process and Product

A detailed discussion about assessing all components that contribute to the written language process and product is not within the scope of this chapter; however, an appropriate evaluation of the multiple skills involved in written language is crucial to identify areas of strength and weakness in speech-language skills. Information obtained from an assessment, combined with clinical knowledge and judgment, contributes to the development of appropriate goals.

An assessment of the written product requires attention to multiple skills and is considered the most challenging domain to assess (Espin, Weissenburger, & Benson, 2004). It also is essential to consider the cultural–linguistic diversity of clients and their families, including those who use nonstandard American English dialects, when conducting a comprehensive speech-language evaluation. Information concerning the assessment of these students' written language skills can be found on the ASHA Practice Portal (ASHA, n.d.b).

Written language can be assessed through administering norm-referenced measures or providing a student with a writing prompt and analyzing the writing sample. An analysis of the written language sample should contain components for productivity (the number of sentences, clauses, ideas, and words); complexity (different clause types, complexity of clauses, words per sentence or clause, grammatically correct sentences); appropriateness for the intended audience and topic; organization (cohesion); mechanics (spelling, punctuation, etc.); and analytic components (revisions, edits) (Paul & Norbury, 2012; Shipley & McAfee, 2016).

The writing sample can be assessed using a terminal unit, or **T-unit analysis** (Kaderavek, 2015; Nelson, 2010; Paul & Norbury, 2012). A T-unit is a main clause with all structure embedded in it or subordinated to it. A mean length of T-unit is a measure of syntactic complexity of the spoken or written syntax of school-aged children (Hunt, 1965; Kaderavek, 2015; Paul & Norbury, 2012). Information obtained from the writing sample is essential for examining syntax and morphology. A detailed step-by-step description of performing a T-unit analysis is provided by Kaderavek (2015). The results of this type of analysis can yield information about a student's strengths and weaknesses, which is essential for writing student-specific goals.

Information detailing the procedures for sampling, eliciting, and analyzing narrative language is presented by Hughes and colleagues (1997). Paul and Norbury (2012) provide extensive information about the assessment of written narrative, expository, and persuasive text. Additional information for the analysis of narrative, expository, and persuasive text is presented by Shipley and McAfee (2016) and Roth and Worthington (2016). Worksheets to assist educational professionals and therapists in this task are also provided by these authors.

Developing Goals

Before the goal writing process begins, it is essential for the educational professionals and therapists to review and be familiar with the CCSS for the student's grade level and the previous grade levels. Familiarity with the standards allows the professionals to determine which skills the student needs to meet the standards. Rudebusch (2012) says the standards should be reviewed through the lens of a speech-language pathologist in terms of syntax, semantics, pragmatics, phonology, and morphology when speech-language intervention is being considered.

Next, all available student data should be thoroughly examined by all professionals who are working with the student. In doing so, the speech-language pathologist will put together a picture of student performance that will provide critical information regarding areas of strength and weakness that is needed for developing goals. Data that should be examined include a variety of classroom writing samples, data obtained from any interventions, criterion-referenced assessments (state assessments), and IEPs from prior school years (Needels & Knapp, 1994; Power-deFur & Flynn, 2012). Whenever possible, the student's actual responses on these assessments should be reviewed to see if patterns emerge. A classroom observation can provide valuable information about the linguistic complexity of instruction and the materials used in the classroom (Needels & Knapp, 1994). The educational professionals and therapists should reach out to the parents or caregivers to obtain information about the literacy support provided in the home and to gain insights into family attitudes toward written language skills.

The speech-language pathologist should also review the student's general file and look for additional information, such as number of days absent or tardy, referrals for instructional support or interventions, grades, home language, and disciplinary actions. This information can provide answers to the following critical questions:

- Have student absences or tardies negatively impacted instruction time?
- If the student is an English language learner, is the student literate in his or her home language, and what literacy supports are in place at home?
- Was the instruction evidence based?
- Did the student receive instruction in content aligned with grade-level standards, and were appropriate instructional materials used?

At this point, the information gathered should provide a picture of the student's strengths and weaknesses and indicate the student's skill level relative to the grade-level standards.

Ehren (2000) says the speech-language pathologist can gain information about student performance across subject matter by collaborating with the classroom teacher. Teachers should be consulted when considering targets and writing goals. The general educator can provide additional information about the student's abilities and needs in the area of written language relative to grade-level standards and can also make comparisons against the performance of peers. Also, since the classroom teacher is in direct daily contact with the student across a variety of subject areas, he or she is the professional with the greatest ability to implement interventions and strategies in a variety of functional written language activities throughout the day.

After the results of the assessment are thoroughly analyzed, it is time to select target behaviors. Hegde and Davis (1999) discuss guidelines that should be kept in mind when choosing target behaviors. The target behaviors should significantly improve the student's social communication, academic achievement, and occupational performance. The chosen target behaviors should be those that are most useful and can be performed and reinforced in the client's home and other natural settings. The target behaviors should also facilitate the expansion of communicative skills. When selecting targets for a client who has a culturally or linguistically diverse background, it is important that the targets be linguistically and culturally appropriate.

Therapists and educational professionals must consider if they will use a developmental or normative strategy, or a client-specific strategy, when selecting targets (Hegde & Davis, 1999; Roth & Worthington, 2016). Typically a developmental approach is used when choosing targets for younger students. This strategy uses normative sequences of development when considering target behaviors for goals. Targets are selected based on the client's age and developmental norms. However, Roth and Worthington (2016) offer cautions when using a developmental strategy. The sample size from which the norms were obtained must be large enough to permit valid generalization of the findings to other populations (Roth & Worthington, 2016). Also, the characteristics of the standardization sample, such as ethnicity, gender, and socioeconomic status, should be similar to the client's characteristics if comparisons are made between the student's performance and the group norms (Roth & Worthington, 2016). This is of particular concern when working with students who are English language learners.

When working with adolescents and adults, the therapy targets are typically based on individual needs and are geared toward increasing functional performance. This strategy for goal selection is called a client-specific strategy. A client-specific strategy uses targets that will make an immediate and significant difference in the client's performance. A thorough analysis of all materials available, and consideration of the student's age, academic needs, and vocational needs, will assist in determining which approach to use. Hegde and Davis (1999) say the client-specific approach is most appropriate for culturally and linguistically diverse clients.

After a picture of the student's present level of performance is developed and targets are determined, the therapists and educational professionals can now begin the goal writing process. Written goals should be in alignment with grade-level standards, but they should not copy the standard (Power-deFur & Flynn, 2012; Rudebusch, 2012). Again, the standards of previous grade levels may need to be checked, depending on the student's level of functioning and IEPs from prior years. Regardless of the written language skill being targeted, the core rules of goal writing should apply. A goal should be realistic, achievable, and measurable (McLeod & Baker, 2017), and it should include the following four critical components (Rudebusch, 2012):

1. Time frame: Amount of time in the goal period (e.g., 12 instructional weeks)
2. Conditions: Specific resources required for the student to attain the goal (e.g., given a third-grade story prompt)
3. Behavior: Performance directly observed and measured (e.g., the third-grade student will write a story)
4. Criterion: How much, how often, or to what extent the behavior must occur for the goal to be achieved (e.g., a two-paragraph composition using both simple and compound sentences and temporal words to signal event order within and among paragraphs, with five or fewer errors)

Rudebusch (2012) and Power-deFur and Flynn (2012) provide thorough discussions on the components of a measurable goal and how to write goals that are aligned with the CCSS. Roth and Worthington (2016) provide detailed information about the elements of a goal and developing a plan of intervention. Flynn (2015) provides detailed information for writing speech-language goals for IEPs that are tied to the CCSS.

When considering the conditions of the task, the educational professionals and therapists should evaluate the classroom-based materials for use within various interventions. The student will more quickly realize that the strategies and skills being developed in speech-language therapy can be applied to daily classroom writing assignments. Materials used by all professionals working with the student should be relevant to the grade-level curriculum (Power-deFur & Flynn, 2012).

The service delivery model and frequency of intervention must be considered when writing goals. Individual public school district policies and state regulations may dictate the frequency of service. Educational professionals and therapists should familiarize themselves with this information and take it into account when writing goals. Some factors to be considered when determining the service delivery model and frequency of services include grade level, number of other services the student receives, student personality, and behavioral characteristics. Service delivery models include the clinical or pull-out model, the consultant model, and the collaborative or pull-out/sit-in model. Cirrin and colleagues (2010) present a complete and thorough evidence-based systematic review of these service delivery models. Their findings do not suggest that one model is better than another, but decisions about frequency and service delivery model should be based on the individual needs of each student in accordance with the Individuals with Disabilities Education Act (IDEA) (2004). The ASHA Practice Portal contains additional information concerning service delivery options (ASHA, n.d.a).

Instructional Strategies

The approach used for teaching and remediating written language is typically included when writing goals. The specific needs and abilities of the client must be kept in mind when determining which approaches will be implemented to remediate areas of need.

Graham and Perin (2007) conducted a meta-analysis to examine approaches to writing instruction. They identified key elements of effective instructional strategies for students in grades 4 to 12 (**TABLE 13-2**). Numerous strategy-based approaches for writing goals are available; they are commonly used because goal formulation is linked to the planned intervention approach.

TABLE 13-2 Key Elements of Effective Instructional Strategies (Grades 4–12)

Key Element	Description
Writing strategies	Explicit instruction in planning, revising, or editing text (Graham, 2006; Graham, Harris, & McKeown, 2013)
Summarization	Explicit and systematic instruction in summarizing texts
Collaborative writing	Student collaboration in planning, drafting, revising, and editing work (Yarrow & Topping, 2001)
Specific product goals	Product goals identifying purpose of assignment and characteristics of finished product (Ferretti, MacArthur, & Dowdy, 2000)
Word processing	Computers used as instructional supports for writing assignments
Sentence combining	Explicit instruction in sentence combining
Prewriting	Prewriting strategies used to generate and organize ideas for writing assignments
Inquiry activities	Analysis of immediate data to develop ideas and content for writing task (Hillocks, 1982)
Process writing approach	Number of interwoven instructional activities emphasizing extended time, personalized or explicit instruction, and student interaction
Study of models	Exemplary models of each type of writing provided as focus of instruction (Knudson, 1991)
Writing for content learning	Writing used as a tool for learning content

Adapted from Graham & Perin (2007).

Self-regulated strategy development (SRSD) is an explicit, highly structured strategy-based approach to teaching writing to students. The objectives of SRSD are to help students develop knowledge of writing and strategies used in the writing process; to facilitate ongoing development of skills needed for self-monitoring and managing their writing; and to promote the development of positive attitudes toward themselves as writers and about the writing process (Graham & Harris, 2005; Harris, Graham, Mason, & Friedlander, 2008). Students are explicitly taught general writing strategies and strategies for writing genres. Students also learn how to utilize self-regulation strategies that assist in managing the writing task. There are six stages of instruction used in this approach:

1. Develop background knowledge: Students collaborate about the topic and discover information.
2. Discuss it: The topic is discussed by the class and a writing strategy is chosen.
3. Model it: Students think aloud about the writing strategy while working.
4. Memorize it: Students think aloud to rehearse and memorize the strategy.
5. Support it: Students use the strategy to write a story.
6. Independent performance: The writing strategy is used independently.

The genre-specific approach (Wong, 2000) focuses on teaching different expository writing genres uses genre-specific rubrics. The rubrics use anchors (e.g., clarity, organization, etc.) and prompt cards for each different expository genre as writing guides (Roth & Worthington, 2016; Wong, 2000).

Assistive and instructional technology can be used as compensatory strategies for students who have difficulties with writing for a variety of reasons. Some examples of assistive and instructional technology are word processing applications and computers; talking word processing programs; word prediction programs; and voice recognition programs (Lerner & Johns, 2015). Word processing applications can be used to make the writing and editing processes less daunting for struggling writers. Clients can use voice recognition systems with dictation software that converts spoken words to text, or they can use word prediction programs that can predict the next word in a sentence, to reduce the amount of cognitive overload involved in writing.

Bouck, Meyer, Satsanti, Savage, and Hunley (2015) provide detailed information on free computer-based technology programs that can be used to support students with written language difficulties. Links to more information and examples of the use and types of assistive technology are available in the "Additional Resources" section of this chapter.

Summary

Writing is the most complex form of language because it requires the integration of many related abilities, such as speaking, listening, and reading. Individuals who have difficulty with writing challenge professionals to accurately identify and isolate areas for effective remediation. Professionals who are responsible for developing remediation goals for these individuals must acquire a thorough understanding of language structure, the cognitive processes required for different types of writing, the typical sequence of writing development, assessment methods, and school curriculum standards. To develop client-specific goals for written language, the results of an appropriate assessment, the individual's cognitive and social–emotional status, and the cultural and linguistic background need be taken into account. Professionals can formulate appropriate goals when they use their knowledge of the process and synthesize the specific information that the client presents.

Case Scenarios

Case Scenario 1

T. J. is an 11-year-old boy in the fifth grade. He attends public school in a middle-class suburban neighborhood. His placement is in a general education class of 22 children.

T. J. comes from an intact family. He has two older siblings—a sister and a brother. His family history is unremarkable. T. J. has no behavioral problems, his health is good, and he is a good athlete. He is well liked and accepted by his peers. He is eager to please and is proud of the work he can accomplish.

Academically, T. J. is on his grade level in all areas except written expression. He seems unable to put his thoughts on paper. He cannot answer essay questions in social studies, and his written reports are very poor. Response to intervention strategies and instruction were implemented, but no measurable progress was noted. For that reason, T. J. was referred to the committee on special education.

📋 Case Scenarios *(continued)*

The mandatory assessments were completed. T. J. was found to have a full-scale intellectual quotient (IQ) of 123 on the Stanford-Binet Intelligence Scales, which is in the high average range. The Woodcock–Johnson III Tests of Achievement and Cognitive Abilities was administered, and although most of his scores showed that his academic skills were in the average range, there were also clear indications of weaknesses in the area of written language. The Test of Written Language (TOWL) supported these findings. His letters were poorly formed, and his work was often illegible. His sentences were judged to be extremely immature and simplistic, and he wrote as little as possible.

What goals would you develop for T. J. in the area of written language?

Case Scenario 2

Seamus is in the fourth grade. He is described as a hard-working student who is well liked by his peers and his teachers. In first grade, he was diagnosed with a language-based learning disability. He is presently placed in a general education class and receives supportive resource room services five times per week. He also attends speech therapy three times per week and remedial reading help three times per week. Despite the added academic support he receives, his reading and writing skills are approximately 1.5 years below grade level. His abilities in the English language arts, especially his semantic and auditory processing skills, show significant deficits.

Seamus's updated formal assessment results were notably better than his classroom performance. His scores were as follows:

- Wechsler Intelligence Scale for Children, Fourth Edition:
  - Full scale: 87
  - Verbal comprehension: 89
  - Perceptual reasoning: 104
  - Working memory: 88
  - Processing speed: 75
- Woodcock–Johnson III Test of Achievement:
  - Broad reading: 102
  - Broad math: 95
  - Oral language: 105
  - Broad written language: 86

📋 **Case Scenarios** *(continued)*

- Test of Auditory Reasoning and Processing Skills (TAPS):
  - ◆ Overall score: 81

    Discuss the differences between classroom performance and formal testing. What goals would you devise for Seamus in the area of written expression? Explain your answer.

REVIEW QUESTIONS

1. Foundation skills for the development of reading and writing include which of the following?
   a. Phonological awareness
   b. Print concepts
   c. Alphabet knowledge
   d. Literate language
   e. All of the above

2. The cognitive processes that allow a student to pay attention, analyze situations, set goals, and organize a plan to complete a task or assignment are called
   a. executive functions.
   b. self-regulation.
   c. the writing process.
   d. executive regulation.

3. What refers to behaviors that help a person guide and monitor his or her performance and stay on track to complete a task?
   a. Executive function
   b. Self-regulation
   c. Writing process
   d. Executive regulation

4. Which of the following means to tell a story and includes fables, realistic fiction, fantasy, personal memoirs, and folktales?
   a. Expository writing
   b. Narrative writing
   c. Persuasive writing
   d. Enumerative writing

5. Which of the following is considered the language of the school curriculum and is the most literate and advanced form of writing?
   a. Expository writing
   b. Narrative writing
   c. Persuasive writing
   d. Enumerative writing

REFERENCES

American Speech-Language-Hearing-Association. (n.d.a). School-based service delivery in speech-language pathology. Retrieved from http://www.asha.org/SLP/schools/School-Based-Service-Delivery-in-Speech-Language-Pathology/

American Speech-Language-Hearing-Association. (n.d.b). Written language disorders. Retrieved from http://www.asha.org/Practice-Portal/Clinical-Topics/Written-Language-Disorders/

American Speech-Language-Hearing Association. (2001). Roles and responsibilities of speech-language pathologists with respect to reading and writing in children and adolescents. Retrieved from http://www.asha.org/policy/PS2001-00104/

American Speech-Language-Hearing Association. (2002). Knowledge and skills needed by speech-language pathologists with respect to reading and writing in children and adolescents. Retrieved from http://www.asha.org/policy/KS2002-00082/

American Speech-Language-Hearing Association. (2004). Preferred practice patterns for the profession of speech-language pathology. Retrieved from http://www.asha.org/policy/PP2004-00191.htm

American Speech-Language-Hearing Association. (2010). Roles and responsibilities of speech-language pathologists in schools. Retrieved from http://www.asha.org/uploadedFiles/Roles-Responsibilities-SLPs-Schools-Poster.pdf

Bashir, A. S., & Singer, B. D. (2006). Assisting students in becoming self-regulated writers. In T. A. Ukrainetz (Ed.), *Contextualized language intervention: Scaffolding pre-k-12 literacy achievement*. Eau Claire, WI: Thinking.

Bauman-Waengler, J. A. (2012). *Articulatory and phonological impairments*. New York, NY: Pearson Higher Education.

Berninger, V. W. (2000). Development of language by hand and its connections to language by ear, mouth, and eye. *Topics in Language Disorders, 20*, 65–84.

Berninger, V. W., Abbott, R. D., Jones, J., Wolf, B., Gould, L., Anderson-Youngstrom, M., . . . Apel, K. (2006). Early development of language by hand: Composing, reading, listening, and speaking connections; three letter-writing modes; and fast mapping in spelling. *Developmental Neuropsychology, 29*(1), 61–92.

Boon, M. (2010). *Understanding dyspraxia: A guide for parents and teachers* (2nd ed.). Philadelphia, PA: Jessica Kingsley.

Bouck, E. C., Meyer, N. K., Satsangi, R., Savage, M., & Hunley, M. (2015). Free computer-based assistive technology to support students with high-incidence disabilities in the writing process. *Preventing School Failure: Alternative Education for Children and Youth, 59*, 90–97. doi:10.1080/1045988X.2013.841116

Cirrin, F. M., Schooling, T. L., Nelson, N. W., Diehl, S. F., Flynn, P. F., Staskowski, M., . . . Adamczyk, D. F. (2010). Evidence-based systematic review: Effects of different service delivery models on communication outcomes for elementary school-age children. *Language, Speech, and Hearing Services in Schools, 41*(3), 233–264. doi:10.1044/0161-1461(2009/08-0128)

Common Core State Standards Initiative. (2017). Preparing America's students for success. Retrieved from http://www.corestandards.org

Ehren, B. J. (2000). Maintaining a therapeutic focus and sharing responsibility for student success: Keys to in-classroom speech-language services. *Language, Speech, and Hearing Services in Schools, 31*, 219–229.

Espin, C. A., Weissenburger, J. W., & Benson, B. J. (2004). Assessing the writing performance of students in special education. *Exceptionality, 12*, 55–66. doi:10.1207/s15327035ex1201_5

Fahy, J. K. (2014). Assessment of executive functions in school-aged children: Challenges and solutions for the SLP. *SIG 16 Perspectives on School-Based Issues, 15*, 151–163. doi:10.1044/sbi15.4.151

Fallon, K. A., & Katz, L. A. (2011). Providing written language services in the schools: The time is now. *Language, Speech, and Hearing Services in Schools, 42*, 3–17.

Feder, K. P., & Majnemer, A. (2007). Handwriting development, competency, and intervention. *Developmental Medicine and Child Neurology, 49*, 312–317.

Ferretti, R. P., MacArthur, C. A., & Dowdy, N. S. (2000). The effects of an elaborated goal on the persuasive writing of students with learning disabilities and their normally achieving peers. *Journal of Educational Psychology, 92*, 694–702.

Flynn, P. (2015). *Speech-language goals that reflect the common core state standards (and extended standards)* [Video]. Retrieved from https://www.asha.org/eWeb/OLSDynamicPage.aspx? Webcode=olsdetails&title=Speech-Language+Goals+that+Reflect+the+Common+Core+State+Standards+(and+Extended+Standards)

Gentry, J. R. (2004). *The science of spelling: The explicit specifics that make great readers and writers.* Portsmouth, NH: Heinemann.

Graham, S. (2006). Strategy instruction and the teaching of writing: A meta-analysis. In C. MacArthur, S. Graham, & J. Fitzgerald (Eds.), *Handbook of writing research* (pp. 187–207). New York, NY: Guilford.

Graham, S., & Harris, K. R. (2003). Students with learning disabilities and the process of writing: A meta-analysis of SRSD Studies. In H. L. Swanson, K. R. Harris, & S. Graham (Eds.), *Handbook of learning disabilities* (pp. 383–402). New York, NY: Guilford.

Graham, S., & Harris, K. R. (2005). *Writing better: Effective strategies for teaching students with learning difficulties.* Baltimore, MD: Brookes.

Graham, S., Harris, K., & McKeown, D. (2013). The writing of students with learning disabilities, meta-analysis of self-regulated strategy development writing intervention studies and future directions: Redux. In H. L. Swanson, K. R. Harris, & S. Graham (Eds.), *Handbook of learning disabilities* (2nd ed.; pp. 405–438). New York, NY: Guilford.

Graham, S., & Perin, D. (2007). *Writing next: Effective strategies to improve writing of adolescents in middle and high schools. A report to Carnegie Corporation of New York.* Washington, DC: Alliance for Excellent Education. Retrieved from http://dl.ueb.edu.vn/bitstream/1247/9990/1/Writing%20Next%20-%20%20strategies%20to%20improve%20writing.pdf

Greenhalgh, K. S., & Strong, C. J. (2001). Literate language features in spoken narratives of children with typical language and children with language impairments. *Language, Speech and Hearing Services in Schools, 32*, 114–125.

Harris, K. R., Graham, S., Mason, L. H., & Friedlander, B. (2008). *Powerful writing strategies for all students.* Baltimore, MD: Paul H. Brookes.

Hegde, M. N. (2010). *Introduction to communicative disorders* (4th ed.). Austin, TX.: Pro-Ed.

Hegde, M. N., & Davis, D. (1999). *Clinical methods and practicum in speech-language pathology* (3rd ed.). San Diego, CA: Singular.

Hendrickx, S. (2010). *The adolescent and adult neuro-diversity handbook: Asperger syndrome, ADHD, dyslexia, dyspraxia and related conditions.* Philadelphia, PA: Jessica Kingsley.

Hillocks, G., Jr. (1982). The interaction of instruction, teacher comment, and revision in teaching the composing process. *Research in the Teaching of English, 16*, 261–278.

Horowitz, S. H. (2007, March). Executive functioning: Regulating behavior for school success. *LD News* [Research Roundup]. Retrieved from http://impactofspecialneeds.weebly.com/uploads/3/4/1/9/3419723/executive_functioning_-_regulating_behavior_for_school_success_-_ncld.org_-_pdf.pdf

Hughes, D., McGillivray, L., & Schmidek, M. (1997). *Guide to narrative language: Procedures for assessment.* Eau Claire, WI: Thinking.

Hunt, K. (1965). *Grammatical structures written at three grade levels.* Champaign, IL: National Council of Teachers of English.

Individuals with Disabilities Education Act of 2004 (IDEA), Public Law 108–446, 118 Stat. 2647 (2004).

Justice, L. M., & Ezell, H. K. (2004). Print referencing: An emergent literacy enhancement strategy and its clinical applications. *Language, Speech, and Hearing Services in Schools, 35*, 185–193. doi:10.1044/0161-1461(2004/018)

Justice, L. M., & Kaderavek, J. N. (2004). Embedded-explicit emergent literacy intervention I: Background and description of approach. *Language, Speech, and Hearing Services in Schools, 35*, 201–211.

Kaderavek, J. (2015). *Language disorder in children: Fundamental concepts of assessment and intervention* (2nd ed.), New York, NY: Pearson.

Knudson, R. E. (1991). Effects of instructional strategies, grade, and sex on student's persuasive writing. *Journal of Experimental Education, 59*, 141–152.

Lerner, J., & Johns, B. H. (2015). *Learning disabilities and related disabilities: Strategies for success* (13th ed.). Stamford, CT: Cengage Learning.

McHale, K., & Cermak, S. A. (1992). Fine motor activities in elementary school: Preliminary findings and provisional implications for children with fine motor problems. *American Journal of Occupational Therapy, 46*, 898–903.

McLeod, S., & Baker, E. (2017). *Children's speech: An evidence-based approach to assessment and intervention*. New York, NY: Pearson.

National Center for Education Statistics. (2012). *The nation's report card: Writing 2011*. Washington, DC: U.S. Department of Education.

Needels, M. C., & Knapp, M. S. (1994). Teaching writing to children who are underserved. *Journal of Educational Psychology, 86*, 339–349.

Nippold, M. A. (2007). *Later language development: School-age children, adolescents, and young adults*. Austin, TX: PRO-ED.

Nippold, M. A., Hesketh, L. J., Duthie, J. K., & Mansfield, T. C. (2005). Conversational versus expository discourse: A study of syntactic development in children, adolescents, and adults. *Journal of Speech, Language, and Hearing Research, 48*, 1048–1064.

Paul, R., & Norbury, C. (2012). *Language disorders from infancy through adolescence: Listening, speaking, reading, writing, and communicating* (4th ed.). Saint Louis, MO: Elsevier Mosby.

Pindzola, R., Plexico, L., & Haynes, W. (2016). *Diagnosis and evaluation in speech pathology* (9th ed.). Boston, MA: Pearson.

Power-deFur, L., & Flynn, P. (2012). Unpacking the standards for intervention. *Perspectives on School-Based Issues, 13*, 11–16. doi:10.1044/sbi13.1.11

Price, J. R., & Jackson, S. C. (2015). Procedures for obtaining and analyzing writing samples of school-age children and adolescents. *Language, Speech, and Hearing Services in Schools, 46*, 277–293.

Pullen, P. C., & Justice, L. M. (2003). Enhancing phonological awareness, print awareness, and oral language skills in preschool children. *Intervention in School and Clinic, 39*, 87–98.

Reid, R., & Lienemann, T. O. (2006). Self-regulated strategy development for written expression with students with attention deficit/hyperactivity disorder. *Exceptional Children, 73*, 53–68.

Richards, R. G. (1999). *The source for dyslexia and dysgraphia*. East Moline, IL: LinguiSystems.

Roth, F., & Worthington, C. (2016). *Treatment resource manual for speech-language pathology* (5th ed.). Clifton Park, NY: Cengage Learning.

Rudebusch, J. (2012). From common core state standards to standards-based IEPs: A brief tutorial. *Perspectives on School-Based Issues, 13*, 17–24. doi:10.1044/sbi13.1.17

Scott, C. (2012). Learning to write. In H. Catts & A. Kamhi (Eds.), *Language and reading disabilities* (3rd ed.; pp. 244–268). Boston, MA: Pearson.

Shipley, K. G., & McAfee, J. G. (2016). *Assessment in speech-language pathology: A resource manual* (5th ed.). Boston, MA: Cengage Learning.

Singer, B. D., & Bashir, A. S. (1999). What are executive functions and self-regulation and what do they have to do with language-learning disorders? *Language, Speech, and Hearing Services in Schools, 30*, 265–273.

Turnbull, K. L. P., & Justice, L. M. (2017). *Language development from theory to practice* (3rd ed.). New York, NY: Pearson.

Ward-Lonergan, J. M., & Duthie, J. K. (2016). Intervention to improve expository reading comprehension skills in older children and adolescents with language disorders. *Topics in Language Disorders, 36*(1), 52–64.

Westby, C. (1991). Learn to talk—talking to learn: Oral-literate language differences. In C. S. Simon (Ed.), *Communication skills and classroom success: Assessment and therapy methodologies for language and learning-disabled students* (pp. 334–357). Eau Claire, WI: Thinking.

Westby, C. E. (2012). Assessing and remediating text comprehension problems. In H. Catts & A. Kamhi (Eds.), *Language and reading disabilities* (3rd ed.; pp. 163–221). Boston, MA: Pearson.

Wong, B. (2000). Writing strategies intervention for expository essays for adolescents with and without learning disabilities. *Topics in Language Disorders, 20*(4), 29–44.

Woods, C. (1997). *Yardsticks: Children in the classroom ages 4–14.* Turner's Falls, MA: Northeast Foundation for Children.

Yarrow, F., & Topping, K. J. (2001). Collaborative writing: The effects of metacognitive prompting and structured peer interaction. *British Journal of Educational Psychology, 71,* 261–282.

ADDITIONAL RESOURCES

Assistive and instructional technology:

Georgia Project for Assistive Technology. Assistive Technology Devices for Writing and Spelling. http://archives.gadoe.org/DMGetDocument.aspx/Writing_Chart_4%E2%80%9310.pdf?p=6CC6799F8C1371F69BD40055318FE41B627D32D2BE14782E2125A78632F8446F

LD OnLine. Assistive Technology for Kids with Learning Disabilities: An Overview. http://www.ldonline.org/article/33074/

Reading Rockets. Assistive Technology Tools: Writing. http://www.readingrockets.org/article/assistive-technology-tools-writing

Understood. Assistive Technology for Writing. https://www.understood.org/en/school-learning/assistive-technology/assistive-technologies-basics/assistive-technology-for-writing

WEBSITES

Common Core State Standards Initiative. www.corestandards.org

Council for Exceptional Children. www.cec.sped.org

Florida Center for Reading Research. www.fcrr.org

Great Schools. www.greatschools.org

Into the Book. http://reading.ecb.org

Learning Disabilities Association of America. www.ldaamerica.org

National Center for Learning Disabilities. www.ncld.org

National Council of Teachers of English. NCTE Beliefs about the Teaching of Writing. www.ncte.org/positions/statements/writingbeliefs

National Writing Project. www.nwp.org

Teachers College Reading and Writing Project. www.readingandwritingproject.com

Understood for Learning and Attention Issues. www.understood.org

BOOKS

Dove, Maria G., and Andrea M. Honigsfeld. *Common Core for the Not-So-Common Learner: English Language Arts Strategies Grades K-5.* Thousand Oaks, CA: Corwin, 2013.

Hughes, Diana L., LaRae McGillivray, and Mark Schmidek. *Guide to Narrative Language: Procedures for Assessment.* Austin, TX: PRO-ED, 2009.

Justice, Laura M., and Helen K. Ezell. *The Syntax Handbook: Everything You Learned about Syntax—but Forgot* (2nd ed.). Austin, TX: PRO-ED, 2016.

Moss, Barbara, and Virginia Shin-Mui Loh. *35 Strategies for Guiding Readers through Informational Texts.* New York, NY: Guilford, 2010.

Nippold, Marilyn A. *Language Sampling with Adolescents: Implications for Intervention* (2nd ed.). San Diego, CA: Plural, 2014.

Roth, Froma P., Deborah Adamczyk Dixon, Diane Paul, Patricia Iafrate Bellini, and American Speech-Language-Hearing Association. *RTI in Action: Grades 3-5: Oral and Written Language Activities for the Common Core State Standards.* Rockville, MD: American Speech-Language-Hearing Association, 2013.

CHAPTER 14

Math Disabilities: Skill Development through Assessment, Goals, and Strategic Instruction

Elizabeth Stein

Key Terms

Achievement assessments
Adaptive reasoning
Conceptual understanding
Curriculum-based measurement
Diagnostic assessments
Dyscalculia

Mnemonics
Procedural fluency
Productive disposition
Strategic competence
Working memory

Introduction

Research suggests that numerical competence is the foundation for more complex math skills. At very young ages, children begin to distinguish different quantities of objects, they learn to count, and they begin to understand that numbers are symbols that represent specific quantities. Children typically enter school with a basic number sense that has been developing naturally since infancy. Math skills are often cumulative in nature—one skill must build upon another for more complex skills to be understood and applied. For example, algebraic applications depend on an understanding of basic math skills and number sense. Essential math skills include basic computations that students need to know in the early elementary grades. Ideally, students need to recall basic number facts for more advanced mathematical thinking (Cantlon et al., 2009).

Math disabilities have their roots in an inability to master foundational skills in the early years of development—prior to entering kindergarten. It is critical that these foundational math skills be taught and practiced often in a child's early years to avoid further cumulative deficit effects.

Types of Mathematical Difficulties

Students with disabilities may experience mathematical difficulties that range from mild to severe. Children may experience procedural difficulties, where they present with frequent errors, as they attempt to follow sequential steps to solve problems. Semantic memory concerns often reveal themselves as students have difficulty remembering math facts. In addition, students may have visual–spatial difficulties, which are demonstrated when students have difficulties writing numerals and equations (Turnbull, Turnbull, & Wehmeyer, 2010).

Because math development skills are cumulative, students who have math disabilities may experience trouble with gaining new skills as they move from grade to grade. For example, a student may have the potential for more abstract mathematical thinking, but if he or she has difficulties with computational skills and lacks a number sense foundation, the student will struggle to reach grade-level math skills. Early intervention is a key factor in supporting students who struggle. Students have a greater chance of reaching their full math potential when their developmental struggles are remediated early. Students who progress through the grades with continued gaps in their math abilities lose confidence and experience adverse emotional responses when approaching math experiences (Bottge, 2001).

Students with math disabilities are typically classified as having a learning or emotional disability, as described in the 13 categories of disabilities in the Individuals with Disabilities Education Act (IDEA). Mathematics disability is an emerging field of research that supports many common characteristics (Watson & Gable, 2013). A math disability can occur in isolation or in combination with reading and writing disabilities. For example, a student who has decoding or comprehension difficulties may exhibit a math disability, characterized by deficits in solving word problems and applying math concepts (Zheng, Flynn, & Swanson, 2013).

Watson and Gable (2013) outline a few common characteristics that may indicate a math disability (**TABLE 14-1**).

Numerical reasoning and computational skills are major areas of weakness for many students who are diagnosed with learning disabilities and exhibit specific math disabilities—or **dyscalculia**. Developmental dyscalculia is defined as a specific learning disability affecting the acquisition of math skills and numerical competencies in the absence of neurological injuries and despite typical intellectual skills. Children with dyscalculia often apply undeveloped strategies and exhibit weak memory storage of math facts (Attout & Majerus, 2015).

TABLE 14-1 Characteristics of Possible Math Disabilities

Math Skill	Characteristics
Number facts	Students have difficulties with basic computations and the memorization of basic facts, such as $5 + 3 = 8$ or $6 \times 3 = 18$. They have great difficulties in recalling facts and procedures needed to systematically complete mathematical problems.
Computation	Students have difficulties remembering previously taught and practiced patterns. Attention difficulties are evident when students solve multistep computational equations because they lose focus or do not remember what to do next.
Knowledge transfer	Students have difficulty connecting the abstract concepts of math with reasonable, realistic solutions. They have difficulty shifting among the multiple demands of a complex math problem.
Spatial organization	In addition to the difficulties in knowledge transfer, students may have difficulties visualizing math concepts and, therefore, need to rely on rote memorization to solve more complex math problems. For example, students have a difficult time describing what a geometric shape would look like if it were rotated and viewed from another angle. Students may also have difficulty understanding how formulas translate into real-world applications. They typically have difficulty expressing their thinking in a neat, organized fashion.
Math language	Many students who have difficulty with reading, writing, listening, or speaking often have difficulty with the language of math. They are confused by the academic vocabulary and have a difficult time translating language into understanding directions or explanations. They typically have trouble remembering definitions and assigned mathematical values, and they have trouble understanding directions.

Working Memory

Working memory refers to how a person processes information in an effort to remember important information. It is the ability to manipulate and prioritize information for later recall. Working memory is an essential cognitive function that is necessary for a wide range of tasks in daily life, such as remembering plans, following directions, performing mental mathematic calculations, engaging in conversations, and recalling an address or telephone number. If information is lost while it is held in working memory, it cannot be stored in long-term memory; therefore, the information will be forgotten (Meltzer, 2010).

According to Watson and Gable (2013), researchers have identified working memory problems as a strong predictor of math disabilities. Students have difficulty determining what is important to remember for future use, and they often have difficulty remembering one thing while performing another (Turnbull et al., 2010). In math disabilities, this is particularly evident in learning that requires the application of background knowledge and following a sequence of procedures, rules, and formulas. A reduced working memory capacity leads students to rely on external supports to make up for their poor storage of math facts. For example, external support strategies could include using finger counting or relying on peers or a teacher for assistance. Seeking external supports is an additional processing step that not only increases computational errors, but also may fatigue and frustrate the student (Attout & Majerus, 2015).

Mathematical Proficiency Assessments

The National Research Council (2001) defined five interconnected strands that, as a whole, constitute mathematical proficiency:

1. **Conceptual understanding**: The integrated and functional understanding of mathematical ideas, which allows students to learn new ideas by connecting them to what they already know. Constructing new understanding to their background knowledge guides and supports retention, accuracy, and fluency of math skills.
2. **Procedural fluency**: The skill of carrying out procedures flexibly, accurately, efficiently, and in a timely manner.
3. **Strategic competence**: The ability to apply strategies to formulate, represent, and solve mathematical problems with accuracy and fluency.
4. **Adaptive reasoning**: The capacity for logical thought, reflection, explanation, and justification to explain the mathematical process and product.

5. **Productive disposition**: The ability and self-confidence to see and apply mathematics as a sensible, useful, and worthwhile process connected to authentic experiences.

Mathematics disabilities are identified in a variety of ways. Typically, the classroom teacher or the parents notice that the child is having consistent difficulty applying the foundation of mathematical thinking skills. The student's classroom performance reveals persistent struggles and poor outcomes during math activities and assessments, as compared to his or her peers. Information about the student's performance is documented in the form of anecdotal notes based on the teacher's observations and the student's work samples to reveal evidence of persistent struggles. Because math skills are developmental in nature, a mathematic disability is not identified with certainty until the upper elementary years. Assessing mathematics ability involves gaining an awareness of how students solve problems, recognize and interpret results, apply math skills to authentic experiences, estimate, perform computations, understand measurement, and create and interpret graphs and charts. Mathematics can be assessed at the individual or group level (Salvia, Ysseldyke, & Witmer, 2012).

Information about students' performance is collected, and patterns in students' performance are analyzed. If a child continues to exhibit learning concerns, a formal referral for a special education assessment might be recommended. Formal and informal assessments are used to identify math skills and concepts that are of specific concern. Formal tests include standardized tests, diagnostic math tests, and individually administered achievement tests that are norm-referenced to compare the student's performance with a reference group of his or her same-age peers. Informal assessments may include curriculum-based measurements and observations. A combination of assessment tools should be used to ascertain the student's performance over time in different settings

Formal Assessments

Diagnostic assessments are norm-referenced tests that provide information about a student's strengths and weaknesses as compared to students of the same age or grade level. Examples include the following:

- The KeyMath 3 diagnostic assessment (Connolly, 2007) measures basic concepts, numerical operations, and applications. Its assessment of a wide range of skills informs instruction for students in grades K–12.

- The Stanford Diagnostic Mathematics Test, Fourth Edition (SDMT4) (Wang, Young, & Brooks, 2004) is a computer-based assessment that is similar to a traditional paper-and-pencil assessment. The SDMT4 measures math competence for students in grades 2–12 on the basic concepts and skills that are necessary for success in mathematics. The emphasis is on problem solving while applying concepts and strategies to seek accurate and meaningful solutions. The test identifies specific areas of difficulty so teachers can plan appropriate instruction.

Achievement assessments broadly measure areas of a student's academic knowledge and application as they compare with the performance of same-aged peers or same-grade level. The math section of achievement tests assesses the accuracy and fluency of a student's computation and problem-solving skills. Examples of achievement assessments include the following:

- Kaufman Test of Educational Achievement (Kaufman, 2014)
- Wide Range Achievement Test 4 (WRAT4) (Wilkinson & Robertson, 2006)
- Woodcock–Johnson III Tests of Achievement (Mather & Wendling, 2009)

Informal Assessments

Curriculum-based measurement specifies procedures for measuring student proficiency within basic skills. It can be used for a variety of assessment-related decisions, including monitoring students for possible additional assessments, identifying students for special services, and developing instructional experiences that meet students' needs. In addition, curriculum-based measurement may be an effective way to guide teachers in monitoring the effectiveness of their instructional decisions. Students respond to teacher-directed questions (probes) that directly connect to classroom lessons and topics. For example, if students are working on reducing fractions or basic multiplication facts, the curriculum-based measurement would include questions that assess their ability to accurately solve those problems. The teacher records the results of students' performance to inform instructional decisions that support and guide students as they continue to strengthen their skills (Hosp & Hosp, 2003).

Performance Assessments

Class work, class assessments, and homework are examples of information the teacher may collect to track students' performance. In addition, the teacher may take notes to document student behaviors when completing math assignments in class. The teacher may also collect information from parents to gain a deeper perspective into the strategy the student exhibits at home. Information from all formal and informal assessments helps the teacher develop an authentic learner profile to support the decision-making process and proactively plan daily instructional experiences.

Student Surveys

Gaining insights into the attitudes and perceptions of students is important when making key instructional decisions. Interest inventories and math interviews are opportunities for teachers and students to connect as they work together to strengthen math skills and applications. Some sample questions include the following (Gargiulo & Metcalf, 2017, p. 387):

- How do you feel about math?
- What do you do when you come across a problem you do not know how to solve?
- What is one thing you are good at when it comes to math?
- What do you not like about math?
- What is one strategy you use?

Error Analysis

In an error analysis, a student completes a few math problems at his or her ability level so the teacher and the student can see how the student approaches problem solving. The student's strengths and specific areas where understanding breaks down become evident. The teacher analyzes both the successful applications and the errors to guide instructional decisions. Ideally, the teacher should include the student in the process of analyzing his or her thinking and strategic applications to guide the student's ability to overcome any areas where learning breaks down.

What Do Math Assessments Tell Us?

The results of any formal or informal assessment in math should empower the teaching and learning process. The results reveal students' abilities and areas of need in the process of mastering and applying the specific foundational and more complex math skills. The ultimate goal is to prepare students for solving real-life problems by transferring and applying key mathematical thinking. Scores on formal and informal assessments are just a part of the process. Gaining meaningful qualitative data on students' performance—such as through performance assessments and student surveys—provide important information in making sure students are gaining mathematical thinking skills that are needed for application in authentic life situations. One important aspect of assessment is making decisions about the next steps in guiding students toward achievement.

Response to Intervention

Response to intervention (RTI) is a general education initiative that ensures high-quality instruction to maximize student learning. It is a cycle of learning that moves along a three-tier process. RTI emerged as a result of the reauthorization of IDEA in 2004 as an alternative way to identify students with learning disabilities. Schools can apply RTI to the pre-referral process to ensure that students are not struggling due to insufficient instruction. RTI ensures that all students are provided with evidence-based instruction within a systematic cycle of instruction and progress monitoring. When the RTI process is embraced, the following procedures are in place (Gargiulo, 2015):

- Universal screening: A district-wide or school-wide assessment is given to all students to identify any students who may have areas of weakness that could negatively impact their grade-level achievement.
- Fidelity of implementation: Instructional practices are implemented according to best practices. The instruction is consistent and specific.
- Tiered instruction: Increasingly intensive instruction is provided, beginning with the general education classroom. If students require more frequent or supplemental instruction, they participate in small-group or individualized sessions to meet their needs.
- Progress monitoring: The students' performance is monitored on an ongoing basis so that effective instructional decisions may be applied.

Determining Eligibility for Special Education Services

In spite of the application of high-quality instructional practices, ongoing progress monitoring, and collaboration, a student may continue to show evidence of learning difficulties. A teacher or parent may refer the student for a special education evaluation to determine if his or her learning needs require more intensive, individualized instruction. After the parent has provided consent for the child to be evaluated, the process of formally gathering information about the student's strengths and weaknesses begins. Both formal and informal assessments are applied to provide a comprehensive view of the student's learning profile. The school's multidisciplinary team, which includes a school psychologist, educational diagnosticians, and other professionals, evaluates the student's areas of strengths and needs. The evaluators put together a complete educational portrait of the student to allow an informed and accurate decision-making process to unfold. The multidisciplinary team meets in a formal committee on special education to determine if the student is eligible for special education services.

Service Delivery Options

To be eligible for special education, the student must meet the requirements of one of the 13 disability categories identified in IDEA. As mentioned earlier, students who exhibit math disabilities are typically classified as having a learning disability. Placement for support is determined through careful identification of the student's least-restrictive environment. According to IDEA, students must be educated alongside their peers, with access to the general education curriculum, to the greatest extent possible (Smith & Tyler, 2010).

Placement Options

The placement options for students who are eligible for special education services include the following:

- General education classroom with a coteacher: Students receive additional support within the general education classroom with two teachers in the room—typically one special education teacher and one general education teacher.
- General education classroom with resource room support: Students receive supplemental instructional support specifically designed to meet their personal needs in a separate setting for a scheduled session each day.
- Full-time in a special education classroom: This option is for students who require more intense specialized instruction to access and meaningfully connect with the curriculum.

Forming Specific Goals

In addition to achieving grade-level expectations, students who have been identified with a math disability have specific goals written in their IEP, which is developed by the special education committee. The IEP states annual measurable goals that address the student's participation and progress in the general education curriculum. The goals are based on the information gathered from assessments and collaborative efforts to determine what specific skills the student must master to have greater academic and learning outcomes.

Present Levels of Performance

So goals can be created and the student can be guided toward achieving those goals, the student's present levels of performance must be considered and documented in the IEP. The student's strengths and needs are mindfully recognized and strategically incorporated during the process of creating meaningful instructional activities and natural learning experiences. As examples, we will consider a third-grade student and a seventh-grade student who present with specific mathematical needs that could be addressed through specific goals and high-quality instruction.

Kyle is a third-grade student whose needs include mastering the language of math and solving multistep word problems. The goal for Kyle is as follows: When given 10 word problems, Kyle will use context clues and visual scaffolds to correctly select the appropriate operation, write the mathematical equation, and solve the equation with 80 percent accuracy over 2 weeks. Kyle's teacher will encourage him to monitor his work by using an answer key to mark his progress. The teacher will also apply an error analysis assessment to help Kyle reflect on the process and identify the strategies he either applied or could apply next time.

Julia is a seventh-grade student whose needs include computing accuracy and applying math concepts and math language within word problems. The goal for Julia is as follows: Julia will write and solve five algebraic expressions for word problems with 90 percent accuracy. The teacher will support Julia by providing short video clips that demonstrate an accurate model, allowing Julia to work in cooperative groups to collaborate with her peers, and assessing her progress through targeted observation and collection of work samples to provide evidence of her thinking and progress over time.

Types of Instructional Approaches

Mastropieri and Scruggs (2002) identified both explicit and systematic instruction as the best practice for guiding students with math disabilities. Explicit instruction includes clear teacher modeling, providing sufficient examples, providing specific feedback, and scaffolding students' learning by gradually releasing responsibility to them for applying their skills independently. Mercer, Mercer, and Pullen (2011) found explicit instruction with mnemonics to be effective when supporting students' understanding of concepts and procedures. **Mnemonics** are strategies that bolster and accelerate memory to guide successful learning outcomes. The use of acronyms is one way to support memory for concepts and procedures.

RIDE Strategy

The RIDE strategy (Mercer et al., 2011) is effective in supporting students as they solve word problems. RIDE can support students who struggle with understanding abstract reasoning and those who lack attention, memory, or visual–spatial skills. Teachers should model each step clearly then guide students to interact through collaboration before applying this strategy independently. It is a good idea for teachers to create an anchor chart, which is a visual aid that can be displayed in the classroom.

The components of RIDE are as follows:

- R: Remember the problem correctly.
- I: Identify the important information.
- D: Determine the operations and unit for expressing the answer.
- E: Enter the correct numbers, calculate, and check the answer.

TINS Strategy

The TINS strategy (Owen, 2003) helps students think systematically to organize the steps needed to solve word problems:

- T: Thought. Think about the context or the story the word problem is depicting. Circle important words and number.
- I: Information. Write down the important information and sketch a quick picture to represent the information. Cross out any unneeded information.
- N: Number sentence. Write a number sentence to represent the problem.
- S: Solution sentence. Write a solution sentence that explains the answer.

STAR Strategy

The STAR strategy (Gagnon & Maccini, 2001) helps students visualize how to solve an equation:

- S: Search the word problem. Ask the following questions: What facts do I know? What do I need to find out? Write down the facts.
- T: Translate the words from the equation into a quick illustration. Choose the variable. Identify the operation or operations. Represent the problem with manipulatives for concrete application (i.e., draw a picture to represent the concrete example), and write an algebraic equation.
- A: Answer the problem.
- R: Review the solution. Reread the problem to see if the answer makes sense. Check the answer for reasonableness and accuracy.

Concrete–Representational–Abstract Approach

The concrete–representational–abstract (CRA) approach (Flores, Hinton, & Strozier, 2014) guides learners to make abstract concepts more visible, tangible, and eventually understood at an abstract level. CRA prepares students to grasp concepts as they move from the concrete level of understanding to more complex and abstract understanding.

The steps of the CRA approach are as follows:

- C: Concrete. Students participate at the concrete level in a hands-on approach. They manipulate objects that represent math problems. For example, they could work with objects like tiles, three-dimensional numbers, three-dimensional objects, fraction bars, and so forth. Students actively explore concepts.
- R: Representational. Students continue to explore, but they use two-dimensional pictures to represent concepts.
- A: Abstract. Students represent the problem using written numbers and symbols.

Summary

Mathematics disability is an emerging field of research. Math disabilities can occur in isolation or in combination with reading and writing disabilities. Math skills develop in a cumulative process. Similarly, math disabilities emerge on a cumulative basis as students move from grade to grade each year because their learning gaps increase. Typically, students with math disabilities are classified as having learning or emotional disabilities. These students have a greater chance of reaching their full math potential when their developmental differences are remediated early.

Informal and formal assessments are used to provide a clear portrait of a student's learning profile. Data from the assessments are used to make meaningful instructional decisions. Explicit and systematic instructional strategies have been proven effective in helping students grasp and apply abstract mathematical concepts. Guiding students through strategies that strengthen their working memory through mnemonics and guiding their understanding of concepts through sequential steps helps them overcome math disabilities and supports their problem-solving success.

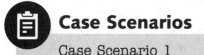

Case Scenarios

Case Scenario 1

Rachel is a seventh-grade student who is struggling in algebra class. Specifically, she is having a difficult time with vocabulary and following multistep directions. In class, she tries to pay attention, but the teacher speaks too quickly. When it is time for students to apply what the teacher modeled, Rachel is lost. She feels defeated and embarrassed as she looks around the room and sees her peers getting to work.

Rachel's teacher decided to review Rachel's IEP goals with the special education teacher. They discuss how they could fine-tune their instructional decisions to support Rachel. They focus on two important goals. One goal addresses guiding Rachel to follow multistep directions. The second goal addresses Rachel's ability to follow up to five multistep real-life problems involving rational numbers. They decide that as one teacher is giving directions verbally, the other teacher will write the directions on the board to provide additional visual cues. In addition, to support Rachel's vocabulary and concept understanding, the teachers decide to add a step before asking the students to apply the information independently. They will invite the students to work with a peer to brainstorm and follow the teacher's modeling. While the students work in pairs, the two teachers will walk around the room and be available to support Rachel and other students who require additional direct instruction.

Case Scenarios (continued)

Case Scenario 2

Daniel is a fifth-grade student who has difficulties with basic math skills. Currently, his goals include solving word problems using the operations of addition and subtraction as well as learning multidigit multiplication. Daniel works at a slow pace because he puts all his effort into trying to apply basic computations. As he struggles, he loses his focus for solving multistep equations and word problems that are presented in class. Daniel's teachers have supported him by giving him extra time to practice basic math facts using classroom games, flash cards, and computer-based math problems. Daniel works hard to practice, but he continues to have difficulty. His teachers are sensitive to the fact that Daniel easily loses confidence. He shares stories of how he is humiliated that his third-grade brother tries to help him with his homework.

The teachers decide to include additional supports in class. They give all the students individual color-coded multiplication charts to use as a visual tool. Because all students have one, Daniel does not feel self-conscious about using it. The teachers also provide additional opportunities for students to practice their math skills by providing extra practice sheets for them to complete during free time throughout the day. The teachers also incorporate more opportunities for students to work together in small groups. One person in the group is designated as the group leader. Each leader is given an answer key with teacher-modeled notes. As the students work in groups, the leader reviews the answers and explanations with their peers. The teachers are preparing Daniel to be a group leader to support both his math skills and his self-esteem.

REVIEW QUESTIONS

1. The main reason students with math disabilities often struggle to learn new math concepts as they progress to new grade levels is because
   a. they have difficulty attending to everything.
   b. they need strategies to guide them through each step.
   c. math learning is cumulative, and students often do not have the foundational skills to help them build on prior conceptual knowledge.
   d. they have emotional or behavioral needs that interfere with all learning.

2. Each of the following may be a characteristic of a math disability *except*
   a. difficulty recalling facts.
   b. difficulty following multistep directions.
   c. difficulty working with peers during group work.
   d. difficulty moving from a concrete understanding to an abstract conceptual understanding.

3. Working memory is a strong indicator of math difficulties mainly because
   a. students do not pay attention to what is important to remember.
   b. students rely on external supports, which easily increases fatigue, inaccuracies, and limited long-term conceptual understanding.
   c. students become distracted and miss key points in the lesson.
   d. students' self-esteem adversely affects their ability to learn math.

4. Instructional strategies that guide students through the mathematical process can strengthen which of the following?
   a. Students' ability to understand the sequence of the mathematical process
   b. Students' ability to apply mathematical concepts and vocabulary
   c. Students' recall of facts and vocabulary
   d. All of the above

5. Which of the following is a main goal of assessing students' mathematical skills?
   a. Strengthen students' cognitive abilities to solve math problems without using a calculator
   b. Guide students to think systematically and to solve real-world problems
   c. Apply mathematical language and vocabulary, and guide the teacher's instructional decisions
   d. B and C

6. Explain the value of early intervention for developing math skills. Why is it so critical that students with math disabilities receive support as early as possible?

7. Review the math skills in Table 14-1 and consider the potential cumulative effects for a student who has difficulties in these areas. How could these difficulties affect the student as he or she progresses to a new grade level each year?

8. Explain the role of memory in learning and applying math skills. Explain how a weakness in working memory may adversely impact a student's ability to apply effective mathematical skills and strategies.

9. Describe the difference between formal assessments and informal assessments. Why is it important to administer and analyze a variety of assessments while shaping a student's learning profile?

10. For one of the case studies, decide how one of the strategies discussed in this chapter could further support the student and guide goal achievement.

REFERENCES

Attout, L., & Majerus, S. (2015). Working memory deficits in developmental dyscalculia: The importance of serial order. *Child Neuropsychology, 21*(4), 432–450. doi:10.1080/09297049. 2014.922170

Bottge, B. A. (2001). Reconceptualizing mathematics problem solving for low-achieving students. *Remedial and Special Education, 22*(2), 102–112.

Cantlon, J. F., Libertus, M. E., Pinel, P., Dehaene, S., Brannon, E. M., & Pelphrey, K. A. (2009). The neural development of an abstract concept of number. *Journal of Cognitive Neuroscience, 21*(11), 2217–2229.

Connolly, A. J. (2007). *KeyMath 3: Diagnostic assessment.* San Antonio, TX: Pearson.

Flores, M. M., Hinton, V., & Strozier, S. (2014). Teaching subtraction and multiplication with regrouping using concrete-representational abstract sequence and the strategic instruction model. *Learning Disabilities Research and Practice, 29*(2), 75–88.

Gagnon, J. C., & Maccini, P. (2001). Preparing students with disabilities for algebra. *Teaching Exceptional Children, 34*(1), 8–15.

Gargiulo, R. M. (2015). *Special education in contemporary society* (5th ed.). Thousand Oaks, CA: SAGE Publications, Inc.

Gargiulo, R.M., & Metcalf, D. (2017). *Teaching in today's inclusive classrooms: A universal design for learning approach.* Belmont, CA: Cengage Learning.

Hosp, M. K., & Hosp, J. L. (2003). Curriculum-based measurement for reading, spelling and math: How to do it and why. *Preventing School Failure, 48*(1), 10–17.

Kaufman, A. S. (2014). *KTEA-3: Kaufman test of educational achievement* (3rd ed.). Minneapolis, MN: Pearson.

Mastropieri, M. A., & Scruggs, T. E. (2002). *Effective instruction for special education* (3rd ed.). Austin, TX: PRO-ED.

Mather, N., & Wendling, B. J. (2009). Woodcock–Johnson III tests of achievement. In J. A. Naglieri & S. Goldstein (Eds.), *Practitioner's guide to assessing intelligence and achievement* (pp. 503–535). Hoboken, NJ: John Wiley & Sons.

Meltzer, L. (2010). *Promoting executive function in the classroom.* New York, NY: Guilford.

Mercer, C. D., Mercer, A. R., & Pullen, P. C. (2011). *Teaching students with learning problems* (8th ed.). Upper Saddle River, NJ: Pearson Education.

National Research Council. (2001). *Adding it up: Helping children learn mathematics.* Washington, DC: National Academies Press.

Owen, M. J. (2003). *It's elementary! 275 math word problems. Book 3.* Toronto, Canada: Educator Publishing Service.

Salvia, J., Ysseldyke, J., & Witmer, S. (2012). *Assessment: In special and inclusive education.* Belmont, CA: Cengage Learning.

Smith, D. D., & Tyler, N. C. (2010). *Introduction to special education: Making a difference, student value edition.* Upper Saddle River, NJ: Pearson.

Turnbull, A., Turnbull, R., & Wehmeyer, M. (2010). *Exceptional lives: Special education in today's schools.* Upper Saddle River, NJ: Pearson.

Wang, S., Young, M. J., & Brooks, T. E. (2004). *Stanford diagnostic mathematics test (SDMT 4).* San Antonio, TX: Pearson.

Watson, S. M., & Gable, R. A. (2013). Unraveling the complex nature of mathematics learning disability: Implications for research and practice. *Learning Disability Quarterly, 36*(3), 178–187.

Wilkinson, G. S., & Robertson, G. J. (2006). *Wide range achievement test 4 (WRAT4).* San Antonio, TX: Pearson.

Zheng, X., Flynn, L. J., & Swanson, H. L. (2013). Experimental intervention studies on word problem solving and math disabilities: A selective analysis of the literature. *Learning Disability Quarterly, 36,* 97–111.

ADDITIONAL RESOURCES

Intervention Central. Curriculum Based Measurement Warehouse: Reading, Math, and Other Academic Assessments. www.interventioncentral.org/curriculum-based-measurement-reading-math-assesment-tests

Math Reasoning Inventory. Online activities and assessments to determine students' abilities in math skills. www.mathreasoninginventory.com

Math Solutions. Professional Learning to Empower Math Achievement. www.mathsolutions.com

RTI Action Network. RTI and Math Instruction: Using RTI to Improve Learning in Mathematics. www.rtinetwork.org/learn/what/rtiandmath

INDEX

Page numbers followed by *f* indicate figures; those followed by *t* indicate tables.